Psychoneuroendocrinology in Psychosocial and Psychotherapeutic Practice

Julia Wiederhofer

Psychoneuroendocrinology in Psychosocial and Psychotherapeutic Practice

A Biopsychosocial Coaching Approach

Springer

Julia Wiederhofer
Heiligenkreuz am Waasen, Austria

ISBN 978-3-658-46274-1 ISBN 978-3-658-46275-8 (eBook)
https://doi.org/10.1007/978-3-658-46275-8

Translation from the German language edition: “Psychoneuroendokrinologie in der psychosozialen und psychotherapeutischen Praxis” by Julia Wiederhofer, © Der/die Herausgeber bzw. der/die Autor(en), exklusiv lizenziert an Springer Fachmedien Wiesbaden GmbH, ein Teil von Springer Nature 2024. Published by Springer Fachmedien Wiesbaden. All Rights Reserved.

This book is a translation of the original German edition “Psychoneuroendokrinologie in der psychosozialen und psychotherapeutischen Praxis” by Julia Wiederhofer, published by Springer Fachmedien Wiesbaden GmbH in 2024. The translation was done with the help of an artificial intelligence machine translation tool. A subsequent human revision was done primarily in terms of content, so that the book will read stylistically differently from a conventional translation. Springer Nature works continuously to further the development of tools for the production of books and on the related technologies to support the authors.

This Springer imprint is published by the registered company Springer Fachmedien Wiesbaden GmbH, part of Springer Nature.
The registered company address is: Abraham-Lincoln-Str. 46, 65189 Wiesbaden, Germany

Acknowledgments

For Markus, Noah, and Lian

Thanks to my husband Markus and my two sons Noah and Lian. For the support, the assistance, the belief in me, the warmth, and endless love.

Thanks also to my parents, my father-in-law, and my siblings.

I would also like to thank Univ.-Doz. DDr. Barbara Friehs and Dr. Martin Gabriele, MSc.

Thank you, everyone, from the bottom of my heart.

Summary

Psychoneuroendocrinology is a relatively young scientific discipline, but it is increasingly being researched that there is a complex interplay between the neurobiological foundations of mental experiences and behaviors on the one hand and the endocrinological processes in the brain and psychosocial environmental influences on the other. Hormones influence our behavior, but our behavior also influences our hormones. Additionally, this book explains how psychoneuroendocrinology is inevitably linked with (behavioral) genetics and what significance this has for all psychological and psychosocial disciplines. Although the research findings of psychoneuroendocrinology are primarily anchored in the field of disease development and are still largely unknown in psychosocial and psychotherapeutic fields of action and have not yet been transferred into therapeutic approaches, it is significant to intertwine psychoneuroendocrinological findings with a coaching concept and to create a biopsychosocial coaching approach—a biopsychosocial coaching approach that is suitable for psychosocial and psychotherapeutic practice. This book presents the basic research of both the scientific discipline of endocrinology and psychoneuroendocrinology in such a way that readers without (behavioral) medical, neurobiological, or endocrinological prior knowledge can understand these complex sciences. To develop a foundation for this biopsychosocial coaching approach, various counseling approaches and psychotherapeutic orientations, methods, and biopsychosocial concepts that can be linked with psychoneuroendocrinological findings are presented and described. Furthermore, this book not only highlights positive aspects but also presents some critical considerations, discussions, and areas of tension, as well as the importance of interdisciplinarity. The aim of this book is to illustrate the complex interactions between psyche, endocrinology, neurobiology, the autonomic nervous system, (behavioral) genetics, and psychosocial environmental factors and to bring the resulting psychoneuroendocrinological findings closer to the readers. Based on interdisciplinary sciences, a modern, scientifically based biopsychosocial coaching approach is presented, which is suitable for both psychotherapeutic and psychosocial practice.

Introduction

"Hormones." The word "hormones" is familiar to almost everyone. One has heard it at some point, and particularly women of childbearing age are regularly confronted with the effects of hormones. But how significant is the influence of hormones on humans really? How much are we influenced by our hormones in everyday life? And do we also have an influence on our hormones? Is the influence of our hormones, possibly for both men and women, much more present than we thought? In which mental illnesses are hormones of particular importance? In contrast to the term "hormones," the term psychoneuroendocrinology is much less known. But why is that? In this book, it is explained, on the one hand, that this scientific discipline is comparatively still very young, and on the other hand, it is also a very complex topic, which originated from endocrinology and thus has a different level of recognition in medicine than in psychological and psychosocial disciplines. And although the answers and insights of this science are so obviously significant for all psychological disciplines as well as psychosocial fields of action, the focus of psychoneuroendocrinology is still on the research of disease development. Psychologists, psychotherapists, and especially psychosocial counselors are less frequently encountered in this scientific discipline than, for example, behavioral medicine specialists, endocrinologists, and neurobiologists. But are the scientific findings of this discipline advanced and established enough to implement them into a practical, psychosocial, and psychotherapeutic coaching concept? Are psychoneuroendocrinological insights helpful and possibly quality-enhancing within psychological interventions? And what is needed to transfer these insights into psychological, psychosocial, and psychotherapeutic practice? In the following, these questions will be answered, and psychoneuroendocrinological insights will be implemented into a coaching concept, and a biopsychosocial coaching approach will be presented, which is suitable for both psychosocial and psychotherapeutic practice. The psychosocial factor plays a central role in this. The "PNES coaching," as I call it, is not presented as a method that promises a healing effect, but it is based on the latest scientific findings and is helpful in making both healthy people's crisis times and mentally ill people's everyday and life management easier. Additionally, PNES coaching is suitable for maintaining health and especially mental well-being, making it also applicable for preventive use.

Furthermore, it is important to note that, in contrast to other psychoneuroendocrinological literature, this book presents, defines, and explains this complex science in such a way that, even if you do not have a basic education in (behavioral) medicine, neurobiology, or endocrinology, you can understand the findings and foundational knowledge of this fascinating science. To this end, technical terms are explained and defined both in the text and in the glossary, and difficult-to-understand scientific literature is supported with simplified explanations to promote understanding. After this science and the basic research are explained and presented, psychosocial counseling approaches and therapeutic orientations are addressed as a foundation for PNES coaching, which can be described as an eclectic-integrative biopsychosocial coaching approach. A toolbox with various methods, approaches, and orientations that can be applied within PNES coaching is presented. The importance of interdisciplinarity is also highlighted.

At the beginning of this book, you will be provided with the foundational knowledge for psychoneuroendocrinology, the so-called endocrinology. Endocrinology is defined, and it is explained what hormones actually are, where they are produced, what their functions are, and much more. This science and its findings are explained in such a way that, even if you have no prior knowledge, you will gain an understanding of this complex science and our endocrine system. Already in the first chapter, it will become apparent what effects hormones can have on our psyche and behavior. Additionally, you will understand the relevance of hormones for our physical as well as mental health. Subsequently, on this foundation, the findings of psychoneuroendocrinology are presented in the second chapter. The scientific discipline is explained, and the connections between our hormones, our feelings, our emotions, our behavior, and even our perceptions are laid out. This chapter explains in detail which hormones are of particular importance for the psyche and, above all, brings closer the fact that not only do hormones influence our behavior, but our behavior also influences our hormones. Furthermore, it is explained and elucidated what significance our nutrition has for the production of important hormones, as well as the connection of psychoneuroendocrinological findings with mental disorders and diseases. This chapter makes it clear how enormously important interdisciplinary cooperation is to transfer these modern scientific findings into clinical practice. Because, in addition to the scientific connections of endocrinology with neurobiology and behavioral medicine as well as psychology and psychiatry, the inseparable connection of psychoneuroendocrinology with (behavioral) genetics and epigenetics is revealed. It is explained that these complex sciences are inevitably linked with modern psychoneuroendocrinology and that these findings are too significant to be ignored based on their complexity or refusal of interdisciplinarity. The importance of gene-environment interaction is explained, and the influences (early childhood) experiences in connection with genetic polymorphisms have on human behavior, as well as the significance that gene-environment interactions have for the development of mental disorders. It is also shown that hormonal influences, such as hypercortisolism of the mother during the perinatal phase, have effects on hormone secretions and, in connection with genetics as well as experiences and environmental influences, on the behavior or psyche of the child and later on the adult. In the third chapter, in particular to gain foundational knowledge about eclectic-integrative concepts and to demonstrate suitable evidence-based methods and training that can be well applied in the following biopsychosocial coaching concept, the psychological and psychosocial counseling process is described. Knowledge is presented, and tools as well as counseling approaches and school-specific orientations are introduced, which form a suitable foundation for the implementation of psychoneuroendocrinological findings in psychological interventions. Interdisciplinary findings are incorporated into the explanations, as critical neuroscientific considerations are presented and the effectiveness of counseling approaches or school-specific orientations is discussed based on contemporary neurobiological scientific findings. It quickly becomes clear that these points of criticism and the suggestion of interdisciplinarity do not excite everyone and that this is a much-debated topic. Nevertheless, it becomes understandable that and/or why some approaches or therapeutic schools do not conform to the contemporary state of science and some approaches, based on current scientific findings, could be described as "outdated." However, neutral towards these critical considerations, the psychological and psychosocial counseling process is subsequently described with the topics of biopsychosocial diagnostics, forms of intervention, methods or training, as well as a successful counseling conclusion and the importance of evaluation. In the final chapter, the goal of this book is then presented: an eclectic-integrative biopsychosocial coaching approach with the implementation of psychoneuroendocrinological findings, which is suitable for both psychosocial and psychotherapeutic practice. At the beginning of this final chapter, it is shown how these psychoneuroendocrinological findings can be transferred into psychosocial and psychotherapeutic practice. Relevant aspects are highlighted, and conclusions are drawn. These form the basis for the following biopsychosocial coaching approach, an eclectic-integrative biopsychosocial coaching approach, in which psychoneuroendocrinological findings are implemented and which is suitable for both psychosocial counseling and psychotherapy.

This book presents a path that highlights various aspects of scientific disciplines. Both successful, effective, and positive aspects as well as critical considerations, discussions, and areas of tension are presented; a path that addresses the importance of interdisciplinarity and illustrates the goal of modern, scientifically based psychological, psychosocial, and psychotherapeutic counseling.

Contents

About the Author

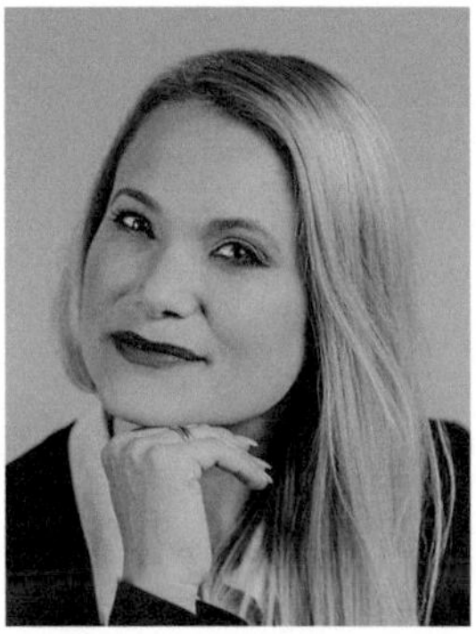

Julia Wiederhofer, Bakk.phil. MA. MSc. The psychosocial counselor, social pedagogue, and educational scientist advised and accompanied children, adolescents, and adults for many years who were traumatized, suffered from psychological disorders, or were in severe life crises. Already during her early research work, she came across findings in psychoneuroendocrinology, which she successfully implemented in her practice. From the experiences of this practice and further research work, she developed this book, which now presents an interdisciplinary, modern, scientific coaching concept. Psychoneuroendocrinological and biopsychosocial findings are linked with evidence-based psychosocial counseling approaches and psychotherapeutic orientations.

List of Abbreviations

ACTH	Adrenocorticotropin
ADH	Antidiuretic hormone, vasopressin
AgRP	Agouti-like protein
APUD (-Zellen)	“amine precursor uptake and decarboxylation”
AVP	Vasopressin, arginine vasopressin, antidiuretic hormone, adiuretin
bzw.	respectively
CCK	Cholecystokinin
CG	Chorionic gonadotropin
CGrP	“calcitonin gene related peptide”
CRF	Corticotropin-releasing factor
CRH	Corticotropin-releasing hormone
d. h.	that is
ebd.	ibid.
et al.	et alia – and others
f.	following
ff.	continuing
FC	Follicular epithelial cells
FSH	Follicle-stimulating hormone
GEP	Gastroenteropancreatic endocrine system
GH	Growth hormone
GHRH	Growth hormone-releasing hormone
GIP	Gastroinhibitory peptide
GIT	Gastrointestinal tract
GnRH	Gonadotropin-releasing hormone
GR	Glucocorticoid receptor
HHGA	Hypothalamus-pituitary-gonadal axis
HHNA	Hypothalamus-pituitary-adrenal axis
IL-6	Interleukin-6
KVT	Cognitive Behavioral Therapy

LH	Luteinizing hormone
MR	Mineralocorticoid receptor
NA	Norepinephrine
NPY	Neuropeptide Y
o. S.	without page number
OXY	Oxytocin
PIF	Prolactin-inhibiting factor
PIH	Prolactin-inhibiting hormone
PNE	Psychoneuroendocrinology
POMC	Proopiomelanocortin
PPP	Pancreatic polypeptide
PRL	Prolactin
PTBS	Post-traumatic stress disorder
SHRP	Stress hyporesponsive period
SRIF	"somatotropin release inhibitory factor"
SST	Somatostatin
T_3	Triiodothyronine
T_4	Thyroxine or tetraiodothyronine
Tab.	Table
TRH	Thyrotropin-releasing hormone
TSH	Thyroid-stimulating hormone (thyrotropin)
u. Ä.	and similar
usw.	and so on
u. v. m.	and much more
vgl.	compare
VIP	Vasoactive intestinal peptide
VTA	Ventral tegmental area
z. B.	for example
zit. n.	cited according to
ZNS	Central nervous system

Fundamentals of Endocrinology

1

At the beginning of this book, the basic research is presented. The fundamentals of endocrinology are conveyed in such a way that you gain an understanding of the importance of hormones and the endocrine system. Endocrinology is defined and explained as a scientific discipline, and then the endocrine system is discussed in general to give you a brief overview of how hormone secretion works and what significance it has. This chapter thus explains what hormones are, the different types of hormones, when, how, and where they are released, and what effects they have on humans. Abbreviations and tech nical terms are not only explained in the text but can also be found in the list of abbreviations and the glossary. I assume that the readers of this book have little to no medical knowledge or training and possess little to no basic knowledge of endocrinology. Therefore, the basic research, the associated findings, and the importance of this discipline for the human psyche are presented and explained as simply as possible. Partially extremely complex technical literature for laypeople, which presupposes basic medical training, is supported by easily understandable definitions so that the findings of basic research are comprehensible even for laypeople. The goal of this chapter is thus to make the findings of this science understandable to you so that they can be applied in an interdisciplinary context. It is intended to show that

> "(…) there is an intense interplay between the neurobiological foundations of mental experiences and behavior on the one hand and endocrinological (…) processes in the brain and other organ systems on the other hand" (Ehlert and Känel 2011, V).

With the findings presented in this first chapter, it becomes apparent how important an understanding of hormonal relationships is for psychosocial and psychological fields of action.

J. Wiederhofer, *Psychoneuroendocrinology in Psychosocial and Psychotherapeutic Practice*, https://doi.org/10.1007/978-3-658-46275-8_1

1.1 Endocrinology: Definition and Explanation of the Scientific Discipline

Before I delve deeper into the endocrine system, the scientific discipline of endocrinology will be briefly defined and explained.

Endocrinology is the study of the function of endocrine glands as well as the secretion of hormones, their effects, and their disorders (cf. Schöller 2016a, n.p.). It is the study of internal secretion, as endocrine means "secreting inward" and describes the release of hormones into the bloodstream or the lymphatic system (cf. Treeck 2009, 4). The foundation for the field of endocrinology is internal medicine. However, many interdisciplinary collaborations are necessary for successful research and work (cf. Medical University of Vienna 2023, n.p.). In the medical lexicon, endocrinology is defined as follows: Endocrinology refers to the science that deals with the functions and regulation of the endocrine system (hormonal system). The focus here is particularly on the pathophysiology of hormone production and hormonal effects as well as disease patterns, as well as the engagement with hormone therapy for non-endocrine diseases (cf. Medical Lexicon 2005, 466). The term internal secretion was coined by Claude Bernard in 1855. He understood it to mean the release of substances in a living organism, which, after being transported through the bloodstream, exert their effects in other cells and organs. In 1905, Ernest Henry Starling first gave these substances a name: hormone. The term hormone comes from the ancient Greek hormaein and means "to drive." However, the birth of endocrinology is considered to be the experiment conducted by the Göttingen physiologist Arnold Adolph Berthold in 1849. In an experiment, he implanted the testes of other roosters into castrated roosters. After the implantation of these testes, the castrated roosters resumed their sexually specific behavior patterns. Berthold correctly concluded that one or more substances exist in the testes, which exert their specific effects elsewhere via the bloodstream (cf. Treeck 2009, 4).

In the classical definition, hormones are so-called messengers that are produced in gland cells and secreted by them into the bloodstream. Through the blood pathways, the hormones reach the corresponding target organs, which have receptors to read the "message" of the hormone. Thus, hormones can then exert their specific effects (cf. Wuttke 1987, 390). This so-called endocrine system (hormonal system) deals with hormones, which are also referred to as chemical messengers, with the communication between organs and cells. The endocrine system is essential for the human organism and is subject to complex control mechanisms. Hormones can exert significant effects even in the smallest amounts or concentrations. The effects of hormones are of enormous importance for development and growth, sexuality and reproduction, metabolism and energy balance, as well as for responses to stress and adaptation to the environment (cf. Medical University of Vienna 2023, n.p.). Disorders of the endocrine system lead to many different diseases such as obesity, thyroid diseases, diabetes mellitus, osteoporosis, and hypertension, as well as diseases of the parathyroid glands, adrenal glands, hypothalamus, and pituitary gland, as well as bone, fat, and sugar metabolism. There are also disorders of gut hormones and immune- and inflammation-mediated endocrinopathies. Endocrinology also deals with questions of biological sex and gender issues, as well as sexuality and reproduction. The diseases can be based on a hormone deficiency or excess, as well as pathological changes in the glands, imbalances in hormonal interaction, and "organ crosstalk" up to tumors (cf. Medical University of Vienna 2023, n.p.). Ultimately, it should be noted here that endocrinology deals with the regulation of vital functions such as water balance, appetite and hunger, energy metabolism, reproduction, and human growth. This scientific discipline is still relatively young and has led to many new insights into human physiology in recent years (cf. Kleine and Rosmarith 2014, 1). In the next section, the endocrine system will be explained in more detail, defined, and its importance for the body and psyche will be presented. The goal is for you to gain a basic understanding of the human endocrine system to better understand the effects that hormones have on the human psyche and behavior.

1.2 The Endocrine System (Hormonal System)

As a basis for the relevant scientific discipline here, psychoneuroendocrinology, it is important that you gain an understanding of the endocrine system. What are hormones, which ones exist, and how are they secreted? Which organs and glands are involved, and can one influence the endocrine system? For the application of this biopsychosocial coaching approach in practice, having a basic knowledge of the endocrine system is considered fundamental.

In the human body, there are two communication systems responsible for the exchange of information between individual organs. On the one hand, this is the nervous system (especially the autonomic nervous system) and on the other hand, the endocrine system. These two systems are closely intertwined in their functions (cf. Birbaumer and Schmidt 2010, 118). There is a close interrelationship between both systems. The brain is an extremely relevant endocrine gland, which influences all functions of the body via the hypothalamus. Likewise, the brain is a target organ for many diverse hormones such as gonadal, thyroid, and adrenal hormones (cf. DGE 2022, n.p.) (Fig. 1.1).

The Brain

Together, the endocrine system and the nervous system coordinate, among other things, organs that are far apart from each other. The nervous system sends its messages via electrical impulses through the nerve fibers to the organs. The endocrine system uses chemical substances, the so-called hormones, to communicate with the various organs. The chemically coded messages of the hormones are "read" by means of so-called receptors. Apart from the technique of these two systems, they can also be distinguished by the speed of information transmission. This is in the millisecond range for nervous transmission,

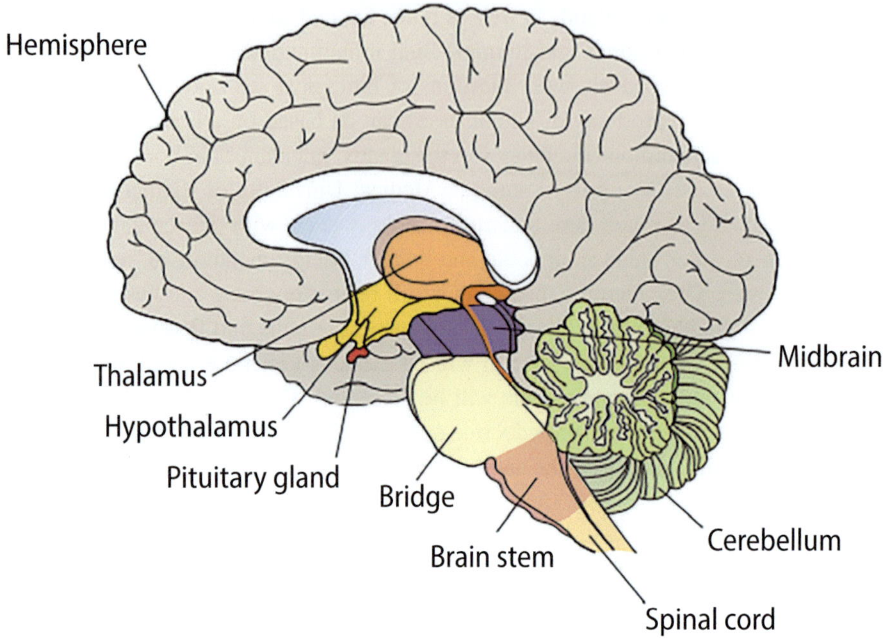

Fig. 1.1 Adult brain. Medial view of the right hemisphere. In: Birbaumer, Niels/Schmidt, Robert F. (2018): Biological Psychology. Special edition. 7th revised and supplemented edition. Heidelberg: Springer Medizin Verlag. 127. *Source:* Birbaumer and Schmidt (2018, 76)

whereas for hormonal information transmission, it can be in the range of minutes to hours (cf. Birbaumer and Schmidt 2010, 118). Above all, however, both systems have one thing in common: "Despite the diversity of their different individual tasks, both have the overarching goal of continuously adapting the body to changing stresses, thus maintaining the 'homeostasis of the internal system'" (Birbaumer and Schmidt 2010, 118). The endocrine system, together with the nervous system, has evolved into a central integration mechanism responsible for communication between cells and organs. The endocrine system is indispensable in the context of reproduction, growth and development, as well as for the response to stress, and adaptation to our environment (cf. DGE 2022, n.p.). The following will now explain what hormones are and what their function is.

What is Meant by Hormones?

In the classical definition of hormones, they are understood as biologically active messengers. They are formed (synthesized) in endocrine glands and, after their release (secretion), reach their target organs (effector organs) via the bloodstream or the lymphatic system. In the effector organs, the hormones trigger an organ- or cell-specific reaction (cf. Treeck 2009, 4).

In general, hormones can thus be described as chemical signal substances. The body produces them in various cells, and they are then transported via the bloodstream to different regions of the body, where they exhibit their various effects. A distinction is made between endocrine and exocrine glands. Exocrine glands produce secretions such as gastric acid, saliva, or breast milk, whereas endocrine glands produce hormones that are released into the blood, tissue, or lymph. The hormone can exert its effect when the target cells have specific docking sites (receptors) for that particular hormone (cf. Ehlert 2011, 4). Hormone production takes place in gland cells, which can form an organ but can also be scattered or grouped in organs that do not produce hormones. Hormones are then released in response to a specific stimulus (cf. Wuttke 1987, 390). Especially in recent years, endocrinology has been expanded by the realization that hormones do not necessarily have to be secreted via the bloodstream to exert their effects. It has now been frequently demonstrated that hormones can also become effective in the immediate vicinity of the hormone-producing cell (paracrine communication). There is also autocrine communication, in which the hormones act directly on their cell of origin (cf. DGE 2022, n.p.). This means that, as a rule, hormones reach their target cells via the bloodstream (cf. Birbaumer and Schmidt 2018, 119). However, it is also possible,

> "(…) that the hormone message can be 'read' by cells that are in the immediate vicinity of the hormone-producing cells. The hormone then diffuses (…). This effect of hormones on neighboring cells is called a paracrine effect. If the hormone acts on its producer cell, this effect is called autocrine" (Birbaumer and Schmidt 2018, 119).

Hormones are capable of triggering strong effects over long distances and in very low concentrations. The effect of the hormones, the duration, and the intensity of the effects are controlled by multiple regulatory circuits and molecular signal transduction chains (cf. Treeck 2009, 4).

Hormone Receptors

> "Hormones, like synaptic transmitters, must bind to receptors to exert their effects. Binding to membrane-bound receptors has a variety of consequences mediated by chains of secondary messengers" (Birbaumer and Schmidt 2018, 120).

As already briefly mentioned, hormones need certain docking sites, called receptors, to exert their effects. These receptors can also be referred to as receiver molecules (cf. DGE 2022, n.p.). For hormones to be effective, they must interact with these "(…) specialized molecules on the surface or inside the target cell" (ibid.). After the hormone binds to its receptor, a so-called signal cascade is triggered, which ultimately leads to the typical response of the target cell (cf. DGE 2022, n.p.). According to the fit-in or lock-and-key principle, a hormone can only show its effect if the target cell is equipped with the respective receptors to which only this hormone can bind (cf. Ehlert 2011, 9). Since the various hormone classes have different fat solubilities, "(…) they dock to different classes of receptors on different cell components" (Ehlert 2011, 9). Membrane receptors and intracellular receptors (steroid receptors) are differentiated (cf. ibid.). They have in common "(…) that they not only exhibit specificity for the respective hormone but also that there are a multitude of subtypes per receptor" (Ehlert 2011, 9).

The following sections will outline and describe various forms of hormones.

1.2.1 Neurotransmitters

The name neurotransmitter is composed of the Greek word neuron = nerve and the Latin word transmittere = to transmit (cf. Spektrum Lexikon der Neurowissenschaft 2000a, n.p.). Neurotransmitters are biochemical compounds or substances that transmit, amplify, and modulate the transmission of stimuli from one nerve cell to another nerve cell or cell at synapses (cf. Walther 2022, n.p.). Hormones can act as neurotransmitters. When a hormone acts as a neurotransmitter, a substance is released that particularly influences another cell. This can be a nerve cell (neuron) or a cell in an effector organ. However, to elicit a specific effect, a sufficiently large amount of the substance is of relevance (cf. Ehlert 2011, 4 f.). The duration of the effect of neurotransmitters generally lasts only milliseconds. The effect is usually limited to the respective synaptic area, but they can also influence cells far from their release site (cf. Spektrum Lexikon der Neurowissenschaft 2000a, n.p.). Chemically, neurotransmitters can be biogenic amines, such as acetylcholine, adrenaline, noradrenaline, serotonin, dopamine, and histamine, as well as amino acids, such as aspartate and glutamate, which are present in more than 50% of the synapses in the central nervous system (CNS), peptides, such as opioids, GABA, and glycine, or nucleotides (cf. Walther 2022a, n.p.).

> "The effect of a neurotransmitter in the brain depends on a variety of influencing factors, so that usually several transmitter and receptor systems are responsible for a specific behavior" (Birbaumer and Schmidt 2018, 94).

Neurotransmitters are of enormous importance for the human psyche and behavior, which can have inhibitory and excitatory functions (cf. Spektrum Lexikon der Neurowissenschaft 2000a, n.p.).

The most important neurotransmitters for the psyche and behavior include:

- **Acetylcholine:** Acetylcholine is considered the best-studied neurotransmitter. It is involved in a variety of processes in the brain (cf. Spektrum Lexikon der Neurowissenschaft 2020b, n.p.). Acetylcholine is relevant for attention, learning, and memory (cf. Birbaumer and Schmidt 2018, 95). It is believed that acetylcholine facilitates the storage of information in the hippocampus and enables higher attention. Additionally, it controls motor centers in the brain, modulates the sleep rhythm, and sensitizes pain receptors (cf. Spektrum Lexikon der Neurowissenschaft 2020b, n.p.).

- **Adrenaline and Noradrenaline:** "Their activation increases performance in attention functions and facilitates learning in emotional situations" (Birbaumer and Schmidt 2018, 95). The release of **adrenaline** is particularly triggered in stressful situations (cf. Spektrum Lexikon der Neurowissenschaft 2020c, n.p.). The mediated effects of adrenaline correspond to "fight-or-flight" reactions (cf. Pschyrembel Redaktion 2020a, n.p.). **Noradrenaline** particularly enhances attention. The noradrenaline level is 2 to 3 times higher than the adrenaline level in resting states and increases with the onset of motor activity (cf. Spektrum Lexikon der Neurowissenschaft 2020d, n.p.).
- **Serotonin:** Serotonin determines the personality structure of a person based on its mood-influencing effects (cf. Birbaumer and Schmidt 2018, 97). Additionally, serotonin is important for the regulation of learning processes and emotions. A lack of serotonin can exacerbate depression (cf. Pschyrembel Redaktion 2020b, n.p.).
- **Dopamine:** "Dopamine is the most important messenger substance in the brain, functioning both motorically and psychologically as the neurochemical basis of incentive and positive psychomotor activity" (Birbaumer and Schmidt 2018, 95). Additionally, dopamine plays a significant role in addictive behavior. A lack of dopamine can lead to the development of endogenous depression, and a change in the dopaminergic system plays a role in various psychotic disorders (cf. Spektrum Lexikon der Neurowissenschaft 2000e, n.p.).

The effect of a neurotransmitter in the brain depends on many influencing factors. Thus, several transmitter and receptor systems are often responsible for a specific behavior (cf. Birbaumer and Schmidt 2018, 94).

Based on the findings presented here, it is clearly evident how enormously relevant neurotransmitters are for the human psyche and behavior, which is why detailed information about these substances will be provided in the following sections.

Neuropeptides can be described as a functional intermediate form between hormones and neurotransmitters. Characteristic of neuropeptides is their effect based on the mediation of slow but long-lasting endocrine as well as paracrine effects. Depending on their chemical structure, messengers can be classified into various classes (cf. Ehlert 2011, 5): "Peptide or protein hormones, amino acid derivatives, steroid hormones, and other substances" (ibid.).

1.2.2 Peptide or Protein Hormones

The majority of all hormones are referred to as peptide or protein hormones and consist of chains of amino acids. If only a few amino acids are linked together, they are referred to as oligopeptides. When 10–100 amino acids are linked together, they are called polypeptides, and when more than 100 amino acids are linked together, they are declared as proteins (cf. Ehlert 2011, 5).

Some important peptide hormones and their sites of formation:

- **Hypothalamus:** Corticotropin-releasing hormone (CRH), gonadotropin-releasing hormone (GnRH), thyrotropin-releasing hormone (TRH), somatostatin (SST), growth hormone-releasing hormone (GHRH, somatoliberin), agouti-related protein (AgRP), urocortin III, and neuropeptide Y (NPY).
- **Adenohypophysis:** Adrenocorticotropin (ACTH), endorphins, follicle-stimulating hormone (FSH), prolactin (PRL), luteinizing hormone (LH), proopiomelanocortin (POMC), growth hormone (GH), and thyroid-stimulating hormone (TSH, thyrotropin).
- **Neurohypophysis:** Oxytocin (OXY), vasopressin (AVP).
- **Gastrointestinal tract:** Cholecystokinin (CCK), somatostatin, gastric inhibitory peptide (GIP), substance P, pancreatic polypeptide (PPP), neurotensin, ghrelin, gastrin, secretin, and vasoactive intestinal peptide (VIP).
- **Pancreas:** Insulin, amylin, and somatostatin.
- **Other sites of formation and their peptide hormones:** Thyroid gland (calcitonin), parathyroid glands (parathyroid hormone), liver (angiotensins), kidneys (renin), adipose tissue (leptin), placenta (β-endorphin), sex organs (follistatin) (cf. Ehlert 2011, 5 f.).

Most hormones are composed of chains of amino acids. This means that they are peptides, which consist of short chains of amino acids, or proteins, which consist of long chains. Furthermore, they are not fat-soluble, and their receptors are embedded in the cell membrane (cf. Birbaumer and Schmidt 2018, 121).

1.2.3 Amino Acid Derivatives

In contrast to peptide hormones, amino acid derivatives are small and can therefore pass through the cell membrane. They consist of the converted amino acid tyrosine (cf. Ehlert 2011, 5). The conversion of the amino acid tyrosine into catecholamines occurs in several synthesis steps, and they then serve both as hormones and as transmitters (cf. Birbaumer and Schmidt 2018, n.p.). Of particular importance here are the catecholamines adrenaline and noradrenaline. They play a role in the transmission of signals in the brain (cf. Bieg et al. 2016a, 7). Like catecholamines, thyroid hormones also have tyrosine as the starting point of their synthesis. These are formed by two molecules of tyrosine and the addition of iodine (cf. Birbaumer and Schmidt 2018, 121).

1.2.4 Steroid Hormones

Steroid hormones consist of fats and are fat-soluble. Thus, they can freely pass through the cell membrane, but they are also not storable. They have 4 interconnected carbon rings and are synthesized from cholesterol. Which steroid hormones are involved depends on the atoms attached to the carbon rings (cf. Ehlert 2011, 5). They exert their effect by "influencing the transcription of DNA" (Bieg et al. 2016b, 6).

Steroid hormones perform a variety of tasks and are classified into glucocorticoids, sex hormones, and mineralocorticoids (cf. Schöller 2016b, n.p.). According to increasing research findings, various steroids (such as glucocorticoids or pregnenolone) are also synthesized in the CNS. These steroids are then called neurosteroids (cf. Hirst et al. 2006; cited in Ehlert 2011, 6). The 5 classes of steroid hormones are glucocorticoids (cortisol), androgens (testosterone, androstenedione, androsterone, dehydroepiandrosterone, and dihydrotestosterone), estrogens (estradiol, estriol, and estrone), progestogens (progesterone, pregnanediol, pregnenolone), mineralocorticoids (cortexone, aldosterone, and cortexolone). The following sites can be named as production sites for steroid hormones: testes, ovaries, adrenal glands, corpus luteum, placenta, and skin (cf. Ehlert 2011, 6). In summary, it should be noted that steroid hormones belong to the 2nd major class of substances, namely the lipophilic (fat-soluble) hormones. Due to their fat solubility, they are able to cross the plasma cell membrane. Steroids include, among others, cortisol and the male sex hormone testosterone (cf. Birbaumer and Schmidt 2018, 121).

1.2.5 Summary and Principles of a Hormone

In summary, it should be noted here that there are various groups of hormones. They are produced in the CNS and/or in the body periphery. Furthermore, some of them can function not only as hormones but also act as neurotransmitters. There are both endocrine and exocrine glands. In contrast to exocrine glands (for example, various salivary glands or sweat from the sweat glands), endocrine glands release their hormones directly into the blood or the intercellular fluid (cf. Ehlert 2011, 7). Hormones have a similar chemical structure in all vertebrates, but their effect can vary depending on the species. The effect of hormones occurs only through binding to cells with corresponding receptors. Hormones influence each other or their effects, they interact with each other. They initiate behavior as well as physiological reactions. This often happens some time after hormone release. Hormones often act gradually. They modulate behavior, and they can trigger a change in behavior. The quantity as well as the type of secreted hormones is influenced by both endogenous and exogenous factors. Our behavior results in hormone releases, just as hormone releases result in certain behaviors. This means that hormones and behavior act reciprocally. Just as each hormone has multiple effects, each behavior also leads to multiple hormone effects. It is also important to mention that the production of hormones occurs in small quantities and the release of hormones is often irregular (pulsatile secretion). The release of hormones can occur rhythmically, for example, according to the circadian rhythm. The quantity as well as the type of secreted hormones is influenced by both endogenous and exogenous factors. Additionally, hormones influence the production and breakdown of fats, carbohydrates, and proteins (cf. Ehlert 2011, 23 f.).

The following will now delve into the morphology of the endocrine system. The most important endocrine glands will be described and their function briefly explained.

1.3 The Endocrine Glands

Ehler and Winkler (2018) state that the endocrine system (hormone system) can be described as a network of glands (cf. Ehler and Winkler 2018, 12). Endocrine glands (Glandulae endocrinae) are glands that do not have an excretory duct and form hormones. They release their secretion into the bloodstream, the intercellular space, or the lymphatic system (cf. Pschyrembel Editorial 2018, n.p.).

Endocrine Glands

- Hypothalamus, pituitary gland
- Thyroid gland, parathyroid glands
- Pancreas,
- Adrenal gland
- Ovaries
- or testes (cf. Ehler and Winkler 2018, 12)

The endocrine cells are located in the heart, kidney, liver, gastrointestinal tract, thymus, brain, and other organs and produce over 30 hormones that are supposed to regulate bodily functions. Inconsistencies in this system, which is considered sensitive, can lead to various medical conditions. These include allergies, headaches, skin impurities, hair loss, menstrual disorders, and loss of libido, but also reduced performance and depression. Furthermore, an unbalanced hormone system can lead to more serious diseases such as diabetes, asthma, Alzheimer's, epilepsy, cancer, and multiple sclerosis. Of particular relevance here is the thyroid gland. The entire metabolism is weakened when it becomes unbalanced. This, in turn, leads to an impairment of all other endocrine glands (cf. Ehler and Winkler 2018, 12). The following sections will provide a closer look at endocrine glands and significant hormones.

1.3.1 Pineal Gland

The pineal gland, also known as the glandula pinealis or pineal gland or corpus pineale (pineal organ), is an endocrine gland located in the epithalamus. It belongs to the circumventricular organs, which are located in the ventricular walls of the brain, but it is assigned to the epithalamus (roof of the diencephalon) (cf. von Werder 2005, cited in Ehlert 2011, 7). The pineal gland can be described as a small, median, cone-shaped protrusion of the epithalamus. It is an end organ of the photoneuroendocrine system, which lies between the two brain hemispheres (cf. Spektrum Lexikon der Neurowissenschaft 2000f, n.p.). It is particularly characterized by its special role in the biorhythm (day-night rhythm) and the production of melatonin in the pinealocytes (pineal cells) (cf. von Werder 2005, cited in Ehlert 2011, 7). Melatonin is produced in the pineal cells in a daily periodic manner, specifically at night or in darkness. This means that the biosynthesis of pineal melatonin follows a circadian rhythm (cf. Spektrum Lexikon der Neurowissenschaft 2000f, n.p.). For humans, rhythms such as the circadian rhythm are of particular importance. Both the psyche and behavior, as well as the daily fluctuation of cognitive performance, diseases, and mortality, show circadian peculiarities (cf. Abbruzzese 2011, 131).

1.3.2 Hypothalamus

The hypothalamus is a section of the diencephalon (interbrain) in the area of the optic chiasm (chiasma opticum). The so-called pituitary stalk connects the hypothalamus with the pituitary gland (hypophysis). Through this pituitary stalk, neuropeptides of the hypothalamus are transported via the bloodstream to the anterior pituitary (adenohypophysis) (cf. von Werder 2005, cited in Ehlert 2011, 7). The hypothalamus is thus a functionally extremely important control organ for the autonomic nervous system as well as for the hormonal system (cf. Spektrum Lexikon der Neurowissenschaft 2000g, n.p.). It is closely connected to the limbic system, but only indirectly to the cortex and thalamus. The hypothalamus is an integration center for circadian, autonomic, and somatomotor functions. It connects autonomic and endocrine functions and controls drive functions as well as endogenous rhythms (cf. Birbaumer and Schmidt 2018, 77 f.).

> "In the hypothalamus, 7 neurohormones are formed, 5 of which act as releasing hormones (liberins) and 2 as inhibiting hormones (statins) on the anterior pituitary" (Birbaumer and Schmidt 2018, 127).

Some neurosecretory cells also extend from the median eminence to the posterior pituitary (neurohypophysis) (cf. von Werder 2005, cited in Ehlert 2011, 7 f.). The hypothalamus "integrates the maintenance of homeostasis with mechanisms of behavioral adaptation" (Spektrum Lexikon der Neurowissenschaft 2000g, n.p.). It can be divided into two main centers: the preoptic area, which is responsible, among other things, for regulating body temperature, and the paraventricular nucleus and the supraoptic nucleus, which produce the peptide hormones oxytocin and vasopressin and release them into the neurohypophysis (posterior pituitary). This is referred to as "classical" neurosecretion. In the median eminence, there are hormone-producing nerve cells that form regulatory hormones. These releasing hormones and inhibiting hormones reach the pituitary gland and influence hormone production there (hypothalamus-pituitary system) (cf. Spektrum Lexikon der Neurowissenschaft 2000g, n.p.). The anterior hypothalamus (the suprachiasmatic nucleus) is significant for chronobiology, as it is considered a central timekeeper. Other centers of the hypothalamus influence "heat, water, and electrolyte balance, heart function, circulation and respiration, sleep/wake rhythm, food and fluid intake, and sexual activity" through connections with brainstem centers (cf. ibid.) (Spektrum Lexikon der Neurowissenschaft 2000g, n.p.). Furthermore, it is integrated into the regulation of emotions and affects as well as memory functions (Korsakoff syndrome). Through the limbic system, emotional components are introduced into the hypothalamus and linked with autonomic functions (cf. ibid.). This leads, for example, to feeling full at the sight of food, eating "comfort food," experiencing "cold sweat" from fear, or getting "cold feet" before an exam (Spektrum Lexikon der Neurowissenschaft 2000g, n.p.).

In summary, it can be stated that the hypothalamus is an important "control center" of our body. It coordinates water and salt balance as well as blood pressure, regulates constant body temperature and food intake. It influences our emotions and sexual behavior and determines the sleep-wake rhythm. Additionally, it is a relevant control organ within the endocrine system, as it regulates the timing and amount of hormone production. Both releasing hormones (which promote the production of other hormones) and inhibiting hormones (which inhibit the release of other hormones) are produced in the hypothalamus. The hormones produced by the hypothalamus reach the pituitary gland (hypophysis) via nerve fibers or blood vessels. Various factors can stimulate or inhibit hormone production in the hypothalamus. These can include emotional stress, our environment, physical exertion, and the biological rhythm. Most hormones are produced and secreted in a specific chronobiological rhythm (cf. BDI 2022, n.p.).

> The hypothalamus "(…) together with the reticular formation of the brainstem, is the 'survival center' of our brain. Through the release of various neuropeptides, the hypothalamus, together with the pituitary gland, is also involved in processes of stress management and interpersonal bonding" (Roth and Strüber 2021, 78).

The following section will therefore take a closer look at the pituitary gland or hypophysis.

1.3.3 Pituitary Gland or Hypophysis

The pituitary gland (hypophysis or glandula pituitaria) is a cherry pit to hazelnut-sized endocrine organ in the central nervous system. It is connected to the hypothalamus via the pituitary stalk and serves, among other things, the release of hypothalamic hormones (cf. Schöller 2019a, n.p.). It is located in a bony indentation, which is also referred to as the sella turcica or Turkish saddle. This is predominantly formed by the sphenoid bone (os sphenoidale) (cf. von Werder 2005, 8). The pituitary gland consists of an anterior lobe (adenohypophysis) and a posterior lobe (neurohypophysis). The adenohypophysis (anterior pituitary lobe) produces several tropins and interleukins (peptide hormones) such as IL-6 in its cells (cf. von Werder 2005, cited in Ehlert 2011, 8). The neurohypophysis (posterior pituitary lobe), on the other hand, does not produce hormones but merely secretes them. The neurohypophysis is a neurohemal organ. Here, neurons end directly at blood vessels, through which hormones are released. The neurosecretory neurons originate in the nuclei supraopticus and paraventricularis (cf. von Werder 2005, cited in Ehlert 2011, 8). In the neurohypophysis, ADH (antidiuretic hormone) and oxytocin (OXY), which are formed in the hypothalamus but not released there, are stored. ADH and OXY are transported via axonal transport to the presynaptic endings of the neurons and subsequently stored there. Even though ADH and OXY are formed in the hypothalamus, they are referred to as pituitary hormones due to their storage and release from the neurohypophysis (cf. Birbaumer and Schmidt 2018, 127).

1.3.4 Adenohypophysis or Anterior Pituitary Lobe

The adenohypophysis (anterior pituitary lobe) is an endocrine part of the pituitary gland. It forms glandotropic hormones (e.g., follicle-stimulating hormone and adrenocorticotropic hormone) as well as glandotropic proteohormones (e.g., prolactin and somatotropin). The adenohypophysis is connected to the hypothalamus via a special vascular system (portal vessels of the pituitary). The activity or regulation of the release (secretion) of the hormones is controlled by releasing hormones of the hypothalamus (cf. Schöller 2019b, n.p.). The peculiarity of the adenohypophysis is that both tropins and interleukins such as IL-6 are produced in its glandular cells (cf. von Werder 2005, cited in Ehlert 2011, 8). The adenohypophysis produces a total of 6 vital hormones. Of these, 4 hormones are glandotropic hormones or regulatory hormones. Their target organs are each a gland. The other two hormones are non-glandotropic hormones, and they are therefore referred to as effector hormones. These two do not act on glands but on the entire organism or other organ systems (cf. Birbaumer and Schmidt 2018, 127).

1.3.5 Neurohypophysis or Posterior Pituitary Lobe

In contrast to the adenohypophysis, the neurohypophysis (posterior pituitary lobe) does not produce hormones itself but merely secretes them. The neurohypophysis is a neurohemal organ. This means that neurons end directly at blood vessels, and hormones are secreted via this pathway (cf. von Werder 2005, cited in Ehlert 2011, 8). It is an outpouching of the diencephalon and is part of the central nervous system (CNS). Like the adenohypophysis, it is also connected to the hypothalamus. The neurohypophysis stores the hormones ADH (antidiuretic hormone) and oxytocin produced there, and these are secreted into the bloodstream by it as needed (cf. Schöller 2019c, n.p.). ADH (antidiuretic hormone) and oxytocin are thus formed in the hypothalamus but not released there. They are stored in the presynaptic endings of the neurohypophysis, and their synaptic release occurs directly into the blood. Even though ADH and oxytocin are formed in the hypothalamus, they are referred to as pituitary hormones due to their storage and release from the neurohypophysis (cf. Birbaumer and Schmidt 2018, 127).

1.3.6 Hypothalamic-Pituitary Hormone System

The so-called pituitary portal system (Fig. 1.2) is a venous system that consists of two capillary beds (one in the median eminence and one in the anterior pituitary). The pituitary portal system connects the pituitary gland and the hypothalamus. Through this system, releasing hormones are transported, which signal the hormone production in the pituitary gland (control of hormone release) (cf. Pschyrembel Editorial 2016a, n.p.).

> "To transport the hypothalamic hormones to their target cells in the anterior pituitary (AP), the organism has developed a special (…) vascular system: A first capillary network absorbs the neurohormones from the axonal terminals of the glandular nerve cells, and a second capillary network in the AP, connected behind it, brings the neurohormones to their pituitary target cells in the fastest way" (Birbaumer and Schmidt 2018, 126).

1.3.7 Thyroid and Parathyroid Glands

The thyroid gland (Glandula thyreoidea) is a vital endocrine gland. It is particularly relevant for metabolism, growth, and the maturation of the body and helps regulate numerous body functions. It continuously secretes a certain amount of thyroid hormones into the blood. When the body requires more energy in various situations, such as in cold conditions, during growth, or during pregnancy, it also produces correspondingly more hormones (cf. IQWiG 2021, n.p.). The thyroid gland (Glandula thyreoidea) along with the parathyroid glands (Glandulae parathyroideae) and the adrenal glands (Glandulae adrenalis) and the gonads are predominantly stimulated by tropins from the adenohypophysis (cf. von Werder 2005, cited in Ehlert 2011, 8). The thyroid gland encircles the

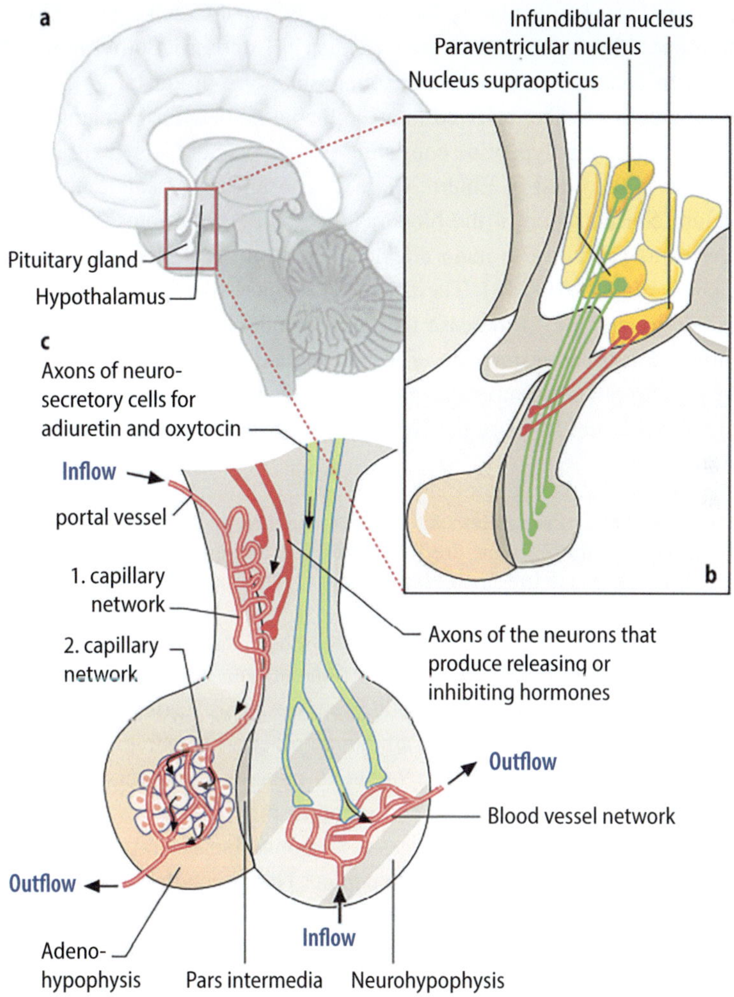

Fig. 1.2 Overview of the location and structure of the hypothalamic-pituitary system. In: Birbaumer, Niels/Schmidt, Robert F. (2018): Biological Psychology. Special edition. 7th revised and supplemented edition. Heidelberg: Springer Medizin Verlag. 127. *Source:* Birbaumer and Schmidt (2018, 127)

trachea in a horseshoe shape below the thyroid cartilage in the lower front third of the neck (cf. Birbaumer and Schmidt 2018, 129). "It is surrounded by a capsule and is movable on the trachea" (ibid.). It is therefore located below the larynx (Larynx) and the trachea (Trachea) (cf. von Werder 2005, cited in Ehlert 2011, 8). "Histologically, it consists of follicles divided into lobular regions, in which the thyroid hormones are contained" (Birbaumer and Schmidt 2018, 129 f.). The hormone-producing cells of the thyroid gland are referred to as follicular epithelial cells (FC) and C-cells. The FC produce the thyroid hormones thyroxine (tetraiodothyronine, T_4) and triiodothyronine (T_3) using stored iodine. In contrast, calcitonin and somatostatin are produced in the C-cells. The 4 parathyroid glands are also referred to as epithelial bodies. In the parathyroid glands, parathyroid hormone (a polypeptide consisting of amino acids) is synthesized by C-cells (cf. von Werder 2005, cited in Ehlert 2011, 8). The release of calcitonin is stimulated by the calcium concentration in the blood as well as by gastrointestinal hormones (for example, by pentagastrin). The main effect of calcitonin is the reduction of blood calcium levels (cf. Ehlert 2011, 18). The thyroid hormones thyroxine (tetraiodothyronine, T_4) and triiodothyronine (T_3) increase the basal metabolic rate in the human organism as they stimulate cellular respiration. They are bound in the thyroid follicles and are released by thyrotropin (a hormonal signal) from the adenohypophysis (thyrotropic feedback loop) (cf. Spektrum Lexikon der Neurowissenschaft 2000h, n.p.). Disorders of thyroid function, such as

> "Hypo- and hyperthyroidism are among the most common endocrine disorders. In adults, the consequences of dysfunctions are fully reversible through therapy, while in infants, hypothyroidism can lead to irreversible brain damage" (Birbaumer and Schmidt 2018, 131).

If thyroid hormones are lacking in early childhood, it leads to what is known as cretinism. These are severe physical and mental retardations. In an adult, dysfunctions are based on the slowing down of all metabolic processes. This leads to a reduction in both physical and mental activity. In adults, all symptoms are reversible through the administration of thyroid hormones. It is important to mention, however, that thyroid function disorders can result in behavioral and mood disorders. Both mood and intellectual performance can be affected. In severe cases, profound behavioral disorders can occur, resembling melancholic depression or dementia. The psychological disorders regress when thyroid function normalizes. It is also observed that depressive and manic-depressive illnesses are often accompanied by a disorder of the thyroid hormone balance. This has led to the frequent use of thyroid hormones as an adjunct therapy for depression (cf. Birbaumer and Schmidt 2018, 131).

1.3.8 Gastroenteropancreatic Endocrine System (GEP)

> "The endocrine gastroenteropancreatic system is the largest endocrine system in the body. The hormones formed here are responsible for the release of digestive juices, intestinal motility, and trophic effects" (Arnold 2007, 378).

It should also be noted that the GEP is considered part of the diffuse neuroendocrine system. The endocrine cells in the duodenum (Duodenum) and in the small intestine (Intestinum tenue) are called APUD cells ("amine precursor uptake and decarboxylation") (cf. von Werder 2005, cited in Ehlert 2011, 8). "These produce CCK (I-cells), secretin (S-cells), gastric inhibitory peptide (GIP) (K-cells), and somatostatin (D-cells)" (ibid.). The pancreas, on the other hand, has both endocrine and exocrine functions. It produces both hormones and digestive enzymes. In the exocrine glandular tissue of the pancreas, the Langerhans cells are located. They consist of various cell types (cf. von Werder 2005, cited in Ehlert 2011, 8). In the Langerhans cells (named after Paul Langerhans), the "hormones glucagon (α-cells), insulin (β-cells), somatostatin (δ-cells), pancreatic polypeptide (PP-cells), and ghrelin (ε-cells)" (von Werder 2005, cited in Ehlert 2011, 8) are produced. It should be noted here that there is highly specific communication between the GIT (gastrointestinal tract) and the brain. This occurs neurally through the enteric nervous system (ENS) as well as biochemically through many hypothalamic-pituitary and gastrointestinal (neuro-)transmitters (cf. Ehlert 2011, 19 f.).

1.3.9 Adrenal Glands

The adrenal glands (Glandula suprarenalis) are paired and lie cap-like over the two kidneys (cf. Schöller 2018, n.p.). They are called adrenal glands only because of their proximity to the kidneys, as they are independent hormone glands (cf. von Werder 2005, cited in Ehlert 2011, 8). Each adrenal gland "consists of the adrenal medulla (Medulla glandulae suprarenalis) and the adrenal cortex (Cortex glandulae suprarenalis)" (ibid.). The adrenal medulla (short medulla) and the adrenal cortex (short cortex) have different functions and are often considered distinct organs (cf. von Werder 2005, cited in Ehlert 2011, 8). The adrenal cortex synthesizes steroid hormones (glucocorticoids, mineralocorticoids, and sex hormones). The adrenal medulla produces catecholamines (cf. Schöller 2018, n.p.). These are the catecholamines adrenaline, noradrenaline, and dopamine, as well as L-tyrosine, which are produced, stored, and released upon cholinergic stimulation (cf. von Werder 2005, cited in Ehlert 2011, 8). In the adrenal cortex, on the other hand, glucocorticoids such as cortisol and cortisone are formed, as well as sex hormones such as estrogens and androgens. Since the adrenal glands are responsible for producing such a high number of hormones, disorders lead to a variety of clinical pictures (cf. Schöller 2018, n.p.).

1.3.10 Gonads

In men, the gonads are called testes (testicles) and in women, they are called ovaries (cf. von Werder 2005, cited in Ehlert 2011, 8). The gonadal or sex hormones, which are formed in the gonads, are steroids. The male sex hormones are called androgens, and the female ones are called estrogens and gestagens. Both sexes produce both female and male gonadal hormones, but in very small amounts in the opposite sex (cf. Birbaumer and Schmidt 2018, 133 f.).

1) Testes or Testicles

In men, the hormones are formed in the testes, specifically in the Sertoli and Leydig cells (cf. von Werder 2005, cited in Ehlert 2011, 8). The testes are a paired male endocrine gland as well as a gonad. They are located in the scrotum (skin sac), and in addition to the production of testosterone in the Leydig interstitial cells, spermatogenesis (development of male germ cells) takes place in the seminiferous tubules (Tubuli seminiferi recti). Furthermore, the seminiferous tubules transport the sperm to the epididymis (cf. Pschyrembel Editorial 2016b, n.p.). The main production of the sex hormone testosterone takes place in the Leydig interstitial cells (cf. von Werder 2005, cited in Ehlert 2011, 8).

Leydig interstitial cells are epithelioid cell groups located in the interstitial connective tissue of the testes, between the seminiferous tubules (tubuli seminiferi recti), and they produce androgens. The synthesis (production) of testosterone occurs through the stimulation of luteinizing hormone (LH). An adult man produces 6–8 mg of testosterone per day (cf. Pschyrembel Editorial 2016c, n.p.). The most significant representative of the produced androgens is testosterone (cf. Birbaumer and Schmidt 2018, 134). The seminiferous tubules are supported by the so-called Sertoli cells. They regulate spermiogenesis and nourish maturing sperm cells. Additionally, they produce hormones (cf. Pschyrembel Editorial 2016d, n.p.).

"The Sertoli cells produce

- the androgen-binding protein
- the transport protein for testosterone, and
- estrogen from testosterone through aromatization" (von Werder 2005, cited in Ehlert 2011, 8).

2) Ovaries

In the ovaries, as in the adrenal glands, the medulla and cortex can be differentiated. In the cortex are the so-called oocytes (female germ cells), which mature into follicles during the reproductive age. These are then released into the fallopian tubes (tubes) during ovulation (follicle rupture) (cf. von Werder 2005, cited in Ehlert 2011, 9). In the first half of the cycle, the so-called maturation phase (follicular phase), the follicles produce estradiol. During this 10- to 14-day maturation phase, the estradiol level steadily increases. During this time, estradiol exerts a dual negative feedback effect on the LH and FSH cells of the pituitary gland (hypophysis). It inhibits their release and makes the LH and FSH-producing cells insensitive to GnRH (from the hypothalamus). Therefore, these hormones are hardly released during this time (cf. Birbaumer and Schmidt 2018, 135). In the middle of the female cycle, the follicle ruptures, and the egg cell is transported to the uterus. The remaining follicle tissue is transformed into the corpus luteum. This corpus luteum produces and secretes corpus luteum hormones (progesterone) and follicle hormones (estrogen) during the second half of the cycle (luteal phase) (cf. von Werder 2005, cited in Ehlert 2011, 9). In the ovulation phase (second half of the cycle; 12th–15th day), the estradiol level finally rises sharply. This causes the negative inhibitory effect on the LH and FSH cells to switch from negative to positive feedback. The LH peak triggers the follicle rupture, releasing a (fertilizable) egg cell (ovulation) (cf. Birbaumer and Schmidt 2018, 135). The LH causes the follicle to begin transforming into the corpus luteum shortly before ovulation. This process is called luteinization (cf. Birbaumer and Schmidt 2018, 135). If pregnancy does not occur and the corpus luteum is not stimulated by hCG (human chorionic gonadotropin), it regresses, leading to menstruation. The theca interna cells then produce testosterone, which is converted to estradiol by the granulosa cells. In the second half of the cycle (luteal phase), both the theca interna and granulosa cells produce progesterone (cf. von Werder 2005, cited in Ehlert 2011, 9). Of the hormones produced in the ovaries, the most significant estrogen is estradiol, and the most significant progestogen is progesterone. Both estradiol and progesterone exert a negative feedback effect on the FSH and LH cells in the third phase of the cycle (especially after ovulation), causing their hormone secretions to decrease. Estradiol and subsequently progesterone prepare the uterine lining for possible implantation. If this does not occur, the lining is shed approximately 14 days after ovulation (cf. Birbaumer and Schmidt 2018, 134–137).

In summary, it can be stated that sex hormones produced in the gonads are steroid hormones derived from cholesterol and that there is a close chemical relationship between them (cf. Birbaumer and Schmidt 2018, 134). "The most important representative of the androgens is testosterone, the most important estrogen is estradiol, and the most important progestogen is progesterone" (ibid.). However, sex hormones are not synthesized solely in the gonads. In men, one-third of testosterone comes from the adrenal cortex, and in women, large amounts of progesterone are produced by the placenta during pregnancy (cf. Birbaumer and Schmidt 2018, 134). Therefore, more on the placenta follows.

1.3.11 Placenta or Afterbirth

The placenta (also called afterbirth) is, like the follicle, an organ that resides in the female body only for a limited time. The placenta is active in the female body only during pregnancy and is expelled as "afterbirth" at birth. It forms after the implantation of the blastocyst (cf. von Werder 2005, cited in Ehlert 2011, 9). The placenta is perfused by both the mother's blood and the child's blood and serves to supply the rapidly growing embryo. The fetus is connected to the placenta via the umbilical cord (cf. Birbaumer and Schmidt 2018, 137). The placenta is the largest organ during pregnancy. It dominates the entire hormonal system during pregnancy (cf. Schleußner 2018, 89–102). The placenta itself produces hormones such as placental GH ("growth hormone"), CRH, various prostaglandins, lactogen, as well as hCG and progesterone (cf. Fowden et al. 2008, cited in Ehlert 2011, 9). The peptide and steroid hormones influence all endocrine functional circuits and regulatory axes. The central pregnancy hormone progesterone relaxes the muscle layer of the uterus (myometrium) and has anti-inflammatory and immunosuppressive functions. These enable the development of the necessary immune tolerance at the interface between the fetus and the mother's organism (fetomaternal interface). Estrogens regulate the maternal adaptation to pregnancy. Placental lactogen, placental growth hormone, and leptin alter maternal metabolism to continuously ensure fetal supply. Placental CRH (corticotropin-releasing hormone) is considered the "placental clock" because it plays a central role in triggering birth (cf. Schleußner 2018, 89–102).

1.3.12 Skin

Finally, the skin should be mentioned as an endocrine organ. Our skin cells are not only influenced by hormones, but they also release hormones themselves, such as:

- Insulin-like growth factors
- Proopiomelanocortin (POMC) derivatives
- Catecholamines
- Cortisol
- Estrogens (cf. von Werder 2005, cited in Ehlert 2011, 9).

It has been found that about 30 different hormones and hormone groups are active in the skin cells of the subcutaneous fat tissue. Hormones play a significant role, especially in development and physiological function. Human skin cells have hormone-specific receptors. These are the targets of various hormones with known effects. However, the skin is not only a recipient but also produces hormones itself (cf. Zouboulis 2013, n.p.).

> "Skin cells have all the biochemical capabilities to produce glucocorticoids, androgens, and estrogens—either from systemic precursors or alternatively by converting cholesterol into the prohormone pregnenolone and subsequently converting it into biologically active steroids. Examples of this are cortisol, testosterone, and estradiol" (Zouboulis 2013, n.p.).

With a total area of 1.5 to 2 m^2, it is not only the largest organ by surface area (cf. Pschyrembel Redaktion 2016e, n.p.), but also the largest endocrine organ in humans (cf. Zouboulis 2013, n.p.).

After describing the endocrine glands, the following section will outline the most important hormones and their places of origin.

1.4 The Most Important Hormones and Their Places of Origin

The following section describes the most important hormones and their places of origin. This means that in this section, you will gain basic knowledge about the most important hormones and their places of origin. The hormones most significant for psychoneuroendocrinology will then be examined and explained in more detail in Chap. 2. The following is a general introduction to the most important hormones for humans.

1.4.1 Neuropeptides of the Hypothalamus: Releasing Hormones (Liberins)

Releasing hormones are also called liberins and are neuropeptides produced in specific nuclei in the hypothalamus. Their neurons terminate in the median eminence. There, under the influence of other hormones and neurotransmitters, the liberins are secreted into the blood vessels that extend to the adenohypophysis. Consequently, the neuropeptides cause the secretion of various tropins there. The releasing hormones include the peptides CRH, TRH, GnRH, and GHRH (cf. Ehlert 2011, 10).

1.4.1.1 CRH—Corticotropin-Releasing Hormone

Corticotropin-Releasing Hormone, abbreviated CRH (synonym: CRF—Corticotropin-Releasing Factor), is a peptide hormone that is produced in the hypothalamus and consists of over 41 amino acids (cf. Pschyrembel Editorial 2020c, n.p.). Stressful situations of all kinds lead to an activation of the hypothalamus, whereupon CRH is increasingly secreted (cf. Birbaumer and Schmidt 2018, 133). Thus, the hypothalamic-pituitary-adrenal axis is involved in the stress response. CRH also stimulates the release of ACTH (adrenocorticotropin) in the adenohypophysis (anterior pituitary), which activates the sympathetic nervous system. CRH also causes the secretion of β-endorphin in pain and stress situations (cf. Pschyrembel Editorial 2020c, n.p.). The release of CRH follows a circadian rhythm. Compared to the evening, a higher release occurs in the morning. The secretion of CRH is to be understood as a direct response to stress (cf. Ehlert 2011, 10 f.).

"The secretion is influenced, among other things, by

- catecholaminergic stimulation,
- a negative feedback of glucocorticoids formed under the influence of ACTH,
- IL-1 β and TNF" (Ehlert 2011, 10).

When an increased CRH release occurs, it results in an increased release of ACTH (adrenocorticotropic hormone) and subsequently the release of cortisol and other glucocorticoids (cf. Birbaumer and Schmidt 2018, 133). CRH is subject to negative feedback by cortisol, which in turn suppresses the synthesis of CRH in the hypothalamus. This prevents an excessive stress response and allows adaptation to chronic stress situations (cf. Spektrum Lexikon der Biologie 1999, n.p.). Since CRH leads to an increased release of ACTH, it results in the synthesis of glucocorticoids, making CRH indirectly responsible for a variety of effects. This includes impacts on metabolism, the immune system, electrolyte balance, and the nervous system (cf. Pschyrembel Editorial 2020d, n.p.). Furthermore, CRH is involved in thermoregulation and the regulation of hunger and satiety (cf. Ehlert 2011, 10).

Closely related to CRH are the so-called urocortins (cf. Ehlert 2011, 10), which are briefly described below.

1.4.1.2 Urocortins

Urocortins are peptides composed of 40 amino acids and have a high chemical similarity to CRH. There are Urocortin I, II, and III. Like CRH, urocortins also bind to CRH receptors (cf. Ehlert 2011, 10 f.). Thus, urocortins belong to the corticotropin-releasing hormone family (cf. Riester 2013, n.p.). However, while CRH is secreted due to stress, urocortin plays a significant role in the recovery from stress (cf. Ehlert 2011, 10 f.). Urocortins are important modulators in anxiety control, the stress response, and associated disorders such as depression (cf. Riester 2013, n.p.).

1.4.1.3 TRH—Thyrotropin-Releasing Hormone

Thyrotropin (synonym: thyroliberin) is a releasing hormone that stimulates the release of TSH (thyroid-stimulating hormone) from the adenohypophysis (anterior pituitary) (cf. Pschyrembel Editorial 2020e, n.p.). Additionally, TRH initiates the thyroid cycle and stimulates the transcription and secretion of prolactin (cf. Ehlert 2011, 11). It is produced in the hypothalamus, with its synthesis being inhibited by thyroid hormones (via a negative feedback mechanism). The release of TRH is stimulated by norepinephrine and reduced by serotonin (cf. Pschyrembel Editorial 2020e, n.p.). TRH is found in almost the entire central nervous system and influences many behavioral functions (cf. Birbaumer and Schmidt 2018, 130). It acts as a neurotransmitter in various locations in the brain and spinal cord (cf. Ehlert 2011, 11).

1.4.1.4 GnRH—Gonadotropin-Releasing Hormone

GnRH (Gonadotropin-Releasing Hormone) is a decapeptide that is secreted at intervals of 30–120 minutes and influences, among other things, the release of the pregnancy hormone hCG (human chorionic gonadotropin) (cf. Ehlert 2011, 11). The gonadotropin-releasing hormone (synonym: gonadoliberin) is synthesized in the hypothalamus. As part of the gonadotropic axis, it stimulates both the synthesis and secretion of LH (luteinizing hormone) and FSH (follicle-stimulating hormone) from the adenohypophysis (anterior pituitary gland) (cf. Pschyrembel Redaktion 2020f, n.p.). LH and FSH release the sex hormones and in turn negatively feedback on both the hypothalamus and the pituitary gland. Thus, the sex hormones are involved in the hypothalamic-pituitary regulatory circuit. LH is primarily responsible for the production of androgens in the male testes.

Androgens and FSH together are responsible for spermatogenesis, i.e., the formation of male sperm cells (spermatozoa), which are located in the seminiferous tubules of the testes. The effects of androgens, particularly testosterone, lead to a masculine appearance (cf. Bierbaumer and Schmidt 2018, 135).

1.4.1.5 GHRH—Somatoliberin

GHRH ("growth hormone releasing hormone") is also referred to as somatoliberin and stimulates the production and secretion of somatotropin (growth hormone) in the adenohypophysis (anterior pituitary gland). GHRH influences sleep behavior. Suppressed release of GHRH leads to a reduction in NREM sleep. A day-night rhythm in GHRH release can be observed, which correlates with wake-sleep behavior (cf. Ehlert 2011, 11). Birbaumer and Schmidt (2018) note that the pulsatile release of somatotropin is regulated by the two hypothalamic hormones GHRH and somatostatin. The growth hormone somatotropin is essential for normal physical development (cf. Birbaumer and Schmidt 2018, 129). Additionally, GHRH is present both in the gastrointestinal tract and as a neurotransmitter in various brain regions (cf. Ehlert 2011, 11).

1.4.2 Neuropeptides of the Hypothalamus: Release-Inhibiting Hormones

In addition to the already mentioned releasing hormones (liberins), various release-inhibiting hormones influence the hypothalamic-pituitary hormone system. The inhibiting hormones include SST (somatostatin), PIF (prolactin-inhibiting factor), and MRIH (melanotropin-release-inhibiting hormone). Their function is sometimes controversially discussed (cf. Ehlert 2011, 11).

1.4.2.1 SST—Somatostatin

SST is considered the antagonist of somatoliberin. It is formed in the hypothalamus and blocks the release of GHRH, which is why it is also called "somatotropin release inhibitory factor." During the day-night release rhythm, SST has a modulating influence on the secretion of GHRH. Furthermore, the formation of SST has been demonstrated in the stomach, small intestine, and pancreas, where it also inhibits the release of several hormones (cf. Ehlert 2011, 11).

1.4.2.2 PRH—Prolactin-Releasing Hormone

Prolactin is an effector hormone that primarily controls the initiation and maintenance of milk synthesis (milk production). Oxytocin, on the other hand, controls milk ejection (cf. Birbaumer and Schmidt 2018, 128). PRH stimulates the release of prolactin (PRL) in the pituitary gland, as do TRH (thyrotropin-releasing hormone) and VIP (vasoactive intestinal peptide). Although it is a potent releaser, it is not considered a liberin like the aforementioned neuropeptides. According to Ehlert, PRH acts as a neurotransmitter and influences energy metabolism, pain processing, and autonomic functions (cf. Ehlert 2011, 11 f.).

Since to date (as of 2023) no biochemical evidence for the existence of PRH has been provided, it is debated whether PRH is actually oxytocin (OXY) (cf. Ehlert 2011, 12). Whether PRH can currently (2023) be biochemically detected is scientifically not yet established. Furthermore, PIF (prolactin-inhibiting factor) is dopamine, a biogenic amine secreted by neuron clusters in the hypothalamus, according to Ehlert (cf. Ehlert 2011, 12). The knowledge that it is chemically dopamine is significant because there are many medications with dopaminergic agonist and antagonist effects that either promote or inhibit prolactin secretion (cf. Birbaumer and Schmidt 2018, 129).

1.4.2.3 MRIH—Melanostatin

MRIH (Melanostatin) is a neuropeptide consisting of 3 amino acids. It has been detected in the hypothalamus, and animal experiments have shown (cf. Ehlert 2011, 12) "(…) that an injection of MRIH into the hypothalamus blocks the release of melanotropin (MSH) from the pituitary gland" (ibid.). As melanostatin, the neuropeptide Y (NPY) acts. This is also responsible for triggering hunger, which in turn is suppressed by leptin (cf. Ehlert 2011, 12).

1.4.2.4 Peptides and Food Intake

In the hypothalamus, a variety of peptides are secreted, which (among other things) are involved in food intake, according to Ehlert (2011). These include AgRP (agouti-related peptide), ghrelin, melanotropins (MSH), as well as the already mentioned hormones leptin and NPY (neuropeptide Y). They are involved in the regulation of food intake in the brain and are produced both in the hypothalamus and in the intermediate lobe of the pituitary gland. The neuropeptides AgRP and NPY have an appetite-stimulating effect, whereas POMC (proopiomelanocortin) and CART ("cocaine- and amphetamine-regulated transcript") are considered appetite-suppressing peptides (cf. Ehlert 2011, 12).

1.4.2.5 Dopamine and Dopaminergic Systems

I would also like to mention dopamine among the neuropeptides of the hypothalamus. Since dopamine is of enormous importance for psychoneuroendocrinology, basic knowledge is presented here, and subsequently, in Chap. 2, dopamine is examined in more detail.

> "Dopamine is the most important messenger in the brain, functioning motorically and psychologically as the neurochemical basis of incentive and positive psychomotor activity" (Birbaumer and Schmidt 2018, 95).

As an introduction, it should be noted that the neurons of dopamine (dopaminergic system) are found in various brain regions, particularly in the midbrain (mesencephalon) (cf. Ehlert 2011, 12). Dopamine is a neurotransmitter of the CNS, which is derived from the amino acid tyrosine. Initially, dopa is formed as an intermediate product. The subsequently converted dopamine is then stored in synaptic vesicles. Dopamine belongs to the catecholamines and is the immediate precursor of norepinephrine and adrenaline as well as melanins (cf. Spektrum Lexikon der Neurowissenschaft 2000i, n.p.). Dopamine controls involuntary movements in the striatum and substantia nigra, thus transmitting commands to the muscles via the nervous system. Therefore, a lack of dopamine leads to Parkinson's disease. Projections in the mesolimbic dopamine system play a crucial role in the development of psychoses and addictive behavior. Furthermore, dopamine reaches the pituitary gland via the bloodstream and inhibits prolactin there, which is why a dopamine deficiency is also associated with hyperprolactinemia (excessively high prolactin levels in the blood) (cf. Ehlert 2011, 12).

In addition to the dopaminergic influence on motor skills, involvement in addictive behavior, and significance for psychotic disorders, dopamine also promotes renal blood flow and modulates intestinal activity (cf. Spektrum Lexikon der Neurowissenschaft 2000i, n.p.). The two most important dopamine systems are the mesolimbic and the nigrostriatal systems (cf. Birbaumer and Schmidt 2018, 95). The mesolimbic and nigrostriatal systems are the main connections, but there are also several other cell systems and fibers where dopamine functions as a transmitter, specifically hypothalamic-pituitary, spinal, and limbic structures. Most fibers of the mesolimbic dopamine system originate in the lateral tegmentum of the mesencephalon (midbrain). The mesolimbic system, among other things, has positive incentive functions, and it is important to mention that an excess of dopamine in mesolimbic brain regions combined with a deficiency in frontal brain regions leads to thought disorders in schizophrenics. The nigrostriatal extrapyramidal dopamine system is closely related to the switching of motor programs. A dopamine deficiency in this system, as already mentioned, can lead to symptoms of Parkinson's disease (cf. Birbaumer and Schmidt 2018, 95). Additionally, I would like to address the function of dopamine autoreceptors here.

> "Dopamine autoreceptors at dopaminergic synapses inhibit the reuptake of dopamine into the synapses, thereby increasing its availability in the synaptic cleft" (Birbaumer and Schmidt 2018, 95).

Cocaine, amphetamine, and Ritalin (methylphenidate) are well-known drugs that are based on the mechanisms of these receptors. All the mentioned drugs increase attention and are highly emotionally stimulating. The addictive effect of these substances unfolds through the mesolimbic dopamine system. In case of an overdose, thought disorders such as paranoia occur (cf. Birbaumer and Schmidt 2018, 95).

In-depth knowledge about dopamine, as well as the enormous importance of dopamine for our behavior, will be presented in Chap. 2 ("Psychoneuroendocrinology").

1.4.2.6 Serotonin and the Serotonergic System

Just like dopamine, serotonin is also of particular importance in psychoneuroendocrinology, which is why an introduction to serotonin and the serotonergic system is provided here. A more detailed explanation and description of the effects, as well as the significance of serotonin for the psyche and mental disorders, is provided in Chap. 2 ("Psychoneuroendocrinology").

> "Serotonin, with its mood-influencing effects, determines a person's personality structure" (Birbaumer and Schmidt 2018, 97).

Serotonin is a neurotransmitter of the central nervous system, which also partially acts hormonally. It is formed in a 2-step reaction from the amino acid tryptophan (cf. Pschyrembel Editorial Team 2020b, n.p.). Serotonin is also referred to as 5-HT (5-hydroxytryptamine). It is produced both in the central nervous system and in the body's periphery (cf. Ehlert 2011, 12), with the majority being produced in the gastrointestinal tract and only about 10% in the central nervous system. Serotonergic neurons control, among other things, emotions, learning processes, the sleep-wake cycle, as well as body temperature, blood pressure, and intestinal peristalsis (activity of the intestinal muscles) (cf. Pschyrembel Editorial Team 2020b, n.p.). Serotonin is of particular importance regarding mental disorders such as depression, but also for various other bodily functions. The enormous number of different effects can be seen in the receptor subtypes for serotonin. There are 14 different 5-HT receptors. These receptors are associated in the central nervous system, for example, with thermoregulation and central blood pressure regulation, learning processes, and depressive mood states (cf. Ehlert 2011, 13). Other receptors are responsible for the "serotonergic regulation of gastrointestinal processes" (Ehlert 2011, 13). Additionally, "serotonergic receptor subclasses are involved in circadian rhythms and adaptation to the day-night cycle" (ibid.). As already mentioned, the transmitter serotonin is not present in large quantities in the central nervous system, but based on its extensive connections, it is of great importance. There are more than 10 receptors for serotonin. In addition to its neuronal effects, serotonin is also important for the regulation of cerebral blood flow and vessel diameter (cf. Birbaumer and Schmidt 2018, 96). The origin nuclei in the rhombencephalon and the fiber systems are in close proximity to the noradrenaline systems. Together with other transmitters, the fibers descending into the spinal cord coordinate pain perception. If the serotonin concentration decreases or there is a loss of serotonin receptors, this is associated with excessively aggressive behavior (cf. Birbaumer and Schmidt 2018, 96). "Androgens (…) also reduce the activity of serotonergic synapses and are responsible for the increased aggressiveness of the male sex" (Birbaumer and Schmidt 2018, 97).

How significant serotonin is for the human psyche and behavior will be further illustrated in the following sections.

1.4.2.7 KiSS Peptides

The so-called KiSS peptides were first characterized in 2001. The most significant KiSS peptide is kisspeptin-54 (cf. Ehlert 2011, 13). Kisspeptin is a peptide hormone and is synthesized in the hypothalamus. It is a trigger of puberty, and it is also suspected to induce the release of gonadoliberin. It should also be mentioned that kisspeptin further suppresses the development of metastases in breast cancer and skin cancer (cf. Pschyrembel 2020 g, n.p.). Kisspeptin-54 is produced in both women and men, but it is secreted by women of childbearing age in 7 times higher amounts than in men. Especially during pregnancy, women reach extremely high concentrations here (cf. Ehlert 2011, 13).

1.4.3 Hormones of the Adenohypophysis

As previously described, releasing hormones (liberins) in the adenohypophysis (anterior pituitary) release tropins, which in turn secrete hormones in various peripheral endocrine glands (cf. Ehlert 2011, 13). The following will outline the most significant hormones of the adenohypophysis.

1.4.3.1 ACTH—Adrenocorticotropin

Under the influence of CRH (corticotropin-releasing hormone), ACTH (adrenocorticotropin) is formed in the adenohypophysis from POMC (proopiomelanocortin). ACTH consists of a total of 39 amino acids, but only 24 of them are physiologically significant. It acts as an agonist of melanocortin receptors in the adrenal cortex, where it stimulates the synthesis of glucocorticoids, mineralocorticoids, and androgenic steroids (sex hormones). Like all hormones of the hypothalamic-pituitary-adrenal axis, ACTH is subject to a circadian rhythm and is secreted in a pulsatile manner with a peak value in the morning (cf. Ehlert 2011, 13 f.). The main function of ACTH is to increase the production and release of glucocorticoids. Additionally, ACTH directly influences insulin production and secretion. ACTH is classified as a stress hormone because stress causes increased release of ACTH (cf. Pschyrembel 2020h, n.p.).

1.4.3.2 TSH—Thyrotropin, T3—Triiodothyronine, and T4—Thyroxine

TSH (thyrotropin) is a peptide hormone that is secreted in the adenohypophysis and stimulates the production of thyroid hormones in the thyroid gland (cf. Pschyrembel 2020i, n.p.). The release of TSH requires TRH (thyrotropin-releasing hormone), which is a hypothalamic releasing hormone. The TSH-producing gland cells of the adenohypophysis are controlled by the liberin TRH (cf. Birbaumer and Schmidt 2018, 130). TSH reaches the thyroid gland through the bloodstream. In the thyroid gland, it promotes cell division, leads to better iodine uptake in the thyrocytes, and the formation and release of the iodine-containing thyroid hormones T_3 (triiodothyronine) and T_4 (thyroxine) (cf. Ehlert 2011, 14). This means: "Hypothalamic TRH releases TSH from the anterior pituitary, which releases T_3 and T_4 from the follicles" (Birbaumer and Schmidt 2018, 130). The increase in concentration of T_3 and T_4 exerts negative feedback on both the hypothalamus and the pituitary gland. Furthermore, TSH is subject to a circadian rhythm, is secreted in a pulsatile manner, and reaches its peak value around midnight (cf. Ehlert 2011, 14). The lowest value, however, is reached in the afternoon. Abnormalities in TSH levels should be clarified through further diagnostics, as this can particularly identify hyperthyroidism or hypothyroidism (cf. Pschyrembel 2020i, n.p.).

Thyroid Hormones

"The main effect of T_3 and T_4 is the influence on energy metabolism, which is also called the calorigenic effect" (Birbaumer and Schmidt 2018, 130).

Thyroid hormones are used as an adjunct therapy in depressive disorders. For example, T_3 can "accelerate the onset of action of tricyclic antidepressants" (Birbaumer and Schmidt 2018, 131) and enhance the effectiveness of these antidepressants. T_4 is prescribed in high doses, especially to women who do not respond to usual medications. Here too, both the symptoms and the course of depression are improved (cf. ibid.).

1.4.3.3 LH—luteinizing hormone, and FSH—follicle-stimulating hormone

LH and FSH are gonadotropins and, like TSH for example, glycoproteins. They are secreted in a pulsatile manner under the influence of GnRH and affect gonadal functions in both the ovaries and the testes. In men, LH stimulates the production of testosterone in the Leydig cells. Subsequently, testosterone, together with FSH, stimulates sperm development (cf. Ehlert 2011, 14).

> "In women, LH stimulation leads to ovarian stimulation of estrogen and progesterone production, induction of ovulation, transformation of the follicle into the corpus luteum, and the resulting increase in progesterone" (Ehlert 2011, 14).

FSH enhances the effect of LH on the production of estrogen in the egg (ovary). This stimulates follicle maturation (cf. ibid.).

Menstrual Cycle

A steep increase in LH production can often be caused by psychological influences and results in the absence of menstruation. Additionally, psychological stress can prevent both menstruation and ovulation (egg release) by weakening or suppressing the LH surge. In diseases such as anorexia, the LH surge is also absent. In this case, it is often due to a lack of nutrition. In summary, it can be stated that if hormone secretion occurs irregularly and not within the given rhythm, both follicle maturation and ovulation (egg release) fail to occur (cf. Birbaumer and Schmidt 2018, 136). The so-called premenstrual syndrome (PMS) is associated with the aforementioned hormonal influences. It appears a few days before menstruation. Irritability and increased aggressiveness as well as depression are symptoms (cf. Birbaumer and Schmidt 2018, 136). Overall, PMS is one of the most common health impairments in women of reproductive age (cf. BMJ Open 2018, n.p.). PMS presents a complex symptomatology that begins 4–14 days before menstruation and subsides only with the onset of bleeding. The symptoms are both psychological and physical. Psychological symptoms include depressive moods, mood instability, anxiety, sleep disturbances, and lack of drive, as well as forgetfulness, affective instability, tearfulness, loss of control, and aggressiveness. General symptoms such as food cravings, headaches, and back pain, weight gain due to fluid retention, bloating, painful and tense breasts, and skin blemishes are also some symptoms. The exact causes of PMS are unclear, but hormonal cycle fluctuations, familial predispositions, and environmental factors are discussed, as well as the interaction of progesterone, especially with serotonin, and an increased sensitivity to progesterone breakdown products (cf. Krause 2022, n.p.). A 2018 study concludes that women who regularly consume alcohol are more likely to suffer from PMS (cf. BMJ Open 2018, n.p.). Birbaumer and Schmidt (2018) note that, even though the causes are still not entirely clear, psychological factors are inextricably and clearly linked with hormonal ones (cf. Birbaumer and Schmidt 2018, 136).

1.4.3.4 GH—"growth hormone"

GH—"growth hormone," also called somatotropin, is a peptide hormone produced in the adenohypophysis that promotes growth in the skeleton and muscles (cf. Pschyrembel Editorial 2020j, n.p.). GH is secreted in the adenohypophysis in a pulsatile manner, based on GHRH stimulation, as well as signals from the amygdala and noradrenergic neurons from the brainstem (cf. Ehlert 2011, 14). Production and release are inhibited by somatostatin and promoted by somatotropin-releasing hormones. Due to the hormone's relevance for growth, it is particularly important during childhood and adolescence. The highest concentration of GH occurs during puberty. A deficiency of this hormone leads to dwarfism, and excessive production results in gigantism (cf. Pschyrembel Editorial 2020j, n.p.). Somatostatin (SST) inhibits GH release as well as IGF-1 ("insulin-like growth factor-1"), which is also produced in the liver and is also known as somatomedin C. However, GH stimulates IGF-1, which in turn promotes bone and cartilage growth, thus GH has an indirect effect here. During pregnancy, the growth hormone is also produced in the placenta. In the pulsatile release of the hormone, no circadian rhythmic secretion pattern is observed, yet nighttime sleep leads to an increased release rate. This is attributed to increased melatonin release during the deep sleep phase (cf. Ehlert 2011, 14). Unlike other tropins mentioned earlier, GH "has no releasing effect on other hormones in an endocrine gland" (ibid.).

In summary, it can be stated that the growth hormone is indispensable for normal physical development. The pulsatile release is regulated by two hypothalamic hormones. These are referred to as somatoliberin (GHRH) and somatostatin (SST) (cf. Birbaumer and Schmidt 2018, 129).

1.4.3.5 PRL—Prolactin

PRL is released in a pulsatile manner during nocturnal sleep. In addition to hormonal secretion patterns and inhibitory mechanisms, various behaviors have a releasing effect. These include sucking and touching the nipples, sexual intercourse, food intake, physical activity, as well as epileptic seizures. In women of reproductive age, PRL has an inhibitory effect on sex hormone secretion. During pregnancy and after birth, prolactin promotes lactogenesis and lactation (cf. Ehlert 2011, 14). PRL is a hormone that controls the initiation and maintenance of milk synthesis in women (cf. Birbaumer and Schmidt 2018, 128).

Through mechanical stimulation of the nipples, among other sensory stimuli, the oxytocin-producing neurons in the hypothalamus can be activated. As a result, oxytocin is secreted into the blood and reaches the mammary gland. In the mammary gland, this increases the milk ejection pressure. Similarly, the uterine muscles are activated (cf. Birbaumer and Schmidt 2018, 129). Studies indicate that prolactin also influences reproductive function in men. PRL is released during orgasm in both women and men. However, excessively high PRL levels lead to impotence and gonadal dysfunction (hypogonadism) in men. Additionally, spermatogenesis can be negatively affected by elevated levels. Similarly, PRL levels increase in men during the transition to fatherhood. This may be evolutionarily beneficial, as it promotes "parental care behavior" in men as well (cf. Ehlert 2011, 15). The release of PRL from the adenohypophysis is inhibited or controlled by only one hypothalamic hormone, PIH. Chemically, this hormone is dopamine (cf. Birbaumer and Schmidt 2018, 129). This means that the secretion of prolactin is based on the "removal of tonic PIH inhibition" (Birbaumer and Schmidt 2018, 129). The knowledge that PIH is chemically dopamine is significant because there are numerous medications with both dopaminergic agonist and antagonist effects. These can either promote or inhibit prolactin release (cf. ibid.). However, it should be noted that only PRL release initiated by TRH (thyrotropin-releasing hormone) can be inhibited by dopamine. PRL secretion triggered by OXY (oxytocin) and VIP (vasoactive intestinal peptide) is not affected by dopamine (cf. Ehlert 2011, 15).

1.4.3.6 POMC—Proopiomelanocortin

The prohormone and protein POMC (proopiomelanocortin) is primarily produced in the corticotropic cells of the adenohypophysis, in the hypothalamus, in the placenta, and in the epithelia. In the fetus, POMC is produced in the intermediate lobe of the pituitary gland. Gene expression is stimulated by CRH and vasopressin (cf. Ehlert 2011, 15).

Proopiomelanocortin is the precursor protein of the peptide hormones:

- Adrenocorticotropin (ACTH)
- β-Lipotropin (β-LPH)
- β-Endorphin
- "corticotropin-like intermediate peptide" (CLIP)
- melanocyte-stimulating hormones (MSH): α-MSH, β-MSH, and γ-MSH (cf. Walther 2022b, n.p.).

The particular significance of POMC is based on the fact that POMC-producing neurons and the various cleavage hormones are involved in stress processing on the one hand, and play a role in the regulation of satiety and thus ultimately in weight regulation on the other. Additionally, POMC acts as both an autocrine and paracrine hormone in immunomodulation or cell regulation, for example, of the skin (cf. Ehlert 2011, 15).

The next section will introduce the most important hormones of the neurohypophysis (posterior pituitary gland).

1.4.4 Hormones of the Neurohypophysis

The following describes the hormones arginine vasopressin (AVP) and oxytocin (OXY). They are considered individually, and their commonalities are also explained. Since oxytocin, in particular, plays a significant role in psychoneuroendocrinology, basic knowledge about oxytocin is provided here and further elaborated in the subsequent chapter "Psychoneuroendocrinology." For now, you will receive an introduction to the two neuropeptides.

AVP and OXY are produced in the neurons of the hypothalamus, but they are not released in the hypothalamus. They are stored and released only in the neurohypophysis, which is why they are also classified as pituitary hormones. Upon the arrival of an action potential from the hypothalamus, AVP and OXY are immediately secreted into the blood (cf. Birbaumer and Schmidt 2018, 127). Furthermore, OXY and AVP have an extremely short half-life, which means that both neuropeptides are hardly detectable outside the brain. The first studies on the measurement of OXY in saliva were published in 2009. However, whether these values actually represent the true OXY release in the brain is questionable (cf. Ehlert 2011, 15 f.).

Of particular interest for this topic are studies by Engel and Schuhmacher (2022), which investigated the role of AVP and OXY in relation to post-traumatic stress disorder (PTSD). Engel and Schuhmacher examined the influence of PTSD symptoms and general traumatic events on possible dysregulations of the endocrine systems (cf. Engel and Schuhmacher 2022, n.p.). Additionally, it is investigated,

> "(…) to what extent the two peptides are involved in phases of symptom changes, that is, both in the development of PTSD symptoms immediately after a traumatic event and in the psychotherapeutic treatment of this disorder" (Engel and Schuhmacher 2022, n.p.).

Therefore, the following section will focus on AVP.

1.4.4.1 AVP—Arginine Vasopressin

Arginine vasopressin (AVP) is also known as antidiuretic hormone (ADH). It is a hypothalamic-pituitary peptide hormone that plays a significant role in the regulation of water balance. It is also important for blood pressure, as AVP increases blood pressure in cases of volume deficiency. This occurs by constricting the blood vessels and reducing water excretion (cf. Pschyrembel Editorial 2020k, n.p.). CRH is involved in the release of ACTH, and AVP also initiates the release of ACTH. AVP is associated with an anxiety-increasing effect in the limbic system as well as with socially aggressive male behaviors (cf. Ehlert 2011, 15).

1.4.4.2 OXY—Oxytocin

Oxytocin (OXY) is, on the one hand, an important hormone for inducing labor to increase uterine contractions (labor-inducing effect) and in connection with lactation (both to trigger milk letdown and to promote milk ejection). On the other hand, it has an anxiolytic (anxiety-reducing) effect and thus particularly promotes bonding behavior as well as positive social interactions. Since OXY has an inhibitory effect on the release of ACTH and cortisol, OXY is also attributed with a stress-reducing effect. OXY secretion occurs through stimulation of the nipple and through stretch receptors in the uterus (cf. Ehlert 2011, 15). Besides the significant role of OXY concerning mother and child, birth, and the milk ejection reflex, oxytocin is also important for both men and women, as it is closely linked to the regulation of sexual approach and bonding (cf. Birbaumer and Schmidt 2018, 128). More about OXY, its significance for the psyche and behavior, and findings from current studies will follow in Chap. 2 ("Psychoneuroendocrinology"). The following provides basic knowledge about other significant hormones from various endocrine glands and organs.

1.4.5 Hormones from Endocrine Glands and Organs

The following provides further information on significant hormones from various endocrine glands and organs. They are produced both in organs and endocrine glands and are indispensable for the human organism.

1.4.5.1 Melatonin—Pineal Gland, Gut, and Retina

An example of a hormone that is produced in both hormone glands and organs is melatonin. Melatonin is formed in the pineal gland (epiphysis or also glandula pinealis) and in small amounts in the gut as well as the retina of the eye from serotonin. Melatonin is secreted in a pulsatile manner, with a significantly pronounced nocturnal increase (10 times higher than during the day) being observed. Daylight inhibits the influence of melatonin production. Melatonin particularly influences our sleep regulation, our mood, as well as reproductive functions. With increasing age, a decrease in melatonin production is observed. Additionally, it has been shown that prolonged exposure to light during the night leads to a reduction in melatonin levels. This, in turn, increases the oncological risk (cf. Ehlert 2011, 16). Furthermore, melatonin plays a role in the first half of the night in the recovery of immune competence (cf. Birbaumer and Schmidt 2018, 146). "Melatonin seems to be the mediator of the circadian effects on the immune system" (ibid.). If melatonin is administered before falling asleep, it helps reduce stress effects. Additionally, it is possible to resynchronize the rhythm with melatonin in the case of jet lag. In antigen-activating T-helper cells, melatonin causes the release of small amounts of endogenous opiates. Animal experiments have shown that tumor growth could be slowed down and the various hormonal effects of stress (or strain) could be neutralized (cf. Birbaumer and Schmidt 2018, 171).

1.4.5.2 Hormones of the Paired Adrenal Glands

A certain basic knowledge about the adrenal glands has already been explained (see above). This section is about the most important hormones of the adrenal glands. The hormones can each be classified according to their site of synthesis. In the adrenal medulla (AM), 80% adrenaline and 20% noradrenaline are synthesized from L-tyrosine. In the 3 layers of the adrenal cortex (AC), various hormones are formed (cf. Ehlert 2011, 16):

- Outer zone (zona glomerulosa): Deoxycorticosterone, the mineralocorticoid aldosterone, which is part of the RAAS (renin-angiotensin-aldosterone system, which serves to regulate potassium and sodium concentration).
- Middle layer (zona fasciculata): Glucocorticoids (cortisol) and sex steroids (androgens such as dehydroepiandrosterone, DHEA).
- Innermost layer (zona reticularis, closest to AM): Androgens. The zona reticularis forms a functional unit with the zona fasciculata (cf. Ehlert 2011, 16).

In summary, it should be noted that the AC has a three-layer structure, with each layer forming a group of hormones. The outer layer (zona glomerulosa) primarily forms mineralocorticoids, the middle and broadest layer (zona fasciculata) primarily glucocorticoids, and the inner layer (zona reticularis) predominantly forms androgens or male sex hormones. Additionally, all hormones of the adrenal cortex are steroids. The most significant representative of the mineralocorticoids is the so called aldosterone, which is involved in the formation of urine in the kidneys. Cortisol is the most important representative of the glucocorticoids. This group of hormones has a multitude of tasks both in metabolism and in the immune system and especially influences human behavior (cf. Birbaumer and Schmidt 2018, 131 f.).

The following describes some of the hormones mentioned here.

1.4.5.3 DHEA—Dehydroepiandrosterone

DHEA is the precursor of androgens (cf. Ehlert 2011, 17). Androgens are the male sex hormones, the most important of which is testosterone (cf. Birbaumer and Schmidt 2018, 134). In men, DHEA is produced 100% in the adrenal cortex (AC). In women, however, about 70% of the hormone is produced in the AC and 30% in the ovaries. The production of DHEA is both age- and gender-dependent and follows a circadian rhythm. The peak of production is reached at around 25 years of age. From this age, the DHEA level continuously decreases, with men having higher levels than women. Additionally, DHEA is detectable in larger quantities only prepubertally. This prohormone is said to have an anti-aging effect. However, there is no evidence that cognitive performance can be increased by it (cf. Ehlert 2011, 17).

1.4.5.4 Cortisol

Cortisol is of enormous importance for the human psyche. Therefore, the chapter "Psychoneuroendocrinology" also provides more details on the mechanisms of action and current studies on cortisol. Here you will now receive a brief introduction to this important hormone.

Cortisol is a natural glucocorticoid and is referred to as a stress hormone. Cortisol secretion is stimulated by ACTH (cf. Pschyrembel Editorial Team 2020l, n.p.). The production follows a daily rhythm, with the highest release values being observed in the morning and continuously decreasing throughout the day. Cortisol is secreted in response to stress and influences a variety of immunological and hormonal processes, with the reactivity of cortisol to psychological or physical stress being slower than the stress-induced secretion of adrenaline and noradrenaline (cf. Ehlert 2011, 17). The effect of cortisol includes providing energy during periods of hunger, inhibiting inflammatory reactions, and having an immunosuppressive effect (cf. Pschyrembel Editorial Team 2020l, n.p.).

To enhance your understanding of the effects of cortisol, particularly in relation to stress, the following section will delve deeper into glucocorticoids, their production, and regulation.

1.4.5.5 Glucocorticoids

Glucocorticoids have a variety of functions, particularly concerning metabolism, the immune system, and human behavior. The secretion of cortisol is regulated by one of the four glandotropic hormones of the adenohypophysis (anterior pituitary gland, APG). These are referred to as adrenocorticotropic hormones, in this case, ACTH, which in turn is regulated by the pituitary releasing hormone CRH. This is referred to as corticoliberin (cf. Birbaumer and Schmidt 2018, 132).

Glucocorticoid Release

> "Hypothalamic CRH releases ACTH from the APG, which releases glucocorticoids, especially cortisol, from the adrenal cortex. This, in turn, has a feedback inhibitory effect on both CRH and ACTH release. Additionally, cortisol secretion is subject to diurnal fluctuations" (Birbaumer and Schmidt 2018, 123).

The metabolic effects of glucocorticoids particularly influence the human glucose requirement. They stimulate gluconeogenesis, as briefly mentioned above. This occurs through the conversion of amino acids into glucose. In times of increased energy demand, glucocorticoids primarily serve to mobilize glucose (cf. Birbaumer and Schmidt 2018, 133). When glucocorticoids are used pharmacologically, i.e., in high doses, they weaken the immune defense. This effect is used in organ transplants as a form of immunosuppressive therapy to prevent the rejection of transplanted tissue. Furthermore, they have anti-inflammatory (antiphlogistic) and antiallergic effects (cf. ibid., 133). They have strong effects on the nervous system, although these are difficult to predict. The excitability threshold is lowered at elevated cortisol levels. Possibly, in epilepsy patients, an increased seizure readiness after cortisol administration can be attributed to this mechanism. Additionally, high doses of cortisol lead to insomnia. Initially, many patients experience euphoria, but over time, depression is a common problem. So-called membrane receptors for cortisol are present in several areas of the brain. The functions of these receptors are highly diverse. Glucocorticoids also have a significant impact on the function of sensory organs, such as the ability to distinguish between sweet and salty. In cases of adrenal insufficiency, patients require much higher concentrations of substances to differentiate between sweet and salty. Similar changes in sensory performance can also be observed in smell and hearing. Given the already outlined metabolic effects of glucocorticoids, it is not surprising that stress situations of all kinds alter the glucocorticoid regulatory circuit. Stress leads, among other effects, to the activation of the hypothalamus and thus to an increased release of CRH. The increased release of CRH subsequently causes an increased release of ACTH, which in turn leads to an increase in cortisol and other glucocorticoids. This stress-induced release of CRH significantly alters the regulatory circuit for these adrenal cortex hormones. In severe stress situations, the induced ACTH release can be so intense (cf. Birbaumer and Schmidt 2018, 133) that "more ACTH appears in the blood than is necessary for maximum cortisol secretion" (Birbaumer and Schmidt 2018, 133). Further connections between stress and stress hormones are discussed in more detail in Chap. 2 ("Psychoneuroendocrinology").

1.4.6 Hormones of the Adrenal Medulla (AM)

The NNM is the inner part of the adrenal gland. When the endocrine cells or the preganglionic axons of the NNM are stimulated, this leads to the release of a hormone mixture of 80% adrenaline and 20% noradrenaline into the blood. The effects of the adrenergic substances released from the NNM are particularly important for the digestive glands of the stomach as well as the pancreas. Adrenaline and noradrenaline, as metabolic hormones, ensure a rapid supply of fuels, especially during physical exertion (cf. Birbaumer and Schmidt 2018, 107). The synthesis of NNM hormones begins with the starting material tyrosine and leads to dopa and dopamine, from which noradrenaline and adrenaline are then synthesized (cf. Ehlert 2011, 17).

Synthesis of Adrenal Medulla Hormones Tyrosine → Dopa → Dopamine → Noradrenaline → Adrenaline

In emergency situations, both physical (such as extreme physical exertion like blood loss or burns) and psychological stress, there are high secretions of adrenaline and noradrenaline from the NNM. Under emotional stress, this can be 10 times higher than the resting secretion. The secretion is controlled by both the hypothalamus and the limbic system. Constantly recurring stress situations or a long-term elevated adrenaline level in the blood can promote the development of various diseases. On the other hand, stress reactions should be regularly trained, i.e., a certain amount of moderate stress has a positive effect on the responsiveness of this system. From this perspective, a life completely without any stress is just as unhealthy as too much stress (cf. Birbaumer and Schmidt 2018, 107).

1.4.6.1 Catecholamines

Catecholamines are hormones and neurotransmitters that, among other things, increase blood pressure and are also involved in metabolism (breakdown of proteins). The natural catecholamines include dopamine, noradrenaline, and adrenaline, with the starting substance for biosynthesis being the amino acid tyrosine (cf. Walther 2022c, n.p.). The catecholamines adrenaline, noradrenaline, and dopamine are classified as biogenic amines. Furthermore, they are also declared as monoamines, like serotonin and histamine. Additionally, noradrenaline, adrenaline, and dopamine are referred to as adrenergic transmitter substances. The effect of these transmitters ends particularly with the reuptake into the presynaptic endings (cf. Birbaumer and Schmidt 2018, 57). Besides the synthesis of catecholamines, which takes place in the central nervous system (neurotransmitter effect), catecholamines are also produced in the NNM. The effect of catecholamines is mediated by binding to adrenoceptors (adrenergic alpha and beta receptors). The catecholamine level rises immediately after the onset of stress (in both psychological and physical stress) (cf. Ehlert 2011, 17). "For this reason, the release of catecholamines is also referred to as the 'first wave,' while the delayed release of cortisol is referred to as the 'second wave' of the endocrine stress response" (Ehlert 2011, 17). In extreme stress stimuli (trauma), if there is a genetically determined vulnerability of the individual, it can lead to increased noradrenaline-induced emotional imprinting and cell loss in the hippocampus. This is referred to as post-traumatic stress disorder (cf. Birbaumer and Schmidt 2018, 152). Since several findings about dopamine have already been presented, the following will focus on noradrenaline and adrenaline. Regarding these two substances, two major systems are distinguished: the noradrenergic and the adrenergic central transmitter system. For psychological functions, the locus coeruleus system is of particular relevance (cf. Birbaumer and Schmidt 2018, 95), which will also be examined in more detail.

1.4.6.2 Noradrenaline and Noradrenergic Systems

As already mentioned, noradrenaline (NA) is a neurotransmitter and hormone that belongs to the group of catecholamines. The biosynthesis proceeds from tyrosine via DOPA and dopamine as the L-form in the adrenal medulla (AM) and in the sympathetic nervous system. Through adrenergic receptors, NA increases blood pressure, circulatory resistance, and heart rate. The effect on the intestines and metabolism, as well as on smooth muscles and the bronchi, is weaker than that of adrenaline (cf. Pschyrembel 2020 m, n.p.). Most noradrenaline systems originate in the locus coeruleus (or nucleus coeruleus). With the medial forebrain bundle (a nerve pathway), they extend into the limbic system and the neocortex. Their activation enhances performance regarding attention functions, and learning in emotional situations is facilitated (cf. Birbaumer and Schmidt 2018, 95). Noradrenaline, like acetylcholine, is considered a classic transmitter in the peripheral autonomic nervous system (ANS) (cf. ibid., 109). NA acts as a transmitter, just like dopamine, in the central nervous system (CNS), such as in the hypothalamus, the limbic system, and the basal ganglia nuclei (cf. Birbaumer and Schmidt 2018, 57). Particularly during emotional stress, there are extremely high releases of noradrenaline. This can be up to 10 times higher in the short term compared to resting releases (cf. ibid., 107). The release of noradrenaline or the release of catecholamines is also associated with anxiety and fear.

> "The activity of the central and peripheral noradrenergic systems is necessary for anxiety and fear reactions; especially the concentration of attention on anxiety stimuli depends on the central NA (noradrenaline) system" (Birbaumer and Schmidt 2018, 728).

Selective attention to intense stimuli is attributed to NA, which improves the signal-to-noise ratio in the cortex. Additionally, NA, together with the release of stress hormones or glucocorticoids, causes memory fixation of fear stimuli (cf. Birbaumer and Schmidt 2018, 728). Corticotropin-releasing hormone (CRH) and noradrenaline (NA) "enhance the fixation of implicit traumatic memories" (ibid., 729). This leads to lifelong fear in post-traumatic stress disorder (PTSD), which results in "flashbacks" (uncontrolled memories) (cf. ibid., 728). Based on the findings presented here, it is clearly evident how significant noradrenaline and its effects are for psychoneuroendocrinology, and what an important role NA can play in the psyche and human behavior. Further insights into noradrenaline will therefore be presented in Chap. 2.

1.4.6.3 Adrenaline and Adrenergic Systems

Like noradrenaline, adrenaline belongs to the group of catecholamines and is produced in the adrenal medulla (AM). It is also synthesized from the amino acid tyrosine (cf. Pschyrembel 2020n, n.p.). In addition to the synthesis of adrenaline in the AM, it is also secreted there. Like NA and dopamine, adrenaline is classified as a biogenic amine, is declared a monoamine, and is also referred to as an adrenergic transmitter substance (cf. Birbaumer and Schmidt 2018, 57). Adrenaline is secreted into the bloodstream as a hormone mixture with NA during arousal. Together, they act as metabolic hormones during physical exertion and ensure the rapid provision of fuels. A long-term elevated adrenaline level in the blood, based on, for example, constantly recurring stressful situations, promotes the development of various diseases (cf. Birbaumer and Schmidt 2018, 107). Adrenaline binds to adrenergic receptors, and its effects correspond to the "fight-or-flight" reactions. It increases blood pressure and heart rate and enhances vascular tone. Adrenaline promotes the rapid provision of energy as it affects glycogen and glucose metabolism. It also causes the bronchi to dilate. The effects of adrenaline are also of enormous importance in the medical field. As a medication, adrenaline is used, for example, in severe acute allergic reactions and shock, in acute cardiac arrest (as part of resuscitation), for hemostasis, or in acute respiratory distress. Overproduction or overdose of adrenaline leads, among other things, to high blood pressure, palpitations, sweating, headaches, and feelings of anxiety (cf. Pschyrembel 2020n, n.p.).

In summary, it can be stated that catecholamines have enormous relevance for the human organism, psyche, and behavior, which is why findings in psychoneuroendocrinology are based on the effects of catecholamines. These will therefore be examined in more detail in the following chapters. However, before that, to better understand the effects of the endocrine system and, based on that, psychoneuroendocrinology (PNE), the most important pathways of hormones will be explained.

1.5 Communication Pathways of Hormones: The Hormone Axes

The hypothalamic-pituitary system is a neuroendocrine control and regulation system that ensures the functional coordination between the endocrine system and the CNS. The releasing hormones formed in the hypothalamus act selectively on various cell groups of the pituitary gland. They stimulate or inhibit the secretion of pituitary hormones. These, in turn, act on different endocrine systems and organs. The "communication pathways" required here are referred to as hormone axes: hypothalamic-pituitary-gonadal axis, hypothalamic-pituitary-thyroid axis, and hypothalamic-pituitary-adrenal axis (cf. Schöller 2016c, n.p.). The hypothalamic-pituitary system can be regarded as the superior center of the endocrine system. Through the interaction of the hypothalamus and pituitary gland, the activity of numerous endocrine glands throughout the body is controlled (cf. Spektrum Lexikon der Neurowissenschaft 2000j, n.p.). Endocrine processes consist of the human organism striving to return to its original state after the release of hormones. This striving for balance is called homeostasis. So-called homeostatic mechanisms are control and feedback processes that serve to restore a physiological balance after activation (cf. Ehlert 2011, 24). Two different principles can be distinguished here:

- **Pulsatile release:** This is a principle of hormonal regulation that is subject to circadian rhythm and is controlled by central timekeepers. It is influenced by the day-night rhythm or by (daylight) exposure.
- **Hormone axes:** These feedback mechanisms are of particular importance for psychoneuroendocrinology. Here, there is a reciprocal communication between the brain and the body periphery (cf. Ehlert 2011, 24).

Hypothalamically controlled hormone axes follow the principle of a cascade. The secretion of a releasing hormone in the hypothalamus, for example, initiates the secretion of further hormones at various brain (pituitary) and body levels (endocrine glands). Ultimately, a biological response results, which is referred to as a "feedforward mechanism" because each step leads to further activation. If continuous further activation were to occur, it would lead to overstrain, causing physiological damage and potentially even death. To prevent this, there is a biological response that uses part of the released hormones to initiate negative feedback. Thus, the further release of hormones is inhibited (feedback principle) (cf. Ehlert 2011, 24).

Depending on hormone synthesis, gonadotropic, thyrotropic, corticotropic, somatotropic, and lactotropic cells are distinguished in the adenohypophysis, which are involved in hormonal circuits (regulatory circuits):

- gonadotropic regulatory circuit (hypothalamic-pituitary-gonadal axis)
- thyrotropic regulatory circuit (hypothalamic-pituitary-thyroid axis)
- corticotropic regulatory circuit (hypothalamic-pituitary-adrenal axis)
- somatotropic regulatory circuit (somatotropic axis) and
- lactotropic regulatory circuit (lactotropic axis) (cf. Spektrum Lexikon der Neurowissenschaft 2000j, n.p.)

A feedforward and simultaneous feedback principle occurs, for example, in the hypothalamic-pituitary-thyroid axis. The hormone axes most studied by psychoendocrinology, which are based on a feedforward-feedback principle, are the hypothalamic-pituitary-adrenal axis and the hypothalamic-pituitary-gonadal axis (cf. Ehlert 2011, 24), which are described below.

1.5.1 Hypothalamus-Pituitary-Adrenal Axis (HPA)

> "The hypothalamus-pituitary-adrenal axis stimulates the secretion of glucocorticoids, which act in the brain via mineralocorticoid receptors and glucocorticoid receptors, where particularly the glucocorticoid receptors regulate psychological processes (…)", (Pschyrembel Editorial 2016f, n.p.).

Emotions, such as depressive moods or anxiety, are regulated as well as cognitive processes, such as memory and learning (cf. Pschyrembel Editorial 2016f, n.p.). The hormones of the HPA (hypothalamus-pituitary-adrenal axis) are extremely sensitive indicators. They respond to both physical and psychological stress. When a stressor (stress trigger) occurs, humans try to regulate and process the stress themselves using coping strategies based on the homeostatic principle. The ability to cope with stress is reflected in the hormone release of the HPA (cf. Ehlert 2011, 25). CRH is stimulated by impulses from the limbic system as well as by cytokines (e.g., IL-1 and IL-6). As a neuroendocrine messenger in the central nervous system (CNS), CRH has important tasks, namely in the adaptation of the organism to both physical and psychological stress. One of the main tasks is, for example, the control of the synthesis and release of the hormone ACTH as well as the release of POMC peptides. CRH is projected into the pituitary stalk via axons, where CRH type 1 receptors reach corticotropic cells of the anterior pituitary.

This initiates both the synthesis and release of ACTH. Subsequently, ACTH reaches the adrenal cortex (AC) via the bloodstream. In the AC, it in turn causes the biosynthesis and release of cortisol, which in turn initiates various processes. At the same time, cortisol also has the task of regulating the activity of the HPA at the pituitary and hypothalamic levels based on a negative feedback loop (cf. Ehlert 2011, 25). It should be noted here that glucocorticoid receptors (GR) and mineralocorticoid receptors (MR) have various effects related to homeostasis:

- **GR activation**: among others, control of energy metabolism, modulation of memory processes, support of behavioral adaptation to stress.
- **MR activation**: In response to stress, homeostatic cellular processes are initiated, and the process of behavioral selection in response to stress is supported (cf. Ehlert 2011, 25).

> "The hormones of the HPA have a variety of psychological and physiological consequences, which can be summarized as permissive (preparatory), suppressive, and stimulating effects" (Ehlert 2011, 25).

CRH acts as a coordinator "(…) of emotional, behavioral, and autonomic adaptation processes to stress, particularly initiating activation processes" (ibid.). CRH effects can be distinguished between indirect and direct. On the one hand, direct CRH effects can be found, for example, in the gastrointestinal tract. On the other hand, CRH has partially indirect releaser functions that are characteristic of the HPA (cf. Ehlert 2011, 26). The stimulation of ACTH is also caused by norepinephrine (NE), serotonin, and acetylcholine. In contrast, dopamine, GABA (gamma-aminobutyric acid), and endogenous opiates have an inhibitory influence (cf. von Werder 2005, cited in Ehlert 2011, 26). Thus, ACTH acts activating (agonistically) and causes the release of mineralocorticoids, androgens, and glucocorticoids (cf. Ehlert 2011, 26). The most relevant hormone of the glucocorticoids is cortisol. Its release, as already mentioned, particularly responds to environmental and stress factors. Since almost every physiological system and nearly every cell responds to these hormonal signals, impairments of the HPA are associated with a variety of physical and psychological disorders (cf. Bullmann 2020, n.p.). For example, dysregulation of the HPA system has been found to be associated with psychological disorders such as post-traumatic stress disorder (PTSD), depression, and chronic fatigue syndrome (cf. Pschyrembel Editorial 2016f, n.p.). However, new meta-analyses show "(…) that disorder-specific dysregulation processes cannot generally be assumed" (ibid.).

1.5.2 Hypothalamus-Pituitary-Gonadal Axis (HPGA)

The HPGA is, in terms of the principle of action, comparable to the HPA axis. It is also based on the feedforward mechanism, but from the brain to the gonads. However, the gonadal hormones provide (mostly) negative feedback to the hypothalamus and the pituitary gland (cf. Ehlert 2011, 26). Here, a clear difference between men and women must be noted. For the HPGA shows relatively constant release patterns in men. In women of childbearing age, however, the feedback system varies significantly during the cycle (cf. Ehlert 2011, 26).

1.5.2.1 Reproductive Control in Men

The hypothalamus-pituitary-gonadal axis (HPGA) in men is controlled by hypothalamic GnRH release. This occurs in pulses with approximately 18 pulses per day—as in women. These pulses initiate gonadotropin secretion, which subsequently leads to the release of sex hormones. The sex hormones are released into the Sertoli and Leydig cells. In healthy men after puberty, the release of hormones occurs approximately consistently, i.e., there are no hormonal fluctuations as in the female cycle. In men, there is no event in advanced age that triggers a hormonal shift; rather, there is a continuous, slow adjustment. This occurs from about the age of 40, based on a lower testosterone level. The negative feedback of testosterone (i.e., the inhibitory influence) on the hypothalamus and the pituitary gland therefore decreases, whereas the GnRH pulse frequency continues to increase. This process is a good example of a normal physiological degradation process. Homeostasis changes slowly and leads to age-related dysregulation (cf. Ehlert 2011, 27).

1.5.2.2 Reproductive Control in Women

In the female cycle, the release of HPGA hormones varies. The coordination of the already described hormonal changes during the cycle is based, on the one hand, on aminergic (nerve ending or synapses) stimulation as well as neuropeptidergic stimulation, which in turn influences the GnRH pulse generator. On the other hand, this is based on the feedback mechanisms of gonadal steroids. Through neurosecretion, GnRH reaches the pituitary stalk and subsequently through the pituitary portal system to the adenohypophysis (anterior pituitary). GnRH stimulation leads to the release of LH and FSH. Additionally, activin stimulates the release of FSH. For the promotion of reproduction, a regular pulsatile secretion of GnRH, LH, and FSH is crucial (cf. Ehlert 2011, 28 f.).

1.5.2.3 Mediators of the Hypothalamus-Pituitary-Gonadal Axis (HPGA)

> "The HPGA is influenced by a number of neurotransmitters: the endogenous opiates (β-endorphin, enkephalins, dynorphin), substance P, CRH, and dopamine have an inhibitory influence. In contrast, GABA, galanin, serotonin, neurotensin, NPY, and NA, among others, have a stimulating effect" (Ehlert and Hanker 2001, quoted in Ehlert 2011, 29 f.).

PRL has an influence on the corpus luteum (yellow body) especially in the second half of the cycle, which in turn affects the effects of estrogen and progesterone (cf. Ehlert 2011, 30). Kisspeptin-54 also has a relevant stimulating influence on the release of GnRH (cf. Murphy 2005, quoted in Ehlert 2011, 30). Leptin has a stimulating influence on kisspeptin-54, which would (partly) explain why women with severe underweight can experience cycle disorders or even complete cessation of menstruation. Based on the decrease in leptin levels, which is lower due to weight, both kisspeptin-54 release and GnRH secretion are reduced. Kisspeptin-54 stimulates both ovulation and the activity of the corpus luteum (yellow body). Finally, pheromones should be mentioned. Various studies have shown that these can be found in axillary sweat. Pheromones also include the steroids androstadienone and estratetraenol, which in turn influence the pulsatile release of LH. It has been shown that LH release can be manipulated by presenting women with concentrated sweat from other women in different cycle phases through olfactory perception (cf. Ehlert 2011, 30).

In summary, it should be noted that endocrine feedforward-feedback control loops are very complex systems. Many endocrine factors influence the modes of action of these systems. It is also important to note that new insights are constantly being gained about the mentioned hormonal axes. Additionally, the complexity of these systems is further complicated by central nervous and immunological influences (cf. Ehlert 2011, 30).

1.6 Summary: Fundamentals of Endocrinology

In this chapter, you were provided with foundational knowledge about endocrine systems, significant hormones, and their mechanisms of action. Endocrinology was introduced to you in such a way that the subsequent psychoneuroendocrinology and its significance for psychosocial and psychotherapeutic practice are easier to understand.

In summary, it should be noted that the importance of the endocrine system is vital for the human organism and has enormous impacts not only on physiological functions but also on the psyche and behavior of humans. The endocrine system, particularly the hypothalamic-pituitary system (neuroendocrine system), is of such significance that an imbalance in this system leads to a variety of clinical pictures affecting both physiology and psychology. It has become evident that endocrinological and neurobiological fundamentals are important for human behavior in general as well as for mental disorders. There is a vital interplay between the brain and other organ systems, which is why the insights presented should not be ignored in psychological and psychosocial practice. The following chapter, "Psychoneuroendocrinology," builds on the foundational knowledge established in this chapter. It will become clearly evident that psychoneuroendocrinological insights are inevitably connected with psychosocial and psychotherapeutic practice.

References

Abbruzzese, Elvira (2011): Chronobiologie des Hormon- und des Immunsystems. In: Ehlert, Ulrike/von Känel, Roland (Hrsg.) (2011): Psychoendokrinologie und Psychoimmunologie. Berlin/Heidelberg: Springer-Verlag GmbH. 129–149.

Arnold, Rudolf (2007): Endokrine Tumoren des gastroenteropankreatischen Systems. In: Rothmund, Mathias/Schumpelick, Volker/Siewert, Jörg (Hrsg.): Praxis der Viszeralchirurgie. Berlin/Heidelberg: Springer Verlag. https://doi.org/10.1007/978-3-642-14285-7_5. [29.04.2023].

BDI (2022): Hypothalamus. In: BDI. Berufsverband deutscher Internist*innen und Internisten e. V. (Hrsg.). München: Monks – Ärzte im Netz GmbH. https://www.internisten-im-netz.de/fachgebiete/hormone-stoffwechsel/hormondruesen-und-moegliche-erkrankungen/hypothalamus.html [27.01.2022].

Bieg, Sabine/Maelicke, Alfred/Schatzl, Martin/Waßmer, Thomas (2016a): Hormone – eine Einleitung. Aminosäurederivate. In: CHEMGAROO-ChemgaPedia: Biochemie. Weinheim: Wiley-VCH Verlag GmbH & Co. KGaA. 1–17. http://www.chemgapedia.de/vsengine/vlu/vsc/de/ch/8/bc/vlu/botenstoffe/hormone_einleitung.vlu/Page/vsc/de/ch/8/bc/botenstoffe/hormone/aminosaeurederivate.vscml.html [22.01.2022].

Bieg, Sabine/Maelicke, Alfred/Schatzl, Martin/Waßmer, Thomas (2016b): Hormone – eine Einleitung. Steroidhormone. In: CHEMGAROO-ChemgaPedia: Biochemie. Weinheim: Wiley-VCH Verlag GmbH & Co. KGaA. 1–17. http://www.chemgapedia.de/vsengine/vlu/vsc/de/ch/8/bc/vlu/botenstoffe/hormone_einleitung.vlu/Page/vsc/de/ch/8/bc/botenstoffe/hormone/steroidhormone.vscml.html [22.01.2022].

Birbaumer, Niels/Schmidt, Robert F. (2010): Endokrine Systeme (Hormone). In: Birbaumer, Niels/Schmidt, Robert F. (Hrsg.): Biologische Psychologie. 7. überarb. und erw. Aufl. Heidelberg: Springer Medizin Verlag. 117–140.

Birbaumer, Niels/Schmidt, Robert F. (2018): Biologische Psychologie. Sonderausgabe. 7. überarb. und ergänzte Aufl. Heidelberg: Springer Medizin Verlag.

BMJ Open (2018): Studie: Alkoholkonsum ist häufiger Verursacher des prämenstruellen Syndroms. In: Deutsches Ärzteblatt. Berlin: Deutscher Ärzteverlag GmbH. https://www.aerzteblatt.de/nachrichten/94733/Studie-Alkoholkonsum-ist-haeufiger-Verursacher-des-praemenstruellen-Syndroms [05.02.2022].

Bullmann, Catharina (2020): Bedeutung der Hypothalamus-Hypophysen-Nebennierenrinden-Achse. Gynäkologische Endokrinologie. 135–139. https://doi.org/10.1007/s10304-020-00324-z [01.05.2023].

DGE (2022): Was ist Endokrinologie? In: Deutsche Gesellschaft für Endokrinologie. e. V. c/o EndoScience Endokrinologie Service GmbH. https://www.endokrinologie.net/endokrinologie.php [25.01.2022].

Ehler, Patrick/Winkler, Anita (2018): Endokrines System. In: Martin, Eckhardt (Hrsg.) (2018): Paracelsus Fachmagazin. Naturheilpraxis – Psychologie – Tierheilkunde. 5/2018. 12–13. https://www.paracelsus.de/magazin/ausgabe/201805/endokrines-system [18.01.2022].

Ehlert, Ulrike (2011): Das endokrine System. In: Ehlert, Ulrike/von Känel, Roland (Hrsg.): Psychoendokrinologie und Psychoimmunologie. Berlin/Heidelberg: Springer-Verlag GmbH. 3–36.

Ehlert, Ulrike/Hanker, Jürgen (2001): Gynäkologie. In: Flor, Herta/Hahlweg, Kurt/Birbaumer, Niels (Hrsg.): Enzyklopädie der Psychologie. Themenbereich D, Serie II Klinische Psychologie. Band 4: Verhaltensmedizin: Spezifische Störungen und Interventionen. Göttingen: Hogrefe Verlag. 435–514.

Ehlert, Ulrike/von Känel, Roland (Hrsg.) (2011): Psychoendokrinologie und Psychoimmunologie. Berlin/Heidelberg: Springer-Verlag GmbH.

Engel, Sinha/Schuhmacher, Sarah (2022): Die Rolle der Neuropeptide Oxytocin und Arginin Vasopressin bei der posttraumatischen Belastungsstörung. In: Freie Universität Berlin. https://www.ewi-psy.fu berlin.de/einrichtungen/arbeitsbereiche/klinisch_psychologische_intervention/forschung/Klin_Biopsychologie/Oxy_Arganin_Vasopressin/index.html [06.02.2022].

Fowden, Abigail/Forhead, Alison/Coan, Philip/Burton, Graham (2008): The placenta and the intrauterine programming. Journal Neuroendocrinology 20(4). 439–450.

Hirst, John/Nguyen, Phuong/Walker, David William/Yawno, Tamara (2006): Stress in pregnancy activates neurosteroid production in the fetal brain. Neuroendocrinology, 84(4), 264–274.

IQWiG (2021): Wie funktioniert die Schilddrüse? In: Institut für Qualität und Wirtschaftlichkeit im Gesundheitswesen (IQWiG) (Hrsg.): Gesundheitsinformation. Verstehen – abwiegen – entscheiden. https://www.gesundheitsinformation.de/wie-funktioniert-die-schilddruese.html [29.01.2022].

Kleine, Bernhard/Rosmanith, Winfried (2014): Hormone und Hormonsystem – Lehrbuch der Endokrinologie. Berlin/Heidelberg: Springer Spektrum Verlag.

Krause, Ute (2022): Prämenstruelles Syndrom (PMS). In: Pschyrembel online. Berlin: Walter de Gruyter GmbH. https://www.pschyrembel.de/pr%C3%A4menstruelle%20Syndrom%20(PMS)/K0M3J/doc/ [30.04.2023].

Lexikon der Medizin (div. Autor*innen) (2005): Lexikon Medizin. Das Nachschlagewerk für Ärzte, Apotheker, Patienten. 4. überarbeitete und erweiterte Auflage. Köln: Naumann & Göbel Verlagsgesellschaft mbH.

Medizinische Universität Wien (2023): Endokrinologie: Allgemeine Informationen. Müller, Markus (Hrsg.): Endokrinologie. Medizinische Universität Wien. Wien: Bundesministerium für Wissenschaft, Forschung und Wirtschaft. In: https://endokrinologie.meduniwien.ac.at/allgemeine-informationen/ [29.04.2023].

Murphy, Kevin (2005): Kisspeptins: regulators of metastasis and the hypothalamic-pituitary-gonadal axis. Journal Neuroendocrinology 17. 519–525.

Pschyrembel Redaktion (2016a): Pfortadergefäße der Hypophyse. In: Pschyrembel online. Berlin: Walter de Gruyter GmbH. https://www.pschyrembel.de/Pfortadersystem%20der%20Hypophyse/K0GRU/doc/ [29.04.2023].

Pschyrembel Redaktion (2016b): Hoden. In: Pschyrembel online. Berlin: Walter de Gruyter GmbH. https://www.pschyrembel.de/Hoden/K09X8 [30.04.2023].

Pschyrembel Redaktion (2016c): Leydig-Zwischenzellen. In: Pschyrembel online. Berlin: Walter de Gruyter GmbH. https://www.pschyrembel.de/Leydig-Zwischenzellen/K0CU8/ [30.04.2023].

Pschyrembel Redaktion (2016d): Sertoli-Zellen. In: Pschyrembel online. Berlin: Walter de Gruyter GmbH. https://www.pschyrembel.de/Sertoli-Zellen/K0KUH/ [30.04.2023].

Pschyrembel Redaktion (2016e): Haut. In: Pschyrembel online. Berlin: Walter de Gruyter GmbH. https://www.pschyrembel.de/Haut/K09HR/doc/ [30.04.2023].

Pschyrembel Redaktion (2016f): Hypothalamus-Hypophysen-Nebennierenrinden-Achse. In: Pschyrembel online. Berlin: Walter de Gruyter GmbH. https://www.pschyrembel.de/Hypothalamus-Hypophysen-Nebennierenrinden-Achse/P05W9/doc/ [01.05.2023].

Pschyrembel Redaktion (2018): Glandulae endocrinae. In: Pschyrembel online. Berlin: Walter de Gruyter GmbH. https://www.pschyrembel.de/Endokrine%20Dr%C3%BCsen/K08TA/doc/ [29.04.2023].

Pschyrembel Redaktion (2020a): Adrenalin. In: Pschyrembel online. Berlin: Walter de Gruyter GmbH. https://www.pschyrembel.de/Adrenalin%20/K01QL/doc/ [29.04.2023].

Pschyrembel Redaktion (2020b): Serotonin. In: Pschyrembel online. Berlin: Walter de Gruyter GmbH. https://www.pschyrembel.de/Serotonin/K0KU3/doc/ [29.04.2023].

Pschyrembel Redaktion (2020c): Corticotropin-Releasing-Hormon (CRH). In: Pschyrembel online. Berlin: Walter de Gruyter GmbH. https://www.pschyrembel.de/Corticotropin-Releasing-Hormon/K05BF/doc/ [30.04.2023].

Pschyrembel Redaktion (2020d): Glukokortikoide. In: Pschyrembel online. Berlin: Walter de Gruyter GmbH. https://www.pschyrembel.de/Glukokortikoide/K08WW/doc/ [30.04.2023].

Pschyrembel Redaktion (2020e): Thyrotropin-Releasing-Hormon (TRH). In: Pschyrembel online. Berlin: Walter de Gruyter GmbH. https://www.pschyrembel.de/TRH/K0MVP/doc/ [30.04.2023].

Pschyrembel Redaktion (2020f): Gonadotropin-Releasing-Hormon (GnRH). In: Pschyrembel online. Berlin: Walter de Gruyter GmbH. https://www.pschyrembel.de/Gonadotropin-Releasing-Hormon/K091B/doc/ [30.04.2023].

Pschyrembel Redaktion (2020g): Kisspeptin. In: Pschyrembel online. Berlin: Walter de Gruyter GmbH. https://www.pschyrembel.de/KiSS-Peptide/A0TMH/doc/ [30.04.2023].

Pschyrembel Redaktion (2020h): Adrenocorticotropes Hormon (ACTH). In: Pschyrembel online. Berlin: Walter de Gruyter GmbH. https://www.pschyrembel.de/Adrenocorticotropin/K01LU/doc/ [30.04.2023].

Pschyrembel Redaktion (2020i): Thyroidea stimulierendes Hormon (TSH). In: Pschyrembel online. Berlin: Walter de Gruyter GmbH. https://www.pschyrembel.de/Thyrotropin/K0N3L/doc/ [30.04.2023].

Pschyrembel Redaktion (2020j): Somatotropes Hormon (STH). In: Pschyrembel online. Berlin: Walter de Gruyter GmbH. https://www.pschyrembel.de/growth%20hormone/K0LL6/doc/ [30.04.2023].

Pschyrembel Redaktion (2020k): Antidiuretisches Hormon (ADH). In: Pschyrembel online. Berlin: Walter de Gruyter GmbH. https://www.pschyrembel.de/Arginin-Vasopressin/K01P6/doc/ [30.04.2023].

Pschyrembel Redaktion (2020l): Kortisol. In: Pschyrembel online. Berlin: Walter de Gruyter GmbH. https://www.pschyrembel.de/Kortisol/K059R/doc/ [30.04.2023].

Pschyrembel Redaktion (2020m): Noradrenalin. In: Pschyrembel online. Berlin: Walter de Gruyter GmbH. https://www.pschyrembel.de/Noradrenalin/K0FDS/doc/ [01.05.2023].

Pschyrembel Redaktion (2020n): Adrenalin. In: Pschyrembel online. Berlin: Walter de Gruyter GmbH. https://www.pschyrembel.de/Adrenalin/K01QL [01.05.2023].

Riester, Anna (2013): Urocortin-abhängige Effekte auf die Struktur und Funktion der Nebenniere in vivo. Dissertation. Ludwig-Maximilians-Universität München: Medizinische Fakultät. DOI: https://doi.org/10.5282/edoc.15635 [30.04.2023].

Schleußner, Ekkehard (2018): Endokrinologie der Plazenta. In: Huppertz, Berthold/Schleußner, Ekkehard (Hrsg.): Die Plazenta. Berlin/Heidelberg: Springer Verlag. 89–102. https://doi.org/10.1007/978-3-662-55622-1_5 [30.04.2023].

Schöller, Dorit (2016a): Endokrinologie. In: Pschyrembel online. Berlin: Walter de Gruyter GmbH. https://www.pschyrembel.de/Endokrinologie/K06TG/doc/ [29.04.2023].

Schöller, Dorit (2016b): Steroidhormone. In: Pschyrembel online. Berlin: Walter de Gruyter GmbH. https://www.pschyrembel.de/steroidhormone/K0LKS/doc/ [29.04.2023].

Schöller, Dorit (2016c): Hypothalamus-Hypophysen-System. In: Pschyrembel online. Berlin: Walter de Gruyter GmbH. https://www.pschyrembel.de/Hypothalamus-Hypophysen-System/K0AFT/doc/ [01.05.2023].

Schöller, Dorit (2018): Nebenniere. In: Pschyrembel online. Berlin: Walter de Gruyter GmbH. https://www.pschyrembel.de/Nebennieren/K0F0A/doc/ [29.04.2023].

Schöller, Dorit (2019a): Hypophyse. In: Pschyrembel online. Berlin: Walter de Gruyter GmbH. https://www.pschyrembel.de/Hypophyse/K0AF1/doc/ [29.04.2023].

Schöller, Dorit (2019b): Adenohypophyse. In: Pschyrembel online. Berlin: Walter de Gruyter GmbH. https://www.pschyrembel.de/Hypophysenvorderlappen/K0A4K/doc/ [29.04.2023].

Schöller, Dorit (2019c): Neurohypophyse. In: Pschyrembel online. Berlin: Walter de Gruyter GmbH. https://www.pschyrembel.de/Neurohypophyse/K0F59/doc/ [29.04.2023].

Spektrum Lexikon der Biologie (1999): Corticotropin-Releasing-Hormon. In: Spektrum der Wissenschaft. Heidelberg: Spektrum der Wissenschaft Verlagsgesellschaft mbH., Springer Nature. https://www.spektrum.de/lexikon/biologie/corticotropin-releasing-hormon/15429 [30.04.2023].

Spektrum Lexikon der Neurowissenschaft (2000a): Neurotransmitter. In: Spektrum der Wissenschaft. Heidelberg: Spektrum der Wissenschaft Verlagsgesellschaft mbH., Springer Nature. https://www.spektrum.de/lexikon/neurowissenschaft/neurotransmitter/8752 [29.04.2023].

Spektrum Lexikon der Neurowissenschaft (2000b): Acetylcholin. In: Spektrum der Wissenschaft. Heidelberg: Spektrum der Wissenschaft Verlagsgesellschaft mbH., Springer Nature. https://www.spektrum.de/lexikon/neurowissenschaft/acetylcholin/69 [29.04.2023].

Spektrum Lexikon der Neurowissenschaft (2000c): Adrenalin. In: Spektrum der Wissenschaft. Heidelberg: Spektrum der Wissenschaft Verlagsgesellschaft mbH., Springer Nature. https://www.spektrum.de/lexikon/neurowissenschaft/adrenalin/166 [29.04.2023].

Spektrum Lexikon der Neurowissenschaft (2000d): Noradrenalin. In: Spektrum der Wissenschaft. Heidelberg: Spektrum der Wissenschaft Verlagsgesellschaft mbH., Springer Nature. https://www.spektrum.de/lexikon/neurowissenschaft/noradrenalin/8872 [29.04.2023].

Spektrum Lexikon der Neurowissenschaft (2000e): Dopamin. In: Spektrum der Wissenschaft. Heidelberg: Spektrum der Wissenschaft Verlagsgesellschaft mbH., Springer Nature. https://www.spektrum.de/lexikon/neurowissenschaft/dopamin/2959 [29.04.2023].

Spektrum Lexikon der Neurowissenschaft (2000f): Epiphyse. In: Spektrum der Wissenschaft. Heidelberg: Spektrum der Wissenschaft Verlagsgesellschaft mbH., Springer Nature. https://www.spektrum.de/lexikon/neurowissenschaft/epiphyse/3605 [29.04.2023].

Spektrum Lexikon der Neurowissenschaft (2000g): Hypothalamus. In: Spektrum der Wissenschaft. Heidelberg: Spektrum der Wissenschaft Verlagsgesellschaft mbH., Springer Nature. https://www.spektrum.de/lexikon/neurowissenschaft/hypothalamus/5891 [27.01.2022].

Spektrum Lexikon der Neurowissenschaft (2000h): Schilddrüse. In: Spektrum der Wissenschaft. Heidelberg: Spektrum der Wissenschaft Verlagsgesellschaft mbH., Springer Nature. https://www.spektrum.de/lexikon/neurowissenschaft/schilddruese/11353 [29.04.2023].

Spektrum Lexikon der Neurowissenschaft (2000i): Dopamin. In: Spektrum der Wissenschaft. Heidelberg: Spektrum der Wissenschaft Verlagsgesellschaft mbH., Springer Nature. https://www.spektrum.de/lexikon/neurowissenschaft/dopamin/2959 [30.04.2023].

Spektrum Lexikon der Neurowissenschaft (2000j): Hypothalamus-Hypophysen-System. In: Spektrum der Wissenschaft. Heidelberg: Spektrum der Wissenschaft Verlagsgesellschaft mbH., Springer Nature. https://www.spektrum.de/lexikon/neurowissenschaft/hypothalamus-hypophysen-system/5895 [01.05.2023].

Treeck, Oliver (2009): Einführung in die Endokrinologie. In: Leidenberger, Freimut/Strowitzki, Thomas/Ortmann, Olaf (Hrsg.): Klinische Endokrinologie für Frauenärzte. Berlin/Heidelberg: Springer Verlag. S. 3–22. https://doi.org/10.1007/978-3-540-89760-6_1 [29.04.2023].

von Werder, Klaus (2005): Klinische Neuroendokrinologie. 2. Aufl. Heidelberg: Springer Medizin Verlag.

Walther, Reinhard (2022a): Neurotransmitter. In: Pschyrembel online. Berlin: Walter de Gruyter GmbH. https://www.pschyrembel.de/Neurotransmitter/K0F6D/doc/ [29.04.2023].

Walther, Reinhard (2022b): Proopiomelanocortin (POMC). In: Pschyrembel online. Berlin: Walter de Gruyter GmbH. https://www.pschyrembel.de/%20Proopiomelanokortin/K0HSS/doc/ [30.04.2023].

Walther, Reinhard (2022c): Katecholamine. In: Pschyrembel online. Berlin: Walter de Gruyter GmbH. https://www.pschyrembel.de/Katecholamine/K0BGT/doc/ [01.05.2023].

Wuttke, Wolfgang (1987): Endokrinologie. In: Schmidt, Robert F./Thews, Gerhard (Hrsg.): Physiologie des Menschen. Berlin/Heidelberg: Springer Verlag. https://doi.org/10.1007/978-3-662-09340-5_17 [29.04.2023].

Zouboulis, Christos (2013): Interview: Die Haut als endokrines Organ – auf dem Weg zur individualisierten Aknetherapie. In: Medscape Deutschland. New York: WebMD LLC Verlag. https://deutsch.medscape.com/artikel/4901535 [31.01.2022].

Psychoneuroendocrinology

2

In this chapter, psychoneuroendocrinology (PNE) is defined and explained. The basic research of this relatively young scientific discipline is presented, and the enormous relevance of these findings for psychosocial fields of action as well as psychological and psychotherapeutic practice is made clear. In doing so, psychoneuroendocrinology describes the reciprocal relationships between experience and behavior and the functions of the endocrine system. These relationships exist, for example, in that acute emotional stress increases cortisol levels in blood and saliva and, conversely, hormones influence human behavior and psychological experience. This happens because hormones can alter the activity of brain areas (cf. Ehlert and Känel 2011, V). In this chapter, the complex interactions between psyche, neurobiology, endocrinology, and the autonomic nervous system are demonstrated and explained, making the enormous importance of hormones for the human psyche understandable for you. I would like to emphasize in advance that the fascinating field of research and work of psychoneuroendocrinology is still relatively new and that there is no foreseeable end to the discovery of new messengers and hormones and their functions, both in animal and human physiology.

Furthermore, this chapter makes it clear that the increasing willingness to consider interdisciplinary perspectives makes human behavior more explainable. In addition, the basic assumption of the biopsychosocial concept of health and disease, psychosomatics, and behavioral medicine is presented, as well as the fact that psyche and soma are inextricably intertwined. The chapter highlights the complexity of this scientific discipline and makes it clear that research here particularly benefits when various disciplines such as psychology, psychiatry, psychosomatics, behavioral medicine, neuroscience, and endocrinology engage in interdisciplinary exchange and transfer or implement the already gained insights into clinical practice (cf. Ehlert and Känel 2011, VI). Furthermore, this chapter explores the connection between psychoneuroendocrinology and behavioral genetics. You will gain a basic understanding of behavioral genetics, the

J. Wiederhofer, *Psychoneuroendocrinology in Psychosocial and Psychotherapeutic Practice*, https://doi.org/10.1007/978-3-658-46275-8_2

heritability (heritability) explained, and thus the connections between genetics, experience, behavior, psyche, and endocrinology are demonstrated. It becomes clear that psychoneuroendocrinology and thus psychosocial and psychotherapeutic practice are inevitably linked with (behavioral) genetics. The insights presented in this chapter are the foundation on which the biopsychosocial approach "PNES-Coaching" is based.

2.1 Definition and Explanation of the Scientific Discipline

In this chapter, psychoneuroendocrinology (PNE) is defined, explained, and its significance for psychological and psychosocial work is presented. The most important hormones for this are introduced, and it is particularly discussed in which areas of life or emotions they are significant. Emotions, stress, attachment, partnership, and aggressive behavior are examined in more detail. It is also clarified where in our lives, both in everyday life and in psychologically challenging times, hormones have significant influences on us. It is also shown how diseases can arise through psychosocial influences. The connection between psychosocial influences, behavior, and the endocrine system is illustrated through the findings of René Spitz, making it clear what PNE deals with. The great developmental psychologist René Spitz noticed that children from extremely stressful or neglected homes did not have age-appropriate growth. The children often showed apathetic behavior. This apathy is a syndrome that is now referred to as learned helplessness. The children's symptoms were attributed by Spitz to their psychological exceptional situation. Years later, it was realized that the children's short stature was related to the insomnia they suffered due to the stress. As mentioned in Chap. 1, the so-called growth hormone (GH) is secreted at night. If the first deep sleep phase is missed, the production and secretion of the growth hormone are suppressed. When the children were taken in by loving and consistent caregivers in a predictable and stimulating social environment, age-appropriate sleep was established, and body growth normalized within a short time (cf. Birbaumer and Schmidt 2018, 142). "This example clearly shows the inseparable feedback loop between psychological-social conditions, the endocrine system, sleep, and behavior (…)" (ibid.).

Henning and Netter state that psychoneuroendocrinology (PNE) deals with the significance of hormones for psychological functions and characteristics. PNE is significant for almost all sub-disciplines of psychology, such as general psychology (hunger, sleep, sexuality, pain, motivation, and emotion), developmental psychology, clinical psychology, differential psychology, but also occupational psychology and social psychology (cf. Henning and Netter 2000, n.p.). The basic assumption is that the physical and social environment is perceived and that we process this perception cognitively, emotionally, and physiologically and subsequently respond to this environmental situation with (individual) behavior. There is an interaction between our physical and psychological processing. In particular, the hormonal reactions to various environmental influences and life circumstances should be mentioned. A focus of this research is on stress and its effects (cf. Ehlert 2011, 33).

2.2 Endocrine System and Nervous System

The following sections will highlight various aspects of the endocrine system and the nervous system, which make it clear that communication between the two systems and interdependent regulation takes place. This, in turn, illustrates that neither of these systems can be considered in isolation.

The endocrine system and the nervous system are structurally related (the pituitary gland is located in nervous system tissue, which in turn regulates the functions of the HPA axis), but they are also related through the signal transmission of the same hormones, such as norepinephrine (cf. Edwards and Mills 2011, 117).

> "Development and psychological processes (the CNS) regulate hormone secretion, and the hormones in turn control or modulate perception and behavior. Neuropeptides play an important role in the control of hormonal processes by the nervous system" (cf. Birbaumer and Schmidt 2018, 142).

But first, a brief introduction to the nervous system to better understand the following: The nervous system is divided into the central nervous system (CNS) and the peripheral nervous system. The peripheral nervous system is further divided into the somatic nervous system, which controls the muscles, and the autonomic nervous system (ANS), which is linked to the organs (cf. Edwards and Mills 2011, 113). The ANS is also referred to as the vegetative nervous system and is the autonomous part of the nervous system. This means that this part of the nervous system largely escapes voluntary control and behaves "autonomously." The ANS is closely related to the central nervous system (CNS) and, together with all endocrine glands and body fluids, forms a functional unit. The ANS regulates vital functions such as breathing, digestion, and metabolism and controls the interaction of individual body parts. In the classification of the ANS, a distinction is made between the enteric nervous system (which controls the functions of the gastrointestinal tract), the sympathetic nervous system, and the parasympathetic nervous system (cf. Falkai 2022a, n.p.). The ANS thus includes the sympathetic nervous system (SNS, sympathetic) and the parasympathetic nervous system (PNS, parasympathetic) (cf. Edwards and Mills 2011, 113). These two are of particular interest "when considering the stress response and recovery from stress" (Edwards and Mills 2011, 113). The sympathetic nervous system plays a significant role in pain perception and is also responsible for the increase in blood pressure (cf. Pschyrembel 2016a, n.p.). The sympathetic nervous system is associated with "fight or flight." It is responsible for rapid energy release and the acceleration of life processes. The effect of the sympathetic nervous system is mediated by adrenergic receptors (transmitters: adrenaline and norepinephrine) (cf. Lexikon der Neurowissenschaft 2000a, n.p.). The parasympathetic nervous system acts in part oppositely. The effect here is mediated by acetylcholine receptors (transmitter acetylcholine, "cholinergic system"). Since the parasympathetic nervous system inhibits energy release and consumption, thus having a dampening effect ("rest and digest"), it also has an energy-conserving effect ("trophotropic system"). Thus, an antagonistic effect to the sympathetic nervous system is often observed (cf. Lexikon der Neurowissenschaft 2000b, n.p.).

The following will outline and explain the neuroendocrine regulatory circuits.

2.2.1 Neuroendocrine Regulatory Circuits

> "Through central nervous processing (…), a stimulus can trigger a behavior and/or a neuroendocrine reaction, and the released hormones act as feedback (…) on behavior and hormone levels. Additionally, hormone reaction and behavior influence both stimulus processing and social interactions" (Birbaumer and Schmidt 2018, 142).

A distinction is made between the developmentally organizing and the activating-mobilizing hormone influence, which acts throughout the entire lifespan. Those hormones that directly or indirectly influence human behavior exert their effect by shaping the synaptic strength of neuronal connections and/or modulating the discharge properties of nerve cells (cf. Birbaumer and Schmidt 2018, 142 f.). Sympathetic neurons release norepinephrine and substance P, thereby stimulating the adrenal medulla to subsequently release adrenaline. The effect occurs due to adrenergic receptors. The ANS has far-reaching effects on the entire organism, leading, for example, to the "fight-or-flight" stress response. This results in increased heart rate, blood pressure, dilation of the trachea and bronchi, and increased availability of glucose (cf. Edwards and Mills 2011, 113). However, the following should be considered: Since the secretion of most hormones is subject to endogenous (internal) time cues or combined endogenous-exogenous (internal and external) time cues, the sensitivity and excitation thresholds in the affected target organs change accordingly. Time cues here mean that hormone secretion is subject to various circadian, episodic, cyclic, and their environmental rhythm setters. This affects both sensory and motor target organs. Exceeding or falling below certain thresholds can thus cause immense changes, affecting both perception and motor skills (cf. Birbaumer and Schmidt 2018, 143). When the brain and endocrine regulatory circuits interact, it is noticeable that, in addition to the effects of neurotransmitters and neuropeptides, other substances also influence the central nervous system, with neuropeptides, especially those hormones composed of amino acids, holding a prominent position because they are produced directly in the brain and act there. Neuropeptides and neurotransmitters act not only in the brain but also in the periphery of the body. In the central nervous system, there are about 100 neuropeptides involved in various functions and having different effects on various psychological functions (cf. ibid., 142). The following briefly outlines some effects (visceral, cognitive, and behavioral effects) of neuropeptides (cf. ibid., 144). Neuropeptides can trigger visceral, cognitive, and behavioral effects, for example, **endogenous opioids.** Endogenous opioids act in the spinal cord, brainstem, hypothalamus, limbic system, ventral tegmentum, and striatum. Depending on the site of action, they have various functions or effects. For example, if they act in the spinal cord and brainstem, they reduce pain perception and lower blood pressure. They also influence the cardiovascular system. If they act in the hypothalamus and limbic system, they inhibit sexual behavior, reduce stress through induced isolation, lower body temperature, and increase food and fluid intake. If endogenous opioids act in the ventral tegmentum and striatum, they cause euphoria and regulate locomotor behavior (cf. Birbaumer and Schmidt 2018, 144). **Oxytocin** is a neurohypophyseal hormone that acts in the thalamus and brainstem. It stimulates maternal behavior, modulates sexual behavior, and reduces memory span. **Vasopressin** acts in the thalamus, limbic system, and particularly in the hypothalamus. It promotes learning and memory and regulates blood pressure. **Somatostatin** is one of the hypothalamic hypophysiotropic hormones; its sites of action are the cerebral cortex and hippocampus. Somatostatin regulates locomotor activity and body temperature and promotes learning and memory. **GHRH** ("growth hormone releasing hormone") are hypothalamic hypophysiotropic hormones that act in the brain. GHRH stimulates food intake and has neuroprotective and antidepressant effects. **CRH** ("corticotropin releasing hormone") acts in the cerebral cortex, hippocampus, hypothalamus, and other parts of the brain. It coordinates the visceral stress response and increases arousal and emotionality. Additionally, CRH inhibits sexual behavior and influences learning. CRHs are hypothalamic hypophysiotropic hormones. Like CRH, **TRH** ("thyrotropin releasing hormone") is a hypothalamic hypophysiotropic hormone. TRH acts in the thalamus, olfactory lobe, and brainstem. It has antidepressant effects and increases body temperature and blood pressure. **LHRH** (luteinizing hormone-releasing hormone) acts in the olfactory and limbic systems and is referred to as a hypothalamic hypophysiotropic hormone. LHRH increases sexual behavior and neuroendocrine responses to primary pheromones. **Prolactin**is an adenohypophyseal hormone. The MPOA (medial preoptic area of the anterior hypothalamus) is mentioned as the site of action. Prolactin inhibits male sexual behavior and promotes female nurturing behavior. **ACTH and α-MSH**are adenohypophyseal hormones. They act in the limbic system and hippocampus. ACTH and α-MSH promote attention, learning, and memory. **Substance P**is one of the gastrointestinal peptides that act in the brain, spinal cord, and also in the hypothalamus. Substance P mediates pain signals, increases arousal and activity, and promotes sexual behavior. The **VIP** (vasoactive intestinal peptide) acts in the cerebral cortex and limbic system. VIP promotes avoidance learning and inhibits anxiety-motivated behavior. VIP is one of the gastrointestinal peptides. **CCK-8** (cholecystokinin) acts in the cerebral cortex, olfactory, and limbic systems and is a gastrointestinal peptide. CCK-8 reduces pain and hunger and induces sleep. **Neurotensin** is one of the gastrointestinal peptides and acts in the limbic system and spinal cord. It reduces body temperature and locomotor activity and promotes sexual behavior. The sites of action of **Insulin**are the olfactory and limbic systems and the hypothalamus. Insulin inhibits hunger and food intake behavior in the CNS. It promotes attention and is a gastrointestinal peptide.

Angiotensin acts in the hypothalamus, causing thirst and influencing drinking behavior, increasing blood pressure, and regulating fluid balance. **Bombesin** influences temperature regulation, inhibits food intake, and increases blood pressure. The hypothalamus and midbrain are mentioned as sites of action. **Bradykinin**acts in the limbic system and spinal cord, transmitting pain. The sites of action of **Neuropeptide Y** are the hypothalamus and thalamus. Neuropeptide Y promotes eating and drinking behavior and reduces blood pressure and body temperature. It also promotes memory. The **delta sleep-inducing peptide** acts in the brain and hypothalamus and has a sleep-inducing effect. The sites of action of**atrial natriuretic factor** are the limbic system and the brain. The atrial natriuretic factor reduces blood volume and regulates fluid balance, thirst, and drinking behavior (cf. Birbaumer and Schmidt 2018, 144).

After discussing some neuropeptides significant for psychoneuroendocrinology, glucocorticoids and their effects on the nervous system will be examined and important information will be presented. The focus will initially be on the effects glucocorticoids have on human senses.

2.2.2 Glucocorticoids and Their Effects on Perception

> "The organization and significance of environmental stimuli, including perception thresholds and the formation of specific associative connections ('binding'), depend on the presence of hormones" (Birbaumer and Schmidt 2018, 145).

As mentioned in Chap. 1, glucocorticoids are produced in the adrenal cortex, with cortisol being particularly relevant for PNE. Glucocorticoids, especially cortisol, are components of a complex regulatory circuit between the brain and the body. Their individual functions go far beyond a simple stress response (cf. Birbaumer and Schmidt 2018, 143). When the splanchnic nerve ("visceral nerve") is stimulated, the adrenal medulla releases adrenaline and noradrenaline. The nerve also stimulates the biosynthesis of adrenaline, a process dependent on glucocorticoids. Adrenaline is produced from noradrenaline by an enzyme called PNMT (phenylethanolamine-N-methyltransferase). PNMT is regulated by glucocorticoids (cf. Edwards and Mills 2011, 117). The interaction between the adrenal medulla and the adrenal cortex provides the physical connections for signal transmission. This also allows for high glucocorticoid concentrations. To maintain adrenaline synthesis, high glucocorticoid concentration is indispensable. Additionally, glucocorticoids exert their effects both in the brain and the nervous system (cf. Edwards and Mills 2011, 117 f.).

> "A distinction must always be made between the central → peripheral effects caused by CRH → ACTH → cortisol and the effects of glucocorticoids directed from the periphery to the center" (Birbaumer and Schmidt 2018, 143).

Considering the brain, glucocorticoid receptors are found in many areas, particularly in the limbic system and especially in the hippocampus. It is assumed that all have various functions for behavior (cf. ibid.).

1) **Sense of smell and taste**

The sense of smell is part of the sensory system and serves the perception of fragrances. It is closely connected to the hypothalamus and the limbic system, or rather, the information that is received through the nose is transmitted to the hypothalamus and the limbic system. However, the sense of smell is not only responsible for the assessment of food, environmental orientation, and social communication or mutual recognition. It also serves as a warning function and thus acts as a protective mechanism (cf. Pschyrembel Editorial 2022a, n.p.). Increasing evidence suggests that the sense of smell also has enormous significance for quality of life and health and exhibits extraordinary performance. Due to the frequently occurring olfactory disorders during the COVID-19 pandemic, there has been increasing clinical interest in the loss of smell and taste. New findings highlight the enormous importance of the sense of smell (cf. Müller and Renner 2022, 8–13). Scents can make one both happy and sad. Additionally, new research has found that the sense of smell is often impaired in neurodegenerative diseases or mental disorders (such as Alzheimer's, autism, and schizophrenia) (cf. Luerweg 2019, n.p.). The sense of smell and the sense of taste are closely connected. After the activation of the taste buds, this sensory perception is transmitted to the somatosensory cortex. Especially in the past, the sense of taste was vital for survival (for example, to identify spoiled food). It is connected to the autonomic nervous system (cf. Pschyrembel Editorial 2022b, n.p.). Due to the neural connections, cortisol, for example, also influences sensory perceptions. When cortisol secretion occurs, it leads to significant perception thresholds. This means that depending on the endogenous or endogenous-exogenous time cues to which most hormones are subject, the sensitivity and excitation thresholds in the respective affected motor and sensory target organs change (cf. Birbaumer and Schmidt 2018, 143). "When certain thresholds are under- or exceeded, this can cause significant changes in perception and motor skills" (Birbaumer and Schmidt 2018, 143). Regarding the sense of smell and taste, significant effects of cortisol on perception thresholds are evident. For example, an increase in cortisol leads to external stimuli requiring a significantly higher intensity to be perceived (cf. Birbaumer and Schmidt 2018, 143). Based on the connection between the sense of smell and taste and the transmission of sensory perception to the hippocampus and amygdala, which are part of the limbic system considered the center for emotions and memories, it seems unsurprising why these two senses can evoke such strong memories and emotions.

2) **Acoustic System**

Birbaumer and Schmidt (2018) are convinced that the acoustic system is obviously influenced by the effect of cortisol (cf. Birbaumer and Schmidt 2018, 143). They justify this as follows:

> "(…) the stapedius reflex, in which, among other things, a stiffening of the stapes in the inner ear dampens the pressure transmission in loud sounds (…), is inhibited by cortisol, which raises the perception threshold for intense sounds" (Birbaumer and Schmidt 2018, 143).

These findings support the general assumption that in short-term stress, the psychological function of glucocorticoids is to "prevent the overshooting of peripheral and central nervous reaction systems" (cf. ibid.) (Birbaumer and Schmidt 2018, 143). This means that after stress, the increase in the perception threshold protects the central nervous system from further escalation of excitation (cf. ibid.).

In summary, it should be noted here that our hormones affect our nervous system, influence our perception and senses, and thus function both as a warning signal and a calming system. The endocrine and nervous systems regulate and control each other, and together they are responsible for both mobilizing the body ("fight or flight") and dampening activity ("rest and digest"), thereby jointly implementing life-sustaining measures. As mentioned in Chap. 1, biological rhythms or endogenous rhythms influence the respective effects. Therefore, the following will delve deeper into these rhythms and the science that deals with this topic ("chronobiology"). Additionally, the findings will be examined and how they relate to psychoneuroendocrinology.

2.3 Chronobiology

> "Chronobiology is the science that deals with the rhythm of life" (Richter 2021, n.p.).

Chronobiology is a young science that has only existed since the mid-20th century. It deals (cf. Abbruzzese 2011, 130) "with the change of the organism as a function of time (…)" (ibid.). Chronobiology is a field of research that deals with the study of biological rhythms. It examines regular, rhythmically recurring factors. These can be rhythms such as the circadian rhythm (sleep-wake cycle), but also the menstrual cycle or breathing as well as heartbeat (cf. Hackermeier 2020, n.p.). Abbruzzese notes that in chronobiology, biological rhythms are discussed, in which various things can be observed from gene expression to behavior. Thus, chronobiology plays a significant role in psychoneuroendocrinology. Most physiological, biochemical, and psychological functions are subject to regular temporal fluctuations (cf. Abbruzzese 2011, 130). The best-researched rhythmic processes are hormone secretion, circadian sleep-wake rhythm disorders, organ activities, and drug effects within a day-night cycle (cf. Hackermeier 2020, n.p.). Normally, the rhythms are divided into constant periods, and clear maxima and minima can be defined. Based on this, we speak of "endogenous rhythms." These are divided into various categories depending on their period length. For humans, circadian, ultradian, and infradian rhythms are of particular importance (cf. Abbruzzese 2011, 130 f.). The **circadian rhythm** has a period length of approximately 24 hours (cf. Abbruzzese 2011, 130 f.). This rhythm is of particular importance to humans because the physiological processes of the human organism are oriented to this circadian rhythm of nature, which is based on the rotation of the Earth (cf. Richter 2021, 87 f.). Here, the day-night behavior, hormone secretion, pain sensitivity, cognitive performance, and body temperature are particularly noteworthy (cf. Abbruzzese 2011, 130 f.). Richter notes that the sleep-wake cycle is the most common cycle and that its disruption or disturbance can lead to numerous psychological and physical disorders (cf. Richter 2021, 87 f.). The **ultradian rhythm** has several cycles per day. Pulsatile hormone secretion is a notable example here. The **infradian rhythm** lasts longer than a day. Here, for example, the menstrual cycle of women or the timing of pregnancy can be mentioned. For other living beings, the circannual rhythm and the circatidal rhythm are of importance. The period length of the **circannual rhythm** is approximately one year. An example of this type of rhythm can be the mating season in certain animals. The **circatidal rhythm** is comparable to ebb and flow. It has a period length of approximately 12.5 hours. This type of rhythm is, for example, important for the foraging of certain crab species. It is important to mention that endogenous rhythms are often "nested" (cf. Abbruzzese 2011, 131). This means "(…) that many parameters simultaneously exhibit multiple rhythms" (ibid.). For example, endocrine parameters are mostly classified as infradian, but at the same time, they show a circadian rhythm, which in turn is divided into "several ultradian pulsatile bursts" (cf. Abbruzzese 2011, 131) (ibid.).

> "The (…) most researched rhythm is the circadian: Almost all physiological as well as psychological parameters show a circadian rhythm" (Abbruzzese 2011, 131).

Due to the importance of endogenous rhythms, they play a significant role in the following sections, particularly the circadian rhythm.

2.3.1 Hormone Secretion and Sleep

The sleep-wake cycle is probably the best-known among circadian rhythms. It is closely linked to the rest-activity rhythm. A healthy person sleeps at least once within 24 hours, for an average of 5–10 hours. With modern measurement methods, 4 sleep stages have been identified within the entire sleep duration. These 4 sleep stages repeat cyclically approximately every 90 minutes, leading to a so-called sleep architecture. At the same time, this is a good example of overlaps of different rhythms. The circadian sleep rhythm is divided into ultradian 90-minute cycles. The subunits are also referred to as "basic rest activity cycles" (BRAC) (cf. Abbruzzese 2011, 134). Birbaumer and Schmidt (2018) note that the regularly changing sleep is indispensable for the endocrine systems as well as for the immune system. Sleep alternates between deep sleep (SWS, "slow wave sleep") and REM sleep ("Rapid-eye-movement" sleep, "dream sleep"). In many significant endocrine systems, significantly higher activity is observed during sleep, such as the growth hormone (GH, "growth hormone") (cf. Birbaumer and Schmidt 2018, 145).

Von Känel (2011) notes that human night sleep, in particular, is characterized by special changes in neuroendocrine hormone activity. In general, it can also be noted that melatonin, growth hormone, and prolactin tend to have an immune-supportive effect. Catecholamines and cortisol are rather declared as immunosuppressive (cf. von Känel 2011, 250). One task of sleep is therefore to stimulate endocrine processes that cannot be triggered during the day. If the sleep rhythm is altered, whether by sleep disorders, developmental changes in the individual, or external influences, this affects both the physiological and psychological regulatory processes of significant hormones as well as the immune system (cf. Birbaumer and Schmidt 2018, 145).

> "In chronobiology, we therefore also speak of 'predictive homeostasis' of sleep, that is, its peculiarity to 'anticipate' regulatory processes expected during the day at night" (Birbaumer and Schmidt 2018, 145).

Richter notes that in individuals suffering from insomnia, abnormalities in circadian rhythms (phase advance or delay) as well as in hormone secretion can be observed. In particular, the abnormalities in melatonin and cortisol release are significant, as these can lead to sleep disorders and contribute to the maintenance of this disorder (cf. Richter 2021, 87 f.) Abbruzzese (2011), on the other hand, notes that it is not completely clear why an organism needs to sleep. However, she is certain that restorative factors and regeneration processes of the body and mind play a significant role. Likewise, the time of low movement serves the repair of nerve cells. Furthermore, sleep serves the consolidation of newly acquired information (cf. Abbruzzese 2011, 134). Birbaumer and Schmidt (2018) are convinced that one of the most important tasks of sleep is to regulate endocrine and immunological processes. This makes it understandable why sleep deprivation in humans (as well as other vertebrates) leads to life-threatening to fatal consequences (cf. Birbaumer and Schmidt 2018, 145). The conclusion here is as follows: "Sleep, especially deep sleep at the beginning of the night, is necessary for the predictive homeostasis of many organ functions" (ibid.).

2.3.2 Growth Hormone (GH) and Cortisol

The growth hormone (GH, "growth hormone") is particularly secreted during SWS ("slow wave sleep"). When REM sleep dominates, later in the night, GH drops to a minimum (cf. Krueger and Obal 2004, cited in von Känel 2011, 251). It is relevant to note here that GH and cortisol have many opposing properties. These are evident not only on the physiological and psychological levels but also in an exactly opposite ultradian periodicity (rhythm that repeats over a 24-hour day) (cf. Birbaumer and Schmidt 2018, 145). Observing GH and cortisol secretion during a 7- to 8-hour sleep, it can be seen that GH is secreted in the first two sleep cycles. Deep sleep itself is not considered a trigger here. Based on the maximum value of GH secretion in the first part of the night, many of the negative effects of sleep deprivation can be explained. This part of sleep or the night is also referred to as the "core sleep" of the circadian periodicity (cf. Birbaumer and Schmidt 2018, 145). Additionally, it is important to mention that individuals who had a deficiency in GH showed a shorter total sleep duration as well as higher sleep fragmentation (cf. Zisapel 2007, cited in von Känel 2011, 251). The negative effects of sleep disorders range from inhibition of body growth and cognitive development to impairment of learning ability. This is based on the fact that GH is involved in the growth of connections between nerve cells in the central nervous system. Stress, depression, and extreme physical activity often lead to sleep disorders, especially disturbances of core sleep, which leads to GH suppression and an increase in cortisol (cf. Birbaumer and Schmidt 2018, 145), whereby the following is important to mention:

> "The relationship between GH and sleep is determined less by a circadian mechanism and more by sleep itself" (Zisapel 2007, cited in von Känel 2011, 251).

At the nadir of the GH level, that is, with the 3rd sleep cycle (but not with a REM phase), the pulsatile ACTH and cortisol secretion begins. In the second half of the night (during the REM phases), the increase in cortisol is slowed down. Cortisol secretion occurs intensively only in the intermediate stages up to waking up (cf. Birbaumer and Schmidt 2018, 145). The following explains cortisol secretion during sleep in more detail.

2.3.3 Cortisol and Immunosuppression

> "The loss of core or deep sleep is accompanied by a weakening of the immune system" (Birbaumer and Schmidt 2018, 145).

As briefly mentioned above, the secretion of cortisol, CRH, and ACTH is minimal during the first half of the night. However, it increases in the second half of the night, with the increase of REM sleep. The peak is reached by the HPA axis at the time of awakening (cf. Meerlo et al. 2008, cited in von Känel 2011, 251). This serves to prepare the organism for awakening and to provide it with the necessary energy (cf. von Känel 2011, 251). But what happens if too many glucocorticoids are released? Glucocorticoids inhibit the release of many cytokines, which means they can be said to have an indirect immunosuppressive effect, whereas the release of GH has an immunostimulatory effect. Based on this relationship, the increasing susceptibility to illness in old age could be explained, as both core sleep and GH production are reduced in old age (cf. Birbaumer and Schmidt 2018, 145).

> "With increasing age, the rise in cortisol during the night occurs earlier, and a nocturnal rise in cortisol is more likely to lead to awakening and suppression of SWS" (von Känel 2011, 251).

The decline in melatonin secretion seems to be partly responsible for the increased activity of the HPA axis. Additionally, an increased 24-hour cortisol secretion is associated with poorer sleep quality (cf. von Känel 2011, 251). This is not only observed in old age but also after prolonged helplessness and depression (cf. Birbaumer and Schmidt 2018, 145). The sleep of depressed patients is significant here, as their sleep is significantly worse than that of healthy individuals. Conversely, prolonged sleep deprivation can lead to the development of depression. Chronic sleep deprivation thus increases the risk of depressive disorders. It is also important to note that studies show chronic psychosocial stress leads to sleep disturbances (cf. von Känel 2011, 260 f.). Additionally, the rise in cortisol exacerbates the destabilization of the cardiac system, which is why cardiovascular disorders are more common in the second half of the night (cf. Birbaumer and Schmidt 2018, 145). Poor sleep can thus help explain the reduced immune competence in old age (cf. von Känel 2011, 261). The question remains, what is different in the endocrine system during an infectious disease. As already stated,

> "(…) normal sleep supports the adaptive immune response to an infectious agent and thus the immune memory" (von Känel 2011, 261).

Fatigue or drowsiness are characteristic symptoms of both viral and bacterial infectious diseases (cf. ibid.). This can be considered a reaction in the acute phase of the infection, ultimately serving the recovery of the organism (cf. Imeri and Opp 2009, cited in von Känel 2011, 262). This is based on the fact that during an infection, the acute phase reaction leads to an increase in stress hormones (cortisol, catecholamines) in the blood. This signals to the brain that the body is undergoing an infection (cf. von Känel 2011, 262). So how does sleep lead to immune competence? This will be discussed in the following section, along with the relationship between psychoneuroendocrinology and psychoneuroimmunology.

2.3.4 Melatonin and Immune Competence

A brief introduction to melatonin was already given in Chap. 1. Here, it is once again demonstrated what significance melatonin has for both psychoneuroendocrinology and psychoneuroimmunology.

> "Melatonin has a somnogenic effect and is considered the actual timekeeper for sleep" (von Känel 2011, 252).

Melatonin is a peptide hormone of the pineal gland, which is released in the dark. It is regulated by the suprachiasmatic nucleus, which most strongly controls the sleep-wake rhythm or circadian rhythm. Light suppresses the release of melatonin (cf. Birbaumer and Schmidt 2018, 146). In contrast to the circadian pacemaker, sleep itself has little effect on melatonin levels (cf. von Känel 2011, 252). However, the suprachiasmatic nucleus not only regulates melatonin secretion but also determines the temporal rhythm of the secretion of stress hormones, thyroid hormones, and sex hormones (cf. Birbaumer and Schmidt 2018, 146). An increase in the need for sleep in the evening occurs about 2 hours after the onset of melatonin production. The peak of melatonin production is reached in the middle of the night, and towards morning the level drops again (cf. Zisapel 2007, cited in von Känel 2011, 252). Ultimately, it should be noted that the influence of melatonin acts synchronizing on endogenous rhythms and contributes to the recovery of immune competence in the first half of the night. In the case of melatonin deficiency, this can lead to sleep disorders and a desynchronization of rhythms and affective disorders (mental health disorders). Overproduction can lead to hypersynchronous, inflexible rhythms such as jet lag (cf. Birbaumer and Schmidt 2018, 146). Demonstrating the connection between melatonin and immune competence is an example of how psychoneuroendocrinology and psychoneuroimmunology are intertwined.

> "Psychoneuroimmunology is understood as the science of the interactions between behavior ('Psycho'), the nervous system ('Neuro'), and the immune system ('Immunology')" (Birbaumer and Schmidt 2018, 167).

The immunological effect of sleep seems to be based on the release of the pineal gland hormone melatonin. Melatonin apparently acts as the mediator of the circadian effects on the immune system. A regular sleep-wake rhythm is thus a prerequisite for sufficient immune competence. Additionally, melatonin, administered before bedtime, reduces stress effects and can also resynchronize the rhythm in cases of jet lag. In animal experiments, the multitude of hormonal effects of stress was neutralized in this way (cf. Birbaumer and Schmidt 2018, 171). It is important to note here that exogenously administered melatonin shortens the time to fall asleep and generally leads to drowsiness (cf. von Känel 2011, 252). Melatonin also causes a slight release of endogenous opioids in antigen-activating T-helper cells, which has slowed the growth of tumors in animal experiments (cf. Birbaumer and Schmidt 2018, 171).

2.3.5 Summary and Intervention

As outlined in this third part of the chapter, sleep is of enormous relevance for both mental and physiological health. It has been shown how behavior ("Psycho"), the nervous system ("Neuro"), and the immune system ("Immunology") are intertwined, and based on this, psychoneuroendocrinology and psychoneuroimmunology cannot be separated from each other. The presented literature shows that healthy sleep is indispensable for a functional immune system, good immune competence, and infection defense, as well as for mental health. Disturbances of a normal sleep-wake cycle inevitably lead to changes in the immune system or affect its functioning, which can be described as reduced immune competence. Changes in the neuro-endocrine-immune system can, for example, negatively influence cardiovascular diseases and depressive disorders. Additionally, sleep loss can lead to increased fatigue and intensified pain in various organic as well as functional diseases (cf. von Känel 2011, 263). But what interventions can be implemented for affected individuals? Von Känel notes that the data on interventions, both psychotherapeutic and behavioral medicine interventions as well as pharmacotherapy, is limited. Measures to restore a normal sleep-wake rhythm with the aim of positively influencing neuroendocrine and immunological deviations are thus difficult to implement. However, he considers it indispensable, especially in the context of psychiatric disorders, to adhere to any sleep hygiene and pharmacological recommendations. Furthermore, it is important to take a 2-hour nap in the afternoon after a sleepless night to lower elevated IL-6 levels and reduce sleepiness (cf. ibid., 263 f.). Mindfulness-based methods (cf. Cole et al. 2009, cited in von Känel 2011, 264) and Tai Chi also have a positive effect on sleep quality (cf. Irwin et al. 2008, cited in von Känel 2011, 264). Additionally, it is advisable to keep a diary of sleep-wake activity for at least a week. Steering behavior so that a person gets enough sleep according to their individual needs, especially night sleep, seems to be a relatively simple measure to promote physiological and mental health. Interventions in this area are thus indispensable to see if regulating sleep leads to a relevant improvement in the health of the client (cf. von Känel 2011, 264 f.).

After providing an insight into psychoneuroimmunology in this chapter, the following section will further delve into psychoneuroendocrinology. However, before further focusing on the relationship between behavior, the nervous system, and the endocrine system, the fourth part of this chapter will present fundamental information regarding the importance of genetics for psychoneuroendocrinology, which, like psychoneuroimmunology and chronobiology, cannot be separated from psychoneuroendocrinology.

2.4 The Importance of (Behavioral) Genetics for Psychoneuroendocrinology

> "All living beings produce offspring of their own kind, so humans only produce humans, with the offspring resembling their parents more than the children of other parents. This transmission of similar traits over generations is what we call inheritance" (Birbaumer and Schmidt 2018, 572).

Parents equip their children with a coded form of hereditary traits, which are referred to as genes. According to Birbaumer and Schmidt (2018), every human probably has around 25,000 genes. These genes collectively form the genome of the individual. The genome consists of 50% maternal and 50% paternal genes. Therefore, children exhibit both similarity and variability. However, it is important to mention that the genetically determined individuality of humans can be altered or further stimulated by environmental influences and learning (cf. Birbaumer and Schmidt 2018, 572). As has been shown several times, psychoneuroendocrinology examines the relationships between behavior and the hormonal system. In a complex interaction between environmental factors or environmental stimuli, all areas of this research discipline are based exclusively on the influence of our genes (cf. de Geus and Wüst 2011, 164). The classification of what part of our behaviors is based on genes and what part on environmental factors is referred to as "Nature (inheritance) or Nurture (environment)." For many behaviors, it can now be empirically demonstrated whether and to what extent they depend on environmental factors as well as genetic factors. Nevertheless, the "either-or" of "Nature or Nurture" is still defended, especially in relation to intelligence and personality traits (cf. Birbaumer and Schmidt 2018, 572). This is still based on the "(…) ignorance of classical and molecular genetics" (ibid.). Genetic factors influence our hormone secretion, how sensitive a receptor is, and they are also of utmost relevance to our behavior. Our genes influence the functioning of neurobiological pathways, which interact with both behavior and the endocrine system. Even the likelihood of being exposed to a particular environmental factor is not free from genetic influences (cf. de Geus and Wüst 2011, 164). Also, in relation to mental illnesses, genes not only have a direct influence on the development of the disease but also an indirect influence by increasing the likelihood of being exposed to stressful life events, which are considered risk factors for mental illnesses (cf. Faller 2003, 80–92). However, it is important to note that there is no gene for intelligence or recklessness, just as there is no warrior gene. It is not the behaviors that are coded by genes, but the proteins (cf. de Geus and Wüst 2011, 164), "which control the formation of neuronal systems" (ibid.). Proteins primarily serve as structural substances in connective and supportive tissues, as well as for the division of cell space, regulation of metabolism, and cell activity. Here, I would like to point out that proteins are made up of amino acids, and most hormones are also made up of amino acids. Furthermore, they serve as sites where signals are received at the target organ (receptors). Additionally, the contractile structures of both smooth and striated muscles are made up of proteins (cf. Birbaumer and Schmidt 2018, 576). Proteins have the ability to respond flexibly to both internal and external stimuli, which is why they represent the true foundation of behavior (cf. de Geus and Wüst 2011, 164).

> Genetic research provides insights into why "under seemingly identical contextual conditions, biopsychological reactions and behaviors vary greatly among different individuals" (ibid.).

The question of how genes influence neurobiological systems also implies the question of where and how behavior is controlled (cf. de Geus and Wüst 2011, 164).

> "Genetic variation largely affects regulatory regions on the DNA, and differences localized here can influence not only how much of a gene product is expressed but also at what time and in which tissue" (ibid.).

Thus, particularly in the brain, genetic differences that, for example, influence the regulation of the expression of a receptor can have relevant effects on behavior (cf. de Geus and Wüst 2011, 164).

> Based on this insight, "genetics is an important tool for uncovering the molecular foundations of behavior, including the foundations of mental disorders" (ibid.).

In summary, it should be noted here that behavior is always attributable to an interplay of genes or hereditary traits and environmental influences. It should be mentioned that in simple motor activities such as breathing, swallowing, sucking, as well as in emotional behavior and character traits, genetic predisposition often dominates. The case where a learned behavior dominates is rare (cf. Birbaumer and Schmidt 2018, 572).

2.4.1 Fundamentals of Behavioral Genetics

> "Almost all variables or 'phenotypes' that are of interest in the field of psychoneuroendocrinology (…) show significant interindividual differences, and the expression of traits in the population is likely to resemble a normal distribution in many cases" (de Geus and Wüst 2011, 164 f.).

At the beginning, it is important here to first explain the terms phenotype and genotype. The term phenotype refers to all characteristics (phenes) present in an individual. This includes its appearance, the entire morphology (shape), and its physiological properties. This term is shaped by the interaction of hereditary (genotype) and non-hereditary traits. The term expressivity is used to describe the degree of phenotypic expression (cf. Schöller 2021a, n.p.). The term genotype, on the other hand, describes the entirety of all hereditary traits of an individual. Dominant and recessive genes or alleles determine the phenotype (cf. Schöller 2021b, n.p.). The divergences between individuals regarding phenotypes are largely attributable to genetic variation, which is stored at the level of DNA molecules ("deoxyribonucleic acid") (cf. de Geus and Wüst 2011, 165) (Fig. 2.1).

DNA molecules are so-called polymers, which have 2 strands that in turn consist of 4 nitrogenous bases (adenosine (A), cytosine (C), guanine (G), thymine (T)). DNA strands are referred to as 3'-end or 5'-end. The twisting of the double strand creates the double helix structure, which together with histones (binding proteins) forms the chromosomes (cf. de Geus and Wüst 2011, 165). The chromosomes are composed of chromatin, which consists of protein and DNA. The genetic material is encoded in this DNA. The two DNA strands are twisted into a double helix, and the base pairing of the two opposing DNA strands occurs by A only forming cross-bridges with T, and C only with G. Based on this, the structure of each strand is completely determined by the opposite strand (cf. Birbaumer and Schmidt 2018, 577).

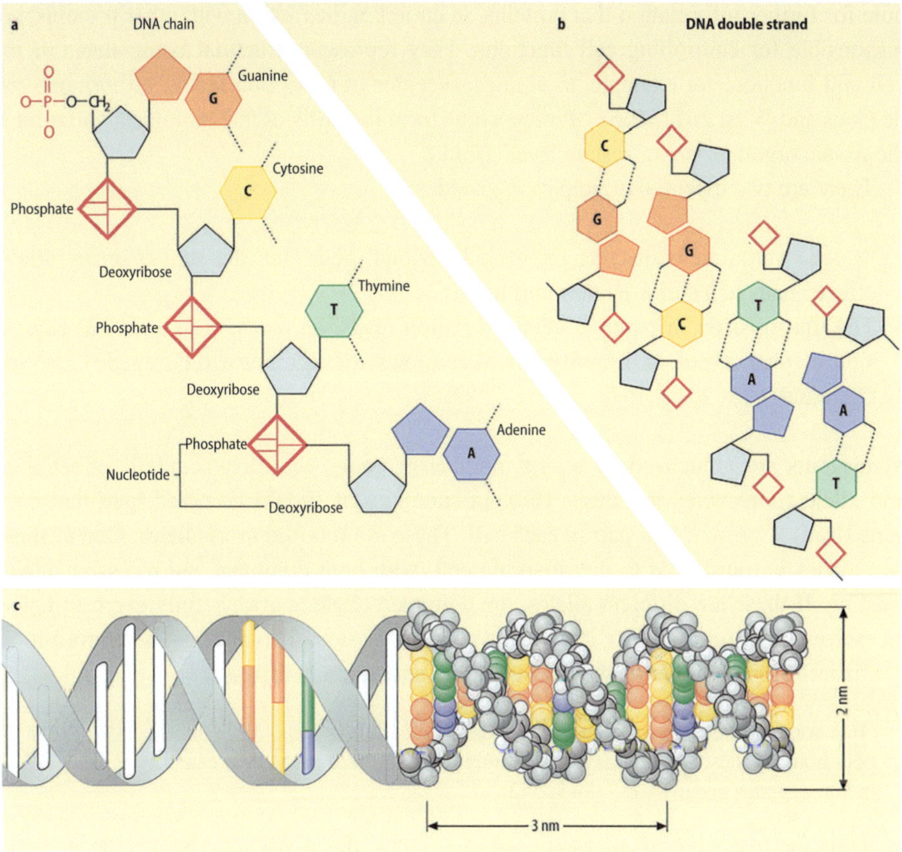

Fig. 2.1 Birbaumer, Niels and Schmidt, Robert F. (2018): Structural model of DNA. In: Biological Psychology. Special edition. 7th revised and supplemented edition. Heidelberg: Springer Medizin Verlag. 577. *Source:* Birbaumer and Schmidt (2018, 577)

> "In the nucleus of human cells, there are 23 pairs of chromosomes (22 pairs of autosomes and 2 sex chromosomes), one of which comes from the mother and one from the father" (de Geus and Wüst 2011, 165).

During the formation of egg or sperm cells (meiosis), more than 8 million recombinations ("mixtures") can arise due to the random distribution of the former 23 maternal and paternal chromosomes (cf. Birbaumer and Schmidt 2018, 583). Thus, the entire human genome is contained in 23 chromosomes (pairs). Each chromosome or its DNA molecule contains around 1000 genes (cf. ibid., 578). The identical loci (locations) of two similar (homologous) chromosomes (maternal, i.e., from the mother, and paternal, i.e., from the father) are referred to as alleles. The genotype of an individual consists of a combination of the two alleles (cf. de Geus and Wüst 2011, 166). Additionally, it is important to note for further information that proteins, in complex interaction with other proteins, are responsible for controlling cell functions. They represent structural components of the cell and function, for example, as storage, receptor transcription factor, or hormone (cf. de Geus and Wüst 2011, 166). "Proteins thus form the basis of any biological variation at the tissue, organ, or organ system level" (ibid.).

There are two essential principles in genetics:

- "Allelic variation is discrete for each individual gene, but the sum of many allelic effects leads to a (semi-)continuous trait.
- The transmission of parental allelic variation leads, on average, to a similar expression of phenotypes in a family, but also allows for significant differences (…)" (de Geus and Wüst 2011, 167).

Many traits are influenced by a large number of genes with diverse allelic effect sizes and allele frequencies (cf. ibid., 168). In summary, it should be noted here that each gene (trait) is present as a pair in each cell. These are referred to as alleles. One of these two alleles is transferred to the offspring cell, with both dominant and recessive alleles existing. If these are different alleles, the dominant allele is always fully expressed. The recessive allele, on the other hand, shows no expression. This process is referred to as dominant-recessive inheritance (cf. Birbaumer and Schmidt 2018, 573).

> "In a dominant-recessive inheritance, the dominant allele is responsible for the phenotype in both homozygous and heterozygous occurrences. The recessive allele can only assert itself in homozygous occurrences" (ibid., 573).

In addition, it is now of enormous relevance that the expression of a trait (gene) is influenced by a multitude of environmental factors. Such factors include, for example, intrauterine factors (such as prenatal stress), nutrition, parenting style, peer connections, accidents, and illnesses, traumatic experiences (such as abuse, war experiences, assaults, etc.), chronic stress, and climate. Furthermore, environmental factors, which are not free from genetic influences, act additively or interactively with other environmental factors or genetic factors on the phenotype. The combination of these effects leads to both biological and psychological traits (cf. de Geus and Wüst 2011, 168 f.).

2.4.2 Twin Studies

> "Research approach in psychology and human genetics, in which identical and fraternal twin pairs are examined regarding the concordance of a trait" (Lieb 2018, n.p.).

The study of familial similarity is a significant tool within genetics. Of particular interest are twin studies (cf. de Geus and Wüst 2011, 170). In contrast to fraternal twins, identical twins share not only their home environment but also their entire DNA. Fraternal twins, like regular siblings, share their home and 50% of their genes. Twin studies are therefore of enormous importance. Adoption studies are also relevant, as they reveal in which areas or traits children are more similar to their biological parents than to their adoptive parents. Such studies have concluded that biological inheritance is not limited to physical appearance but also includes psychological, character, and mental aspects. These include, for example, (anti-)social behavior, intelligence, religiosity, political views, and risk-taking; additionally, the 5 main factors of personality, known as the "Big Five": conscientiousness, openness to experience, agreeableness, introversion/extraversion, and neuroticism (cf. Henderson 2010, 88 f.). Wüst and de Geus note that twin studies are significant because they can demonstrate that "psychobiological phenotypes are significantly influenced by genetic factors" (de Geus and Wüst 2011, 171). When siblings grow up in the same household, the shared environmental conditions potentially include important factors (cf. ibid., 170). These include, for example, socioeconomic status, school, neighborhood, parenting style, and nutrition, etc. Monozygotic twins (MZ; identical twins) are genetically identical with rare and few deviations. In monozygotic twins, the fertilized egg splits before implantation in the uterus, the reasons for which are not yet fully understood. If more than one egg is released by the ovaries, they are fertilized by different sperm, resulting in dizygotic twins (DZ; fraternal twins). Dizygotic twins are no different from regular sibling pairs. They have an average genetic concordance of 50%. Twins of different sexes are always dizygotic twins (cf. de Geus and Wüst 2011, 170). Particularly significant results are obtained from studies with monozygotic twins who were raised apart (cf. Birbaumer and Schmidt 2018, 587).

2.4.3 Gene-Gene, Gene-Age, Gene-Gender, and Gene-Environment Interactions

Environmental factors or influences from the surroundings can influence genetic potential in such a way that it is more strongly realized, which in turn can lead to overestimations regarding genetic variance. Heritability estimates can thus be significantly distorted by the mutual influence of environment and genes (cf. Birbaumer and Schmidt 2018, 589).

> "From a genetic perspective, practically all psychobiological phenotypes are complex. This means that it is highly likely that many genes, each with a small effect, have an influence and that these effects are in turn modulated by other genes, age, gender, and environmental factors" (de Geus and Wüst 2011, 173).

Based on this, it makes sense to implement gene-gene, gene-age, gene-gender, gene-environment interactions, as well as possible higher-order interactions, in all genetic studies or analysis procedures (cf. ibid.).

2.4.4 The Importance of Genetic Factors for the Regulation of the Hypothalamus-Pituitary-Adrenal Axis (HPA Axis)

> "At all levels of stress regulation, pronounced differences between individuals can be observed" (de Geus and Wüst 2011, 174).

This applies to personality traits and response styles as well as to psychological and biological reactions to acute stress and long-term stress consequences (cf. ibid.). Long-term or chronic tension can lead to dysregulation of the physiological stress response. This, in turn, can have neurobiological consequences and lead to both somatic and psychiatric disorders (cf. Krähenmann and Seiferitz 2019, n.p.). HPA axis regulation is relevant for a number of somatic and psychological disorders. For example, numerous twin and family studies demonstrate that diseases such as depression and schizophrenia have significant heritability (cf. de Geus and Wüst 2011, 174). In schizophrenia, this is about 80%, and in depression, it is 30-45% (cf. de Geus and Wüst 2011, 174). Furthermore, the concept of "endophenotype" has also been successful in diseases such as alcoholism or Alzheimer's (cf. Maier and Zobel 2004, n.p.). Additionally, it has been shown that various sets of genes increase the risk for certain types of disorders. Thus, much of what is collected in the field of psychoneuroendocrinology can be attributed to the concept of endophenotypes. The endophenotype concept assumes that neuropsychiatric disorders are based on genetic foundations. In particular, neuroendocrine stress regulation and thus the HPA axis are increasingly coming into focus in psychiatric and medical genetics. Regarding stress regulation, genetic correlations with the "cortisol awakening response" can be demonstrated. Here, it is shown that the cortisol level measured after awakening is under significant genetic influence. During the course of the day, however, the influence is predominantly based on environmental factors. Although the HPA axis responds quickly to changing environmental influences, it can still be assumed that genetic factors are of significant importance for some aspects of HPA axis regulation (cf. de Geus and Wüst 2011, 174 ff.).

2.4.5 Gene-Sex Interactions

There is an increasing number of studies on gene-sex interactions. These suggest (cf. de Geus and Wüst 2011, 180),

> "(…) that the same genetic variant can be associated with HPA axis regulation in different or even opposite ways" (de Geus and Wüst 2011, 180).

It should be considered here that the cellular environment differs significantly between men and women. In particular, the effects of sex steroids and their receptors should be considered. These influence both peripheral bodily and central nervous effects and include both brain development in early life stages and current effects of stress regulation (cf. ibid., 181).

> "In this sense, gene-sex interactions can be interpreted as a special form of gene-environment interaction" (Abney et al. 2006, cited in de Geus and Wüst 2011, 181).

2.4.6 Conclusion

The importance of psychobiological processes for both somatic and psychiatric disorders, the endophenotype approach, and the increased focus on environmental factors in genetic research lead to the conclusion that genetics is of considerable relevance for modern psychoneuroendocrinology. Genetics can also benefit from the concepts and findings of psychobiology. This is particularly evident in psychobiological stress research (cf. de Geus and Wüst 2011, 184),

> "(…) whose core competence is both the characterization of the biological systems relevant to stress regulation in terms of endophenotyping and the description of stress-related environmental factors" (de Geus and Wüst 2011, 184).

This section has now made it clear how enormously important genetics is for the psyche and behavior of humans. Behavioral genetics is inevitably connected with everything that a person is, their personality, their interactions and environmental influences, psychological disorders, and their resilience. Since this scientific discipline cannot be separated from psychoneuroendocrinology, the influence of our genes will be repeatedly addressed in the following sections and is ultimately part of this biopsychosocial coaching approach.

2.5 Emotions and Hormones

As has been stated several times, hormones have strong effects on our emotions. The following will examine these effects on our emotions in more detail. The different emotions associated with the corresponding hormones will be shown and described. The basics of the respective hormones were already explained in Chap. 1, and now the connections of the hormones relevant to psychoneuroendocrinology with emotions and their individual effects on social interactions will be presented.

2.5.1 Oxytocin and Its Importance for Emotions, Behavior, and Attachment Disorders

1) **Attachment and Attachment Disorders**

Attachment primarily refers to the emotional bond between parents and their child (cf. Spektrum 2000a, n.p.). Modern attachment research is based on the foundations laid by John Bowlby, Mary Ainsworth (1951), and René A. Spitz (1965). This attachment research demonstrated the existential dependence of the child on "mothering figures," who, as primary caregivers, are sensitively and continuously available to the child during the first years of life (cf. Beckrath-Wilking and Biberacher 2013, 94). According to John Bowlby, humans are equipped with instinctive behavioral systems to ensure the reproduction of the species (cf. Spektrum 2000a, n.p.). Additionally, the child seeks comfort, protection, and security from the proximity to its mother, making the attachment figure a safe haven from which the child can explore the world. A secure attachment is the foundation for developing trust in one's abilities and for building resilience against external events. The phenomenon that toddlers use their attachment figures as a secure base is vital for their survival. Even in adulthood, a secure attachment remains a retreat for comfort and reassurance in times of trouble (cf. Beckrath-Wilking and Biberacher 2013, 94). Today, it is known that attachment behavior and hormones cannot be separated; they are invariably linked. Primarily, both the formation and maintenance of social bonds are learned. However, attachment reactions are based on various hormones, and conversely, there are typical hormonal reactions determined by specific attachment behaviors. The development of attachment behavior begins immediately after birth, which indeed appears like a non-homeostatic drive. However, attachment behavior is largely determined by learning processes immediately after birth (cf. Birbaumer and Schmidt 2018, 146). The quality of the parent-child attachment has a significant impact on the child's development as well as on their later physical and mental health. Relationship experiences in the family of origin are also important. They affect the strengths of parenting competence. Poor attachment or relationship with parents can have consequences for mental health and lead to later partnership problems. It can also result in negative professional experiences and economic problems such as unemployment or poverty, as well as limited social resources (cf. Falkai 2022b, n.p.). For any living beings that must survive in groups, both permanently and temporarily, a physiological and neurochemical basis must be present. This is based on the premise that there must be a motivation for social bonding, independent of reproductive and sexual drives, as a prerequisite for living together in groups (cf. Birbaumer and Schmidt 2018, 146). The emotional bond between parents and child develops over the course of their time together. Loving touches, eye contact, holding the child, and emotional speaking promote attachment (cf. Spektrum 2000a, n.p.). This is related, as will be explained later, to the hormone oxytocin (OXY). The psychologically relevant effects of OXY are most clearly seen in the early parent-child relationship. Here, OXY is released in both parents and child during their interactions (cf. Roth and Strüber 2021, 140). The maturation and development of our brain are not complete at birth and are influenced by the degree of use and our experiences. In particular, the maturation of the prefrontal cortex is influenced by good early attachment experiences (cf. Beckrath-Wilking and Biberacher 2013, 98). But what happens when this biologically anchored attachment is separated or dissolved? From an attachment-theoretical perspective, the loss or absence of a secure attachment base must be regarded as the earliest and most harmful psychological trauma. Abrupt separations or losses, for example, that are not cushioned by a reliable environment that provides security, have similarly harmful effects as trauma from violence (cf. Brisch 2009, cited in Beckrath-Wilking and Biberacher 2013, 95). If attachment is dissolved through separation in humans, helplessness and hopelessness, comparable to symptoms seen in severe depression, are the result. Consequently, helplessness and hopelessness trigger the opposite physiological processes to attachment reactions, thus inhibiting each other (cf. Birbaumer and Schmidt 2018, 146). It is also of enormous importance that "(…) the innate physiological processes for attachment behavior are prerequisites for learning processes" (ibid.). These learning processes predominantly determine the attachment drive and attachment skills, especially in adolescence and adulthood. All early attachment experiences are stored in human memory and continuously compared with current social situations throughout life (cf. ibid.).

> "With the loss or separation of social bonds, damage to learning and memory processes occurs" (Birbaumer and Schmidt 2018, 146).

This means that with a separation or a loss of attachment, stored attachment expectations in the memory are violated, which in turn leads to helplessness and depression (cf. ibid.). Early attachment traumas have permanently damaging effects. They negatively influence the ability to modulate arousal, stress resilience, and the ability to form healthy relationships. The experience-dependent maturation of the brain, particularly that of the prefrontal cortex, is impaired. This has lifelong consequences for learning and relationship abilities, self- and affect regulation, self-reflection and mentalization functions, as well as stress management competence. Early uncontrolled stress situations shape the stress processing system in such a way that it can lead to limitations in learning ability and attention, but also to increased pain sensitivity and a tendency to somatization. Stressors already affect humans prenatally. These can be strong efforts by the mother as well as unprocessed and lingering or even trauma experienced during pregnancy (cf. Beckrath-Wilking and Biberacher 2013, 98 f.).

> "Attachment traumas experienced in early childhood, lack of empathy, and disregard for basic child needs with alternating neglect and overprotection not only result in insecure to disorganized attachment styles but also in lifelong increased stress vulnerability and attachment disorders as fixed early psychopathology" (ibid., 99).

According to Ainsworth, the following attachment styles are distinguished (cf. Beckrath-Wilking and Biberacher 2013, 96):

- securely attached
- insecure-avoidant attached
- insecure-ambivalent attached
- disorganized attached (ibid.)

Secure Attachment
In secure attachment, the child brings a fundamental trust in the reliability and availability of the attachment figure. This allows the child to build a stable "self-image" and have a secure base to explore the environment. As adults, people with secure attachment behavior can effectively use counseling and therapy in crisis situations (cf. Beckrath-Wilking and Biberacher 2013, 96).

Insecure-Avoidant Attachment
Insecure-avoidant attached children no longer show their fear and insecurity and do not seek physical closeness or comfort from caregivers. These children also do not expect a positive outcome in a crisis situation. This is based on rejecting and dismissive parental behavior, especially in situations characterized by fear and distress. Due to the painful experiences, the child no longer wants to approach the caregivers to minimize the risk of rejection, which is seen as an avoidance strategy. The child distances themselves, responds only briefly, and shares little about themselves to avoid a devaluing reaction. As adults, these individuals often appear distant in relationships, avoid closeness to others, and consider themselves strong people (cf. ibid., 96 f.).

Insecure-Ambivalent Attachment
For these children, the attachment figure is unpredictable. They cannot anticipate how the attachment figure will react in various situations, making them restless and nervous. Separations particularly burden these children, and they behave contradictorily towards the attachment figure. They seek closeness to the caregiver even before the separation but are simultaneously angry and upset with them (approach-avoidance behavior). The child does not develop confidence in the availability of the mother, making even a one-hour separation a significant threat to the child. These children appear clingy and immature for a long time. In adults, this often manifests as confused relationships. They often seem less objective, confused, and contradictory. They are anxious and passive in relationships, angry with attachment figures, and often trapped in relationships. Additionally, these individuals have difficulty integrating and categorizing their various emotions (cf. Beckrath-Wilking and Biberacher 2013, 97).

Disorganized Attachment

The style of disorganized attachment shows the breakdown of attachment (cf. ibid.).

> "Children with a disorganized attachment pattern exhibit contradictory and confusing attachment behavior, are torn between seeking proximity and distance, freeze in their movements, and show sudden outbursts of aggression" (Beckrath-Wilking and Biberacher 2013, 97).

This attachment pattern is often based on a traumatic history with at least one parent. Often, these are based on unresolved separations, which lead to transgenerational transmission. The child finds itself in an insoluble conflict, on the one hand having to seek protection from the parental figure and at the same time having to protect itself from them, resulting in an approach-avoidance conflict. The child develops control strategies, feels responsible for the well-being of the attachment figure, behaves overprotectively, or tries to appear punitive towards the caregiver, which leads to insults from the child (cf. Beckrath-Wilking and Biberacher 2013, 97 f.).

> "This attachment style predisposes to later severe psychopathology such as attachment disorders and dissociative disorders" (Main and Solomon 1986, quoted in Beckrath-Wilking and Biberacher 2013, 98).

It seems that hostile and anxious behaviors of the mother with the child often occur in connection with unresolved traumas of the mother. Ultimately, it should be noted that a secure attachment is a stable foundation for the child and thus promotes stress resilience, providing protection against the consequences of trauma. Additionally, it offers a basis for a stable personality as well as the promotion of a functioning stress processing system (cf. Beckrath-Wilking and Biberacher 2013, 98 f.).

2) **Oxytocin and Attachment Behavior**

As already mentioned, the hormone (neuropeptide) oxytocin (OXY) is particularly important for attachment behavior. It has also been stated that OXY has multiple functions. The secretion of OXY is triggered by many physiological stimuli (cf. Roth and Strüber 2021, 139). As mentioned in Chap. 1, the functions of OXY include, for example, the triggering of milk ejection in the female breast as well as uterine contractions during childbirth and sexual intercourse. It is mainly produced in the PVN (paraventricular nucleus) and the SON (supraoptic nucleus) of the hypothalamus. OXY is then transported to the neurohypophysis (posterior pituitary) via neurons and stored there (cf. Birbaumer and Schmidt 2018, 146). Stimuli that promote secretion into the bloodstream include, for example,

> "(…) the birth of a child, sucking at the mother's breast, sexual activity, skin contact, various forms of stress, as well as positive and negative social interactions" (Landgraf and Neumann 2012, quoted in Roth and Strüber 2021, 139).

Additionally, the release of oxytocin is highly conditionable and can be triggered, for example, merely by memories of positive social experiences (cf. Roth and Strüber 2021, 139). In addition to this described primary production pathway, OXY can also be found in the limbic system and in the autonomic nuclei of the brainstem (cf. Birbaumer and Schmidt 2018, 147).

> "These extrahypothalamic fibers and nuclei are partially independent of the hormonal pathway to the pituitary and into the bloodstream" (ibid.).

In parents, the hormone promotes parental behavior (cf. Roth and Strüber 2021, 140). It is also worth mentioning that short-term stress is associated with an increase in cortisol, vasopressin, and oxytocin, which promotes maternal and paternal caregiving behavior and attachment, before and after birth (cf. Birbaumer and Schmidt 2018, 147).

> "Through its effect on dopaminergic cells of the reward system, it strengthens the mother's attachment to her child and her willingness to be there for it" (Roth and Strüber 2021, 140).

OXY influences various brain structures, thereby inhibiting aversive reactions to the child and promoting understanding and empathy for the child's emotions. Depending on how caring the parents are with the child, the oxytocin concentration in the parental blood increases in the first months after birth. In the mother, a high oxytocin concentration is noticeable through warm speech (motherese), the expression of positive emotions, and loving touches. The paternal oxytocin concentration, on the other hand, is noticeable through stimulating behavior, such as touches or showing objects (cf. Roth and Strüber 2021, 140). Interestingly, parents with high oxytocin concentrations in their blood also have children with high oxytocin levels (cf. Feldman et al. 2010, cited in Roth and Strüber 2021, 140). In the child's body, OXY has a stress-dampening effect. This can be observed when the child is exposed to a stressful situation. Both physical comfort and telephone contact with the mother result in a high oxytocin concentration and a reduced secretion of the stress hormone cortisol. Children who have to cope with the stressful situation alone, on the other hand, react with a low OXY concentration and a high cortisol secretion (cf. Pollak et al. 2010, cited in Roth and Strüber 2021, 141). Warm maternal behavior and loving stimulation by the father thus seem to increase the release of OXY in the child, thereby reducing the release of stress hormones. This would explain why parental comfort can bring about a calming effect on the child. In addition to the positive influence in acute stress situations, the early childhood OXY released in interactions also seems to have long-term effects on the brain (cf. Strüber 2016, cited in Roth and Strüber 2021, 141).

> It seems that OXY "promotes the networking of brain structures of the upper limbic level with each other and with those of the middle limbic level" (Strüber 2016, cited in Roth and Strüber 2021, 141).

This promotes a conscious and reflective processing of feelings as well as emotion regulation. In summary, it should be noted that particularly loving parental contact promotes the release of OXY. Especially sensitive mothers create the conditions for positive early childhood OXY release. Studies have shown that maternal contact promotes OXY release and thus reduces cortisol concentration. Children who had to cope with stress situations alone, on the other hand, showed a low release of OXY but a high cortisol concentration. In addition, a high early childhood release of OXY has a long-term positive influence on the limbic system and thus on emotion regulation. However, OXY is not only of great relevance for the parent-child bond. OXY is also released in social interactions in adulthood and influences both behavior and emotions (cf. Roth and Strüber 2021, 141 f.). The following will therefore address the effect of OXY in adulthood, how it influences our emotions and behavior, and how the release of OXY can be stimulated.

3) **Oxytocin in Adulthood: Social Bonding and Partnership**

OXY is also responsible for the development of the feeling of attachment in adulthood. This is often associated with sexual activity in adults. The availability of OXY at the synapses increases in both sexes through the stimulation of the sexual organs during sexual activity. Animal experiments have also shown that microinjections of OXY increase sexual interest. Furthermore, OXY increases in the period after orgasm (in the refractory phase). It is also important to note here that both the development and maintenance of social bonds depend on the presence of oxytocin in the central nervous system (cf. Birbaumer and Schmidt 2018, 147). In addition to the peripheral effects that OXY has, it is also important to mention that based on the effects that OXY triggers in the brain, it also has many psychological effects (cf. Roth and Strüber 2021, 140).

> "Without the oxytocin gene, social amnesia occurs, while oxytocin together with endogenous opioids makes social contact rewarding" (Birbaumer and Schmidt 2018, 147).

Here, both OXY and ADH (vasopressin, the antidiuretic hormone) are of significance. Even though these two have completely different peripheral functions, both promote sexual behavior and social bonding. In animal experiments, it was shown that mice lacking the genes for the synthesis of these two neuropeptides exhibit social amnesia. This means that they either cannot or do not want to recognize their partner. Additionally, monogamous animals, those that remain connected to a partner for life, show a significantly higher number of oxytocin receptor binding sites in limbic and hypothalamic brain regions. Similarly, intraspecific aggression is lower in monogamous species. It thus appears that OXY in the central nervous system rewards social contacts of all kinds (not just sexual contacts) in cooperation with opioid peptides and opioid structures (cf. Birbaumer and Schmidt 2018, 147).

> "(…) the positively reinforcing effect of intracranial stimulation of opioid brain structures in the social context during the formation of bonds is likely generated by the combined effect

> of OXY (oxytocin) and beta-endorphins. In any case, both neuromodulators increase in the reward structures in such social situations" (ibid.).

As already mentioned, OXY also influences behavior in adulthood. In studies where OXY was administered via nasal spray, it was found that it significantly reduces quarrelsomeness and increases positive communication. Likewise, the activities of the sympathetic nervous system, which are primarily responsible for stress-related fight-or-flight reactions, are inhibited by OXY. The parasympathetic nervous system, on the other hand, which is mainly responsible for protective and maintenance functions, is promoted by OXY. In general, it should be noted here that people who exhibit higher activity of the parasympathetic system have a stronger sense of connectedness on the behavioral level and show a greater tendency towards positive emotions. Additionally, studies with oxytocin nasal spray have shown that OXY promotes divergent and creative thinking and has a beneficial effect on social behavior, trust, empathy, and compassion (cf. Roth and Strüber 2021, 142 ff.). However, it is important to mention that this effect is influenced by biological sex, early experiences, and mental illnesses. Because even though OXY is often referred to as the happiness and love hormone, it can also amplify negative traits such as schadenfreude and envy. This is possibly related to the fact that OXY increases attention to social signals (cf. Roth and Strüber 2021, 144).

> "Oxytocin researchers from Mannheim and Freiburg concluded that oxytocin improves the recognition of emotional and social signals and promotes the willingness to take risks regarding cooperative and trusting behavior. This increases the motivation to engage in social interactions" (Domes et al. 2011, cited in Roth and Strüber 2021, 144).

As already mentioned, the effect of the hormone is influenced by many factors. In addition to those already listed, the influence of genes in connection with experiences also counts. Since this is of enormous importance, the following section will explain how OXY is intertwined with genes and experiences and what diverse effects this has.

4) **Oxytocin and the Influence of Genes and Experiences**

The individual genetic makeup of a person influences the functioning of their oxytocin system and thus also their behavior (cf. Roth and Strüber 2021, 144). Here, I would like to particularly address the A-allele of the rs_{53576} polymorphism (A/A genotype) and the G-allele (G/G genotype) of the oxytocin receptor polymorphism.

The A/A Genotype

> "A specific variant of the gene for the oxytocin receptor (the so-called A-allele of the rs_{53576}polymorphism) is on average associated with a lower expression of prosociality, empathy, trust, positive affect, optimism, mastery, and self-esteem" (Roth and Strüber 2021, 144).

Individuals who carry this allele exhibit greater stress sensitivity and have difficulty understanding other people against a background of noise. A/A genotypes are less likely to seek social support in stressful situations, and their stress response is not inhibited by social interaction. Maternal behavior is also influenced by the A-allele. Mothers with this gene tend to respond less empathetically to their infant than mothers with a different genotype. It seems they are less sensitive to messages from the baby. This is shown by a lower physiological reactivity of the mother in response to the baby's crying. However, it should be mentioned that the A-allele can produce resilience against the effects of early negative experiences (cf. Roth and Strüber 2021, 144–147).

The G/G Genotype

Unlike individuals with the A allele, individuals with the G allele benefit from social support from their partner in stressful situations. Furthermore, they exhibit only a low subjective stress sensitivity and a lower cortisol release in response to stress. The G allele could be a genetic variant that is more affected by the impacts of environmental influences. G/G genotypes show a greater risk of developing emotional dysregulation and a disorganized attachment representation as a result of child abuse compared to the A allele (cf. Roth and Strüber 2021, 144–147). This clearly shows the diverse influences that experiences, in connection with genetic makeup, have on the oxytocin system of individuals.

The Influence of Experiences on the Oxytocin System

Experiences can influence the oxytocin balance in the long term, especially experiences that the child has with the mother. For example, high maternal care leads to increased oxytocin function in children, and reduced maternal care can decrease the functionality of the oxytocin system in the long term (cf. Insel et al. 2003, cited in Roth and Strüber 2021, 145). In some people who have had early negative experiences, an experience-related reduced oxytocin function is still evident in adulthood, with a particularly sensitive period here. Many children who were neglected early but have lived well-protected in an adoptive family for several years do not respond to physical contact with the mother with increased oxytocin secretion. This shows that early neglect, in particular, significantly impairs the normal development of the oxytocin system. Studies show that women, in particular, who experienced abuse during their childhood have significantly lower oxytocin concentrations in the cerebrospinal fluid as adults. The greater the number of diverse categories of abuse, such as emotional, sexual, and physical abuse, emotional or physical neglect, the lower the concentration of OXY (cf. Heim et al. 2009, cited in Roth and Strüber 2021, 145 f.). However, it is important to mention that there are also children who, despite early neglect, have a normally functioning oxytocin system. It can be assumed that, based on their genetic makeup and the connection with additional positive environmental conditions, such as a surrogate mother in close proximity, they have developed sufficient resilience (cf. Roth and Strüber 2021, 145). The influence of early experiences can not only affect the oxytocin system but also lead to a change in oxytocin receptors (cf. Alleva et al. 2013, cited in Roth and Strüber 2021, 145). This leads to a reduced effect of oxytocin. Not all people are equally positively influenced by OXY, as early negative experiences can also weaken the effect of, for example, the administration of OXY via nasal spray. It is highly likely that the cause of this reduced sensitivity to intranasal oxytocin is based on a change in the functionality of the oxytocin receptor. Since the production of receptor protein is influenced by epigenetic markings, epigenetics could be the cause (cf. Roth and Strüber 2021, 145 f.).

> According to a study, "people who report low maternal care have higher methylation of the gene for the oxytocin receptor than people who recall high care" (Burkhardt et al. 2015, cited in Roth and Strüber 2021, 147).

Methylation is an epigenetic mechanism or an epigenetic change that prevents the reading and formation of receptor proteins (cf. Roth and Strüber 2021, 147). These epigenetic changes are, in turn, linked to specific behaviors and certain characteristics. For example, people with low DNA methylation (which presumably leads to a high occurrence of the receptor protein) (cf. Cochran et al. 2016, cited in Roth and Strüber 2021, 144) "are more likely to show a secure attachment style (…) and an improved ability to recognize emotional facial expressions" (ibid., 147). Early negative experiences that have influenced oxytocin function can also affect later stress management. As already mentioned, oxytocin can inhibit the secretion of the stress hormone cortisol. Early negative experiences, such as early parental separation, can reduce this function of OXY in the long term (cf. Roth and Strüber 2021, 147).

> "The early traumatic experience therefore seems to be associated with increased stress sensitivity" (ibid.).

As already mentioned, vasopressin is closely related to oxytocin, so the following will address the effects of vasopressin on behavior and emotions.

2.5.2 Vasopressin and Its Importance for Emotions and Behavior

Vasopressin is an antidiuretic hormone and is also referred to as arginine vasopressin. Like oxytocin, it is synthesized in the paraventricular nucleus and supraoptic nucleus of the hypothalamus. However, it is produced by different cells and is secreted into the bloodstream via the pituitary gland (cf. Roth and Strüber 2021, 148). There are 3 different types of receptors that are activated by vasopressin. These are referred to as V_{1a}, V_{1b}, and V_2, with the V_{1a} receptor being particularly developed in the brain and primarily located in the cortex, amygdala, and basal ganglia (cf. Roth and Strüber 2021, 148).

1) **Vasopressin and Oxytocin**

Vasopressin and oxytocin receptors are often arranged in a complementary pattern; however, vasopressin and OXY can activate each other's receptors. Vasopressin receptors are more likely to be found in medial areas, and oxytocin receptors in the lateral areas of the central amygdala. Like oxytocin, vasopressin is secreted in particularly stressful as well as social situations. However, OXY generally has an anxiety- and stress-relieving effect, whereas vasopressin enhances anxious behavior. Similarly, vasopressin acts on the stress system in a manner opposite to oxytocin (cf. Roth and Strüber 2021, 148).

> It "(…) increases attention to environmental stimuli and the activity of the sympathetic nervous system (fight or flight) and decreases the activity of the parasympathetic nervous system (rest and digest)" (ibid.).

The opposing effects of OXY and vasopressin are also evident in the cortisol system. OXY inhibits cortisol production, whereas vasopressin stimulates it. However, vasopressin and OXY also have similar effects. For example, both OXY and vasopressin promote social recognition (cf. Roth and Strüber 2021, 148 f.). Scientists assume that OXY "is more responsible for the acquisition of social memories (…)" (ibid., 149), whereas vasopressin "mediates the consolidation of these memory contents" (ibid.). Additionally, both OXY and vasopressin enhance bonding processes, close relationships between parents and their child, as well as pair bonding (cf. ibid.).

2) **Vasopressin and the Effects on Biological Sexes**

Furthermore, vasopressin has various effects on biological sexes. In studies where vasopressin was administered as a nasal spray, it increased the impression in men that unfamiliar faces appeared threatening. Women, on the other hand, interpreted friendliness and caring into the faces. Similarly, in interactive game situations: in men, vasopressin enhanced cooperation with others, whereas in women, this behavior was not promoted (cf. Roth and Strüber 2021, 148 f.).

3) **Vasopressin and the Influence of Genes and Experiences**

> "Various polymorphisms of the vasopressin receptor gene can influence the effect of vasopressin and thereby behavior" (Roth and Strüber 2021, 149).

For example, a specific gene variant of the V_{1a}receptor influences altruistic behavior in a gambling situation. Another allele appears to be associated with successful or unsuccessful partnership relationships. Male carriers of the $_{334}$ allele are more frequently affected by crises within marriage than others, and the likelihood of divorce is also higher in these individuals (cf. Heinrichs 2009, cited in Roth and Strüber 2021, 149). The activity of the amygdala or certain personality traits such as novelty seeking or harm avoidance are also influenced by this individual genetic variant of the vasopressin receptor. This genetic variant can also influence the risk of developing depression (cf. Roth and Strüber 2021, 149).

4) **Vasopressin and Early Experiences**

As with OXY, the functioning of the vasopressin system is influenced by early experiences. The basal release of vasopressin is reduced in children who were neglected early on. Early experiences also shape the response of the vasopressin system to stress. A study was conducted with male rat pups, in which they were separated from their mother for three hours daily during the first two weeks after birth. As a result, these animals responded to social stress situations with increased vasopressin synthesis. As adult animals, they also exhibited increased aggression towards other male conspecifics when their territory was threatened. Furthermore, it was observed that these animals had more vasopressin receptors in the hypothalamus (cf. Roth and Strüber 2021, 149 f.).

2.5.3 Dopamine and Its Significance for Emotions and Behavior

Basic knowledge about dopamine has already been presented, such as the fact that dopamine is formed from the amino acid tyrosine by "dopaminergic" cells (cf. Roth and Strüber 2021, 114). In the following, however, I would like to delve deeper into dopamine and its significance for our behavior, as well as the associated reward system. Additionally, the influence of genes and experience will also be discussed here. As already mentioned in Chap. 1, the amino acid tyrosine is ingested with food and subsequently synthesized into dopamine by dopaminergic cells. This occurs in the substantia nigra, the frontal cortex, but also in the amygdala. In the substantia nigra, a significant dopaminergic fiber bundle, which is important for the control of voluntary movements, is sent to the dorsal striatum (nigrostriatal dopamine system). Additionally, dopaminergic neurons are located in the VTA (ventral tegmental area of the midbrain), which send their fibers to the frontal cortex (mesocortical dopamine system) and to the amygdala as well as to the nucleus accumbens (mesolimbic dopamine system) (cf. Roth and Strüber 2021, 114). The released dopamine stimulates specific receptors and influences the activity of the affected cell. So far, 5 different dopamine receptors have been identified, which are designated as D_1-, D_2-, D_3-, D_4-, and D_5receptors. Depending on which receptors dopamine binds to, it acts either excitatory (i.e., depolarizing) or inhibitory (i.e., hyperpolarizing). If it binds to D_1 and D_5 receptors, it acts excitatory. This means that these receptors enhance the effect of the affected inhibitory or excitatory synapses. If dopamine binds to D_2-, D_3-, and D_4 receptors, it acts inhibitory. This, in turn, means that they reduce the effect of the synapses. Under the influence of dopamine, an inhibitory (inhibiting) circuit can thus be specifically enhanced in its inhibitory effect or specifically disinhibited, as is the case in the basal ganglia, for example (cf. Roth and Strüber 2021, 114).

1) **Dopamine and Reward**

If the activity of brain structures is influenced by dopaminergic cells, then motivation and goal-directed behavior are the focus. Based on this, it is assumed that the activity of dopaminergic neurons conveys significant information about rewards. For example, if one chemically blocks the $D_1$and D_2 receptors, rewards lose their reinforcing effect on learning processes. For a long time, it was thought that dopamine is the brain's hedonic signal and is responsible for feelings of joy and pleasure (cf. Roth and Strüber 2021, 114 f.). Today, it is known that the function of dopamine is much more complex, as liking, which conveys the pleasure of the reward, is primarily based on the effect of endogenous opioids. Dopamine, on the other hand, is responsible for wanting, meaning it conveys an incentive value for certain stimuli and thus creates an expectation of reward, which can be understood as the basis for motivated action. Dopamine can therefore be seen as the signal that, for example, after seeing a cake (cue), fulfills an expectation of reward, which may be stronger or weaker than anticipated. If the reward is as expected, the activity of the dopaminergic neurons remains the same (tonically slow). In the case of a higher or lower reward than expected, the activity of the dopaminergic neurons is either increased or decreased. If an unexpectedly high reward occurs, a phasic (fast and high) dopamine response follows. This means that from then on, this high activity accompanies the cue and thus signals its reward value (cf. Dayan et al. 1997, cited in Roth and Strüber 2021, 115). Furthermore, certain dopaminergic cells signal the degree of uncertainty of a reward. This means that the greater the uncertainty about whether the cue actually announces a reward, the higher the reward. The target cell can therefore receive two types of signals: A rapid and high dopamine secretion informs that a reward is now expected. A moderate, slow dopamine secretion signals uncertainty, as it is not clear whether the reward will occur. The reward value and the uncertainty factor together influence motivation, i.e., whether one is motivated to perform a behavior (buy the cake) or not (cf. Roth and Strüber 2021, 117 f.). However, it is important to mention that the individual's risk awareness also plays a role here. Gambling is a good example. If the reward value is high, but the uncertainty about whether the reward will occur is also high, cautious individuals with high risk awareness will not be motivated to act or, in the case of gambling, to play. Particularly risk-prone individuals, on the other hand, respond to this pattern with particularly high behavioral readiness. This is because, for them, the slow dopamine signal of uncertainty itself already has a rewarding effect. This leads to increased risky behavior. In the example of gambling, this means that these individuals are willing to bet very high amounts despite great uncertainty about whether a win will occur (cf. Fiorillo et al. 2003, cited in Roth and Strüber 2021, 118). Additionally, a further property of dopaminergic cells was recently discovered. In animal experiments, it was shown that when animals receive a reward after a longer series of actions, the dopamine concentration increases during the search. Applied to humans, this could also provide a sustained drive to act and, for example, be the reason for not getting discouraged or making a coffee when fatigue sets in (cf. Roth and Strüber 2021, 118 f.).

2) **Dopamine and addictive drugs**

In addition to natural things in life that bring joy, addictive drugs (including alcohol and nicotine) especially stimulate the reward system. This increases the dopamine concentration in the nucleus accumbens as well as in the orbitofrontal and ventromedial cortex. Cocaine, for example, prevents the reuptake of dopamine into the cell, resulting in a significant increase in dopamine concentration in the synaptic cleft. Chemical opiates bind to the receptors of endogenous opioids, which also leads to an enhanced dopamine signal. The difference between natural rewards and addictive drugs is that addictive drugs cause dopamine release in the reward system even when they are consumed repeatedly and predictably, meaning even when the reward is as expected. Since pleasure-inducing mechanisms quickly adapt, the natural feeling of pleasure soon diminishes (cf. Roth and Strüber 2021, 115 ff.).

3) **Dopamine and punishment**

In recent years, it has become apparent that some dopaminergic cells also signal aversive (unpleasant) events such as reward withdrawal or punishment. This occurs through a slow and sustained reduction in spontaneous activity, which is likely due to the influence of inhibitory neurons in the VTA. This leads to an increase in withdrawal behavior and the avoidance of a particular stimulus. Additionally, a negative event, punishment, or reward withdrawal causes the dopamine-releasing cells in the VTA to be inhibited, resulting in the suppression of motor behavior (cf. Roth and Strüber 2021, 118 f.).

4) **Dopamine and the Influence of Genes and Experiences**

Genetic makeup and experiences can influence the individual functioning of the dopaminergic system and thus determine personality traits. A specific variant of the gene for the dopamine D_4 receptor, for example, is associated with the trait of openness and tendencies to be curious, imaginative, artistic, perceptive, and intellectual. This also applies to a specific variant of the gene Catechol-O-Methyltransferase (COMT), which is a protein involved in dopamine degradation (cf. Cicchetti et al. 2011a, 364). Gene variants of these and other components of the dopaminergic system have been associated with attention performance, violent, impulsive, or risky behavior, as well as sensation-seeking. In individuals with mental disorders such as ADHD (Attention Deficit Hyperactivity Disorder), specific gene variants of the dopaminergic system have also been found (cf. Roth and Strüber 2021, 119 f.). It is now also recognized that early experiences can sustainably influence the function of the dopamine system. Stress experiences, particularly during perinatal development (the perinatal period ranges from the 28th week of pregnancy to the 7th day of life), seem to be of relevance. These include physical, physiological, and toxicological stressors. These lead to increased cortisol release, which in turn shapes the dopamine system. Based on this, early experiences can influence traits such as impulsivity. Both over- and under-functioning of the dopamine system have been observed in connection with early experiences (cf. Gatzke-Kopp 2011, 794). Depending on whether over- or under-functioning prevails, this has various effects on the individual's behavior (cf. Roth and Strüber 2021, 121). In rodents, it has been found that if the animals are frequently or repeatedly separated from their mother or exposed to periods of social isolation before weaning, it leads to reduced dopamine function in the medial prefrontal cortex. Behaviorally, this results in reduced impulse control and a diminished response to rewards (cf. Braun et al. 2000, cited in Roth and Strüber 2021, 121). In general, it can be said that the influence of various genetic variants for the dopamine receptor shows the relevance of gene-environment interaction. Children, for example, who are equipped with a specific gene variant of the dopamine D_4receptor, react particularly sensitively to the mother's sensitivity. This means that if a mother is not very sensitive in dealing with this child at the age of 10 months, the child will tend to exhibit oppositional and aggressive behavior at the age of 3 years (cf. Bakermans-Kranenburg and van Ijzendoorn 2006, 406). However, if the mother is particularly sensitive, these children show particularly peaceful behavior. Children with a different gene variant do not react to the mother's sensitivity to the same extent (cf. Roth and Strüber 2021, 121 f.). These findings are also highlighted by Jay Belsky's differential susceptibility hypothesis (1997). Belsky notes that the connection between genetically determined variation and environmental influences must be included in the explanation of externalizing behavior in children (cf. Belsky 1997, 182). According to Belsky's hypothesis, some children, due to their genetic makeup or temperament, react more sensitively to certain positive and negative environmental influences than others. These children benefit more from a positive environment than others. However, these children are also more frequently negatively affected by difficult early life conditions (cf. Roth and Strüber 2021, 121).

After already showing in this section to what extent aggressive behavior can be related to hormones, the following will now delve deeper into the topic of aggression in connection with hormones.

2.5.4 Hormones and Aggressive Behavior

First, the term aggression will be defined, because even though aggression is a common term, especially in psychological and educational contexts or in psychosocial fields of action, there are nevertheless various forms of aggression, which makes a difference, particularly with endocrine influences.

To define aggression, Selg first notes that aggression describes behavior and does not represent a motive. Aggression does not mean an aggression-affine affect, such as anger, rage, or hatred. It is also significant that accidental harm is not considered aggression. Vandalism, on the other hand, is considered aggression (cf. Selg 2000, n.p.).

> "Aggressiveness can be understood as the relatively enduring readiness of a person (or animal) to engage in aggressive behavior" (ibid.).

Already from this definition of aggression, it can be concluded that there are probably various types or intentions of aggression, and it is important to classify them. Before I explain the hormonal connections with aggression in this section, the types of aggression will be listed. Subsequently, relevant hormones will be explained, neurobiological as well as relevant neurochemical connections will be presented, and the connection of aggression with genetics will be shown.

2.5.4.1 Classification of Aggression

Here, a brief overview of the different forms of aggression is given.

Selg notes that with the term aggression, there is not merely "the" aggression or "the" aggressiveness, but it is important to differentiate between various forms. For example, it is important to distinguish between direct and indirect aggression, where slander can be cited as an example of indirect aggression. There is also individual and group aggression, where war can be cited as an example of group aggression, as well as self- and other-directed aggression, which can be counted among the external-formal categories. Motivationally, it is necessary to separate positive and negative aggressions. Here, for example, hostile, affect-accompanied (expressive), and instrumental aggressions can be mentioned, where it is about success or gain and the suffering of the victim is accepted. Above all, it is especially important to distinguish serious from playful aggression, particularly in children (cf. Segl 2000, n.p.).

Birbaumer and Schmidt point out that, in addition to anger and overt aggression, several diverse categories of antagonistic forms of aggression are distinguished (cf. Birbaumer and Schmidt 2018, 739):

Forms of Aggression	Explanation/Description
Predatory aggression	Triggered by hunger and by stimuli from the prey
Inter-male aggression	e.g., jealousy among men, often triggered by androgens
Inter-female aggression	e.g., jealousy among women, androgens also detectable, reason e.g., territorial competition
Fear-induced aggression	Defensive reaction, after an attempt to flee
Maternal aggression	To protect the young, e.g., in territorial conflicts; sometimes also occurring in animals without young
Irritation aggression (reactive aggression)	Spontaneous and targeted, after frustration and pain
Sexual aggression	Triggered by mating stimuli (in male animals), function unclear
Instrumental aggression	Purpose-oriented, targeted, "cold-blooded"

(cf. Birbaumer and Schmidt 2018, 740)

Dietrich and Walter (1972) summarize aggression as a term for a behavior whose intention is to cause direct or indirect harm to another individual. Most often, this individual is a conspecific (cf. Dietrich and Walter 1972, 18). Based on the definitions and classifications presented, reactive (irritation) aggression and instrumental aggression can be considered the most significant categories (cf. Birbaumer and Schmidt 2018, 740). Reactive aggression is triggered by the withdrawal of positive stimuli (frustration) or by painful stimuli, whereas instrumental aggression can be triggered by many stimuli. However, all stimuli have in common that they promise positive reinforcement for aggression. Biting and teeth-clenching are considered common behavioral expressions of all categories of aggression. This can be seen as an innate elementary aggression reaction (cf. Birbaumer and Schmidt 2018, 740).

2.5.4.2 The Neurobiology of Aggressive Behavior

To understand the psychoneuroendocrinology of aggression, it is primarily important to present a neurobiological basis of aggressive behavior. This promotes the understanding of aggression in general, but especially the understanding of the importance of hormones in connection with aggression.

1) **Hypothalamus**

The hypothalamus has already been mentioned several times in this book. Perhaps you have also looked up the definition in the glossary again. It controls vegetative functions such as food and water intake, temperature and blood pressure, osmolarity, circadian rhythm, sleep, sexual, and reproductive behavior. The significant hormone oxytocin is secreted in the hypothalamus, and it triggers ovulation and puberty. Thus, it is considered the highest regulatory center and is responsible for vital body functions, which are regulated by various hormones.

The extent to which the hypothalamus is associated with aggression is explained as follows.

> "The lateral-medial hypothalamus acts as a coordinating pattern structure for reactive aggressive behavior. It is primarily modulated by limbic structures (amygdala, hippocampus, 'limbic' anterior thalamus) and controls the sensorimotor expression of aggression in deeper brain structures" (cf. Birbaumer and Schmidt 2018, 741).

A precise localization of aggressive behavior in one or more brain structures is not possible based on the heterogeneity of aggressive behavior. However, similar to other emotions, some nodes of neural connections can be outlined here as well. These nodes can show that aggressive behavior is to be seen as hierarchically organized (cf. ibid., 740 f.).

The lateral and medial hypothalamus play a central role as an integrating structure for aggressive behavior. Animal experiments have shown that stimulation of the lateral hypothalamus leads to predatory aggression. In contrast, stimulation of the medial hypothalamus causes affective aggression. Stimulation of the dorsal hypothalamus leads to flight. If obstacles are present, this subsequently leads to fear aggression. Thus, the hypothalamus contains a pattern structure that can be seen as a kind of tendency, which, when activated (by environmental stimuli), can lead to the occurrence of aggressive behavior (cf. Birbaumer and Schmidt 2018, 741).

2) **Amygdala**

The amygdala is an almond-shaped region located in the middle of the brain in front of the hippocampus. It is connected to various brain regions that are associated with sensory and physiological or behavioral processes. The amygdala is associated with both positive and negative emotion regulation. It is also of central importance for memory and learning processes (cf. Choleris et al. 2020, n.p.).

The extent to which the amygdala is now associated with aggression is explained below.

> "The basolateral (excitatory) and medial (inhibitory) nuclei of the amygdala are responsible not only for fear behavior but also for dominance-maintaining aggression. Fear and aggression areas overlap" (Birbaumer and Schmidt 2018, 742).

In humans, the function of the amygdala for aggressive behavior is particularly shaped by its contribution to classical fear conditioning in socialization. If a person does not learn adequate anticipatory fear, aggression tendencies cannot be inhibited. This is visible, for example, in criminal psychopaths. Punitive and inconsistent upbringing leads to poor development of the amygdala, which in turn leads to low activatability of the amygdala. This, in turn, brings a higher risk of combat behavior (antagonistic behavior) and psychopathy (cf. ibid.).

3) **Medial and lateral orbital prefrontal cortex**

The prefrontal cortex is part of the neocortex. It is located in the anterior cortical part of the frontal lobe. The prefrontal cortex includes: the lateral prefrontal cortex, the medial prefrontal cortex, and the orbitofrontal prefrontal cortex. It has, among other things, reciprocal connections with other cortical and subcortical areas such as the temporal lobe, thalamus, and hypothalamus. There are also connections with the brainstem and limbic areas such as the amygdala. Its function implements higher cognitive processes, taking into account the individual's emotional state. It is of enormous importance for human personality. Therefore, damage to the prefrontal cortex results less in a reduction of intelligence than in a change in personality (cf. Spektrum Lexikon der Neurowissenschaft 2000c, n.p.). It is also responsible for the following emotions:

> "The medial prefrontal cortex is activated during feelings of guilt and empathy, while the lateral orbitofrontal cortex responds to violations of expectations with inhibition or activation of aggression in the subcortical aggression system" (Birbaumer and Schmidt 2018, 743).

Impairments of these two brain areas often lead to an increase in the likelihood of both reactive and instrumental aggression, with the lateral orbitofrontal cortex appearing to be capable of both inhibition and disinhibition. Depending on whether expected reward or punishment (such as frustration) occurs or does not occur, aggression is stimulated (reward expectation violated) or aggression is inhibited (reward received). The medial prefrontal cortex is responsible for the activation of feelings of guilt. However, this results from the ability to empathize with other people. Therefore, the medial prefrontal cortex must not be impaired in order to feel empathy. For example, people with high psychopathy scores show no medial-frontal activation at all (cf. ibid., 742).

4) **Summary**

In summary, it should be noted that anatomically, the amygdala, prefrontal and orbital frontal cortex, as well as the rostral and superior temporal cortex, are responsible for social behavior and regulate and modulate it (cf. Birbaumer and Schmidt 2018, 743). Aggressive behavior has various functions in the social context and is primarily learned. However, in addition to environmental stimuli, such as a male competitor, there is also a lowering of intra-organismic thresholds for those stimuli. This occurs particularly in the nuclei of the medial hypothalamus (cf. ibid., 147 f.), which "serves as the highest coordination structure for aggressive behavior" (Birbaumer and Schmidt 2018, 148). Thus, there are various forms of aggression, which in turn correlate with various neurophysiological processes. Since physical aggression has largely lost its function in our society, predatory, warlike, and criminal aggression, as it particularly occurs in young men, is of particular importance here (cf. ibid.). "The lowering of the threshold for predatory aggression takes place in the medial hypothalamus" (Birbaumer and Schmidt 2018, 148). The following will illustrate the connection between aggression and hormones.

2.5.4.3 Aggression and Sex Hormones

Now that aggression has been defined and classified, the relationship between both male and female sex hormones and aggression will be discussed here. Sex hormones not only coordinate our sexual behavior, as is often assumed, but they also modulate both cognitive and emotional processes. For example, gender-specific violent behavior is often associated with testosterone (cf. Hausmann and Jordan 2010, 118).

> "Sex hormones influence neuronal processes on the one hand through binding to intracellular receptors, which modulate gene expression as transcription factors. On the other hand, they can modulate the activity of ligand-gated ion channels through rapid non-genomic mechanisms" (ibid.).

The effects that sex hormones have on aggressive behavior or the extent to which they promote aggressive behavior will be outlined below.

1) **Testosterone and Aggression**

Since testosterone, like other steroid hormones, crosses the blood-brain barrier and there are numerous androgen receptors in the CNS, numerous effects of testosterone on the psyche have been described in both men and women. In particular, aggressiveness has been associated with elevated testosterone levels in the past (cf. Berner et al. 2010, 43). This relationship will be discussed below.

> "The relationship between testosterone production and aggression is only weakly positive in adults" (Birbaumer and Schmidt 2018, 148).

Both testosterone and estrogens occur in the central nervous system only as neuromodulators. However, they can cross the blood-brain barrier and thus bind to the appropriate receptors in various brain regions (cf. ibid.).

Estrogen and testosterone receptors are widespread and reach their highest concentration particularly in the hypothalamus and limbic system (cf. Birbaumer and Schmidt 2018, 148). This system, also referred to as the "paracrine heart of the neuroaxis" (paracrine because it is not a purely endocrine system), centrally intervenes in the control of behaviors necessary for the survival of the species. This means it controls homeostatic and non-homeostatic drives, fight-flight behavior, the increase in excitability of motoneurons, bonding, reproduction, territoriality, and antagonistic (aggressive) behavior. These are all essential brain systems that cluster in and around the hypothalamus and use male and female sex hormones as neuromodulators (cf. ibid., 686). However, age also plays a role in aggressive behavior, as the majority of violent acts are committed by young men who have particularly high testosterone production. Examples of castration also show that testosterone is associated with antisocial behavior in adults, as blocking testosterone secretion leads to a significant reduction in physically aggressive behavior. However, it remains unclear to what extent this is also due to the dampened mood and lethargy after castration (cf. Birbaumer and Schmidt 2018, 148).

> "Reversible and irreversible castration lowers the likelihood of aggressive acts. However, the effect depends on many factors and cannot be attributed solely to androgen inhibition" (ibid., 744).

However, it is undisputed that a minimal level of testosterone must be present both before and after birth for aggressive behavior to occur at all (cf. Birbaumer and Schmidt 2018, 148).

2) **Estrogen and Aggression**

Time and again, estrogen levels in women are associated with fluctuations in psychological well-being, such as during the menstrual cycle, pregnancy, postpartum period, and perimenopause. Additionally, basic research has shown that estrogens have neuro- and psychoprotective properties. Clinically, there is evidence of antipsychotic effects, stress-protective effects, improvement in cognitive functions, improvement in affective symptoms, and a reduction in aggressive and suicidal behavior (cf. Riecher-Rössler 2011, 152). The following will illustrate the relationship between estrogens and aggressive behavior. "Estrogens inhibit aggression when present in the hypothalamus" (Birbaumer and Schmidt 2018, 744). Female aggression is significantly rarer. In certain animal species with high testosterone levels, such as some hyena species, increased aggression also occurs. However, it should be noted that female organisms with elevated testosterone levels are generally physically superior. Successful aggression increases androgen levels in both humans and mammals. This means that in humans, sustained social dominance increases androgen production. Administering female sex hormones, particularly estradiol, to animals inhibits aggression. This is independent of whether the estradiol is administered directly into the hypothalamus or into the bloodstream. However, this is not sufficiently researched in humans (cf. ibid., 148).

3) **Prenatal Androgens and Aggression**

Androgens are male sex hormones that belong to the steroids. The most significant hormone of the androgens is testosterone. Biosynthesis occurs in the testes (Leydig cells) and the adrenal cortex. Androgen or testosterone production is controlled by the pituitary gland, which causes the development of male sex organs and secondary sexual characteristics. Additionally, the "psychological" gender is shaped by central nervous testosterone receptors (cf. Spektrum Lexikon der Neurowissenschaft 2000d, n.p.). Bahner wrote as early as 1974:

> "Androgens have the greatest influence on a man's health, behavior, and well-being. Disorders of androgen secretion cause profound changes in numerous organs, many functions, but above all in the personality of the man" (Bahner 1974, 187).

The circulation of androgens during pregnancy undoubtedly affects human behavior. This is particularly true for sexual orientation, but it is not confirmed for aggressive reactions. However, it has been found that androgens have various influences on the brain and behavior depending on the timing of pregnancy (cf. Birbaumer and Schmidt 2018, 148). In general, it should be noted that the relationship between androgens and the various forms of aggression is complex (cf. ibid., 744).

> "Without sufficient prenatal androgen effects on the brain, the testosterone increasingly secreted during puberty loses its aggression-promoting effect" (Birbaumer and Schmidt 2018, 744).

Without the presence of androgens in the fetus and immediately after birth, the neural connections necessary for aggressive behavior do not develop. If androgens have acted on the brain prenatally in sufficient quantities, they unfold their aggression-promoting effect from puberty onwards. In aggressively bred mice, it was observed that they are less anxious, learn faster, are more sympathetically activated, and have increased adrenal cortex adrenaline secretion. This is also true for female mice. This means they also possess autosomal genes for aggression, which become active when androgens are administered. However, it is particularly interesting that after social isolation, when the animals interact socially again and form social bonds, the genetically induced variation almost completely disappears (cf. Birbaumer and Schmidt 2018, 744).

2.5.4.4 Neurochemistry and Aggression

Since the influence of sex hormones on aggressive behavior was explained in Chap. 1, further substances that are associated with aggressiveness are presented here. The following explains which chemical processes in connection with active hormones in the nervous system influence aggressive behavior.

1) **Serotonin and Aggression**

The neurotransmitter serotonin (5-HT) has been associated with aggression in both animals and humans. The focus here is particularly on the modulation of aggression. Various states of aggression are regulated differently by the 5-HT system, and various 5-HT receptors also seem to be involved (cf. Olivier 2010, 382).

> "Reduction of synaptic activation for serotonin and reduction of serotonin reuptake into the presynaptic terminal in the aggression systems increases the risk of impulsive, aggressive, and suicidal behavior" (Birbaumer and Schmidt 2018, 743).

Serotonin influences both aggressive and suicidal behavior in humans. An increase in 5-HT receptor binding sites, for example, reduces aggression, while a decrease increases aggressiveness. This decrease in 5-HT binding sites in the brain leads to reactive aggressiveness and suicidality. It appears that 5-HT receptor activation contributes to increased impulsivity. The 5-serotonin transport molecule (SERT) is a good predictor of aggressive behavior (cf. ibid.). "Both together, SERT decrease and low serotonin receptor binding, predict violent suicidal behavior" (Birbaumer and Schmidt 2018, 743). Roth and Strüber (2021) note that lower serotonergic activity is associated with increased impulsive-aggressive behavior, suggesting that serotonin would inhibit aggression. However, it is temporarily suspected that serotonin only counteracts aggression, hostility, and quarrelsomeness when there is a personal tendency towards aggressive behavior. Serotonin does not minimize aggression here but impulsivity (cf. Roth and Strüber 2021, 125), "(…) i.e., the willingness to express latently present aggressive tendencies" (ibid.). If the serotonin level is low, the individual reacts with impulsive aggression. Impulsivity here does not only refer to aggressive behavior but can also be described as a tendency towards unplanned, rapid reactions. Possible consequences are not considered (cf. Roth and Strüber 2021, 125).

2) **Gamma-Aminobutyric Acid (GABA) and Aggression**

GABA is a significant inhibitory neurotransmitter in the central nervous system. The inhibitory effect of GABA is exerted on specific GABA receptors. These are classified into $GABA_A$, $GABA_B$, and $GABA_C$ receptors. About 30% of the synapses in the brain are controlled by GABA, which is why it is used, for example, in the treatment of epilepsy. For pharmacology, the $GABA_A$ receptor is particularly important (cf. Spektrum Lexikon der Neurowissenschaft 2000e, n.p.).

> "$GABA_A$ activation in the orbitofrontal cortex and amygdala lowers the threshold for aggressive acts. Alcohol and diazepam are the most common causes of increased risk of antisocial acts" (Birbaumer and Schmidt 2018, 744).

All substances that bind to the $GABA_A$receptor lead to a lower threshold for instrumental and reactive aggression. These are substances such as alcohol, benzodiazepines (Valium), but also blood pressure-lowering substances such as propranolol. A combination lowers the threshold even further. After alcohol consumption and diazepam, those affected can no longer recognize angry, aggressive, or sad faces, which in turn lowers the threshold for aggressive behavior. This effect is even more pronounced in psychopaths. Alcohol and diazepam lead to a reduction in NA activation in the amygdala. However, NA activation in the amygdala is a prerequisite for anticipating and retaining fear-relevant stimuli, which is a prerequisite for overall socialization. Thus, it can be noted that alcohol and benzodiazepines promote aggression via the orbitofrontal cortex and the amygdala (cf. Birbaumer and Schmidt 2018, 743 f.). DeBold, Miczek, Tornatzky, and van Erp also note the connection between benzodiazepines, alcohol, and $GABA_A$ receptors and explain the aggression-promoting effect. They note that this pharmacological modulation of the $GABA_A$ receptor with benzodiazepine agonists and neuroactive steroids leads to a dose-dependent biphasic change in aggressive behavior. In addition, experiments with rats that had already shown aggressive behavior under alcohol provocation showed that they self-administered alcohol before further social confrontations (cf. DeBold et al. 2002, 139).

After discussing hormones, neurochemistry, and neurobiology of aggression, the following will also discuss the connection between genetics and aggression and show to what extent genetics influence endocrine aggression-promoting substances.

2.5.4.5 Genetics of Aggression

The question of what roots aggression and violence have has been controversially discussed for a long time, particularly the approach of whether genetics or environmental factors represent the more decisive foundation. For example, if both the father and the son are imprisoned for violent crimes, the public occasionally speculates about an "aggression gene." To address the question of the respective effectiveness of genetic and environmental factors, a complex study design is required. Twin studies, in particular, are used here (cf. Wahl 2010, 92).

> "In humans, aggressive, antisocial behaviors are primarily environmentally determined. However, genetically determined risk factors, especially a reduced central serotonin level, have been identified" (Birbaumer and Schmidt 2018, 740).

As mentioned in previous sections, aggressive behavior is primarily learned behavior and not a homeostatic drive. The likelihood of occurrence depends, among other things, on constitutional-hormonal conditions. The exact extent to which aggressive behavior is inherited in humans is not known, but twin studies show that there is only a small hereditary component. However, a defective gene on the X chromosome was found in a group of 14 extremely aggressive men. They had a reduced amount of monoamine oxidase A, which in turn indicates a lack of serotonin in the brain. This supports the hypothesis that serotonin is involved in the inhibition of aggressive behavior. Furthermore, it has already been shown how prenatal and postnatal androgen levels influence brain development, which is largely genetically determined (cf. Birbaumer and Schmidt 2018, 740).

In summary, it can be stated that aggression is influenced by many factors. These include endocrine influences as well as genetic, neurobiological, and chemical substances, as well as psychosocial environmental factors. Primarily, however, aggressive behavior is learned, and even in genetically manipulated aggressive mice, this behavior disappears through social interactions and social bonds.

2.6 Stress and Helplessness

Stress is a well-known word that is often heard, both in scientific and private contexts. To explain what stress does to the human organism and to an individual, it is first necessary to clarify what stress actually is. Before I delve into diseases and current studies on the topic of stress, the question will be addressed: What is stress?

2.6.1 Definition and Explanation of Stress

The term "stress" (Latin: strictus: tight) is defined and explained differently in various disciplines, making a general definition of stress rather difficult. The term itself was adopted from English and means pressure, strain, and tension in a technical-physical context (cf. Busse et al. 2006, 3). Ehlert (2011) notes that the word stress is often misused because when environmental demands lead to an individual being burdened and therefore stressed, the wrong term is used according to her explanations. Here, an attempt is made to explain how an individual reacts to the mentioned demand. It is initially about the difference between what triggers stress, i.e., what is the stressor, and what is the stress response. Even if the term is often used incorrectly here, it is still ubiquitous and often heard in everyday use (cf. Ehlert 2011, 33). Busse, Plaumann, and Walter (2006) note here that in everyday life, the term stress is predominantly associated with psychosocial stress. Situations are described that, for example, cause disturbances, irritations, and/or fear and lead to an impairment of both physical and psychological well-being (cf. Busse et al. 2006, 3).

> "The term stress implies a theoretical assumption about the mutual influence process of environmental conditions and personal prerequisites" (Ehlert 2011, 33).

As a result, every situation is analyzed and individually assessed by each individual to estimate the threat and the available coping strategies. This individual assessment process leads to automatic cognitions, assumptions, attitudes, and expectations, which in turn lead to physiological processes, emotions, and ultimately behavior. If the individual frequently experiences situations in which they feel overwhelmed due to a lack of or completely absent coping strategies, it can lead to maladjustments on both physiological and psychological levels. These, in turn, can lead to functional or manifest diseases and disorders (cf. ibid.). Stress can be seen as a so-called psychogenic immunosuppressor, making stress a significant topic, especially in psychoneuroimmunology.

> "Even the pre-Socratics and later Hippocrates saw the emergence of disease as a consequence of the loss of harmonious balance between the organism and the environment" (Birbaumer and Schmidt 2018, 150).

The concept of general equilibrium is replaced in the 20th century by Walter Cannon (1871–1945) with the term homeostasis. Hans Seyle (1907–1982) developed the concept of stress, and both saw stress as a (cf. ibid.) "nonspecific response of the organism to the disturbance of homeostatic balance and as an attempt to restore this balance" (Birbaumer and Schmidt 2018, 150).

However, subjectivity is also significant here.

> "As early as Mason (1968) it was pointed out that situations subjectively experienced as significant, novel, unpredictable, and uncontrollable act as particularly intense stressors, which, in addition to the experience of psychological stress, are associated with a marked activation of endocrine systems" (Mason 1968, quoted in Ehlert 2011, 34).

Since the stress reactions to various stimuli were similar, Seyle spoke of a general adaptation syndrome. He emphasized that the subjectively experienced stress determines whether there is a disturbance of body homeostasis and disease, or whether adaptation occurs. Seyle divided the stress reaction into three phases: alarm, resistance, and exhaustion. Since the exhaustion phase, which is accompanied by the depletion of hormones and changes in receptors, occurs rather rarely, today we distinguish more between short-term and long-term effects of stress or strain. Pathophysiological consequences thus occur after prolonged, chronic stressors and stressors that recur too frequently, as well as without physiological necessity (for example, when there is no possibility of escape) as with psychological-social stressors. In summary, it should be noted here that stress only leads to disturbances of homeostatic bodily processes after a longer period. Furthermore, the stress adaptation syndrome, previously considered general, is dependent on the context, the stress stimuli, and the coping behaviors (cf. Birbaumer and Schmidt 2018, 150).

Furthermore, it should be noted that there are various perspectives on stress:

Biological Perspective:

- Physical reactions are the focus of this perspective.
- The physical or psychological homeostasis (balance) is examined.

Sociological Perspective:
- It deals with deviations from subjective set points.
- Psychological motives and needs (e.g., recognition, security, contact, and self-actualization) are examined.
- The focus is on stressors (strains) where certain stress reactions require different coping strategies.

Psychological Perspective:
- It particularly considers the emotional and cognitive processing of stress.
- The effect on the intensity and quality of stress reactions is examined.
- Subjective perception, interpretation, and evaluation are crucial.

Salutogenetic Perspective:
- It deals with (health-related) protective factors that the individual can draw on in stressful situations.
- Coping with the stressful situation depends on individual and external resources (cf. Busse et al. 2006, 4).

2.6.2 Short-term and Long-term Stress

Before addressing stress management, the difference between short-term and long-term stress as well as the role of the HPA axis is first explained. Natural stressors can be divided into low and high stress depending on individual resilience and, in terms of the duration of the stress, into acute or chronic. Short-term natural stressors differ from long-lasting stress conditions mainly in the intensity of the stress. Short-term natural stressors include, for example, "daily hassles" such as missing the tram, individually important events such as failing an exam, but also traumas such as a car accident, rape, war experiences, and surviving an avalanche. However, Ehlert notes here that trauma can only be spoken of if there is a feeling of life threat to oneself or others, as well as helplessness, intense fear, and horror (cf. Ehlert 2011, 34). In short-term coping, the organism activates the hypothalamic-pituitary-adrenal axis (HPA axis). A rapid, energy-mobilizing stress response and the inhibition of long-term energy storage are necessary. The activation of the HPA axis occurs within minutes, while the activation of the sympathetic nervous system and catecholamine secretion occurs within seconds. In addition, insulin secretion is inhibited, and glucose is made more available in the muscles. This leads to increased sugar levels under stress. Together with the cardiac sympathetic excitations, the efficiency of muscle work (especially for the fight-flight system) is optimized (cf. Birbaumer and Schmidt 2018, 150). Long-lasting stress conditions, on the other hand, with varying stress, can be, for example, an unsatisfactory job, neglect in childhood, impending unemployment, one's own chronic serious illness, or caring for a chronically ill relative (cf. Ehlert 2011, 34). In short-term stress, energy reserves are mobilized, whereas in long-term stress, energy reserves are suppressed. This is the case, for example, with sexual reproduction efficiency (through suppression of sex hormones) as well as with pain perception (stress analgesia) and long-term inflammatory processes, as they would only hinder short-term adaptation (cf. Birbaumer and Schmidt 2018, 150).

In summary, it should be noted here that stressors influence the homeostatic regulation of various hormone axes. This mainly leads to changes in the hypothalamic-pituitary-adrenal axis. Significant hormonal dysregulations can occur, for example, Ehlert (2011, 34) mentions:

> "(…) an increased or decreased basal hormone secretion, an altered feedback of peripheral hormones to the pituitary and hypothalamus, or a down-/up-regulation of hormone receptors" (ibid.).

The Hypothalamic-Pituitary-Adrenal System

Noradrenergic (NA), cholinergic (Ach), and serotonergic influences on the hypothalamus affect the release of corticotropin-releasing factor (CRF), which induces the release of ACTH from the anterior pituitary (AP). ACTH, in turn, stimulates the glucocorticoid release from the adrenal cortex. At the same time, it excites the inhibitory NA neurons of the hypothalamus. The glucocorticoids themselves inhibit the release of both CRF and ACTH and the activity of the adrenal cortex. Stress and helplessness stimulate CRF release, and circadian rhythms determine the fluctuations of the baseline hormone curve (cf. Birbaumer and Schmidt 2018, 151). The consequences of these stress-induced endocrine changes are associated with psychological maladjustments. This can manifest in vital exhaustion and burnout, functional somatic disorders, and psychiatric disorders, or even with comorbidity of physical illness (cf. Ehlert 2011, 34).

2.6.3 Stress Management ("coping")

First, the question arises as to what is actually understood by stress management ("coping"). According to Lazarus and Folkman (1984), stress management ("coping") is understood as a regulatory process triggered by the individual after he/she has assessed a situation as stress-relevant. The person subsequently mobilizes coping efforts, which are part of an appraisal-action chain. This is embedded in the overall dynamics of the stress process and attempts to fulfill an adequate function between environmental conditions and personal characteristics. This can either mean an adaptation of the stressor (assimilation) or a change in environmental conditions (accommodation). How effective the coping attempt is, is excluded by Lazarus and Folkman, as it does not depend on success whether it is understood as coping or not (cf. Bodenmann and Milek 2018, 560). Ehlert (2011) notes that there are definitely factors that protect the individual from permanent psychobiological maladjustments. Here, for example, social support or a pronounced optimism and sense of coherence are mentioned. They seem to have stress-reducing effects in situations of psychological stress (cf. Ehlert 2011, 33 f.). As already mentioned, the effect of stressors, or how they affect the individual's nervous system and hormones, depends on subjective-psychological conditions and primarily on the availability of adequate coping behavior. How people respond to various stress stimuli depends on various factors that interact with each other (cf. Birbaumer and Schmidt 2018, 149). Birbaumer and Schmidt (2018) summarize these as follows:

- "objective, physical intensity of the aversive stimuli,
- subjective-psychological intensity of the aversive stimuli (appraisal and attribution of cause),
- possibility of avoidance and coping ("coping") with the stimulus situation,
- previous experience with stress (immunization versus "being overwhelmed"), the learning history of a person (e.g., early neglect, abuse),
- duration and frequency of stress stimuli,
- constitutional psychological and physiological factors ("stress sensitivity", personality),
- tonic baseline (activation) state of the organism before and during stress stimuli (including circadian and ultradian and other periodicities and sleep stages),
- social support and bonding ("social support"),
- motor "discharge possibilities" (e.g., regular, non-competitive sports)" (Birbaumer and Schmidt 2018, 149).

This enumeration clearly shows that the subjective appraisal of the CNS is the decisive parameter for the dimension of the stress reaction. An objective measurement is therefore not possible without capturing the individual central nervous causal factors (cf. ibid.). To promote individual stress management, there are a variety of preventive stress programs or trainings, for which, however, there is usually no empirical evidence of effectiveness. For example, the "Stress Inoculation Training" (SIT) by Meichenbaum (2003) is considered scientifically sound and empirically evaluated. SIT is suitable both therapeutically and preventively, but even Meichenbaum points out that the instructional phase alone hardly achieves positive effects, but successes only occur when individuals practice and actively train an adequate handling of stress in everyday life (cf. Bodenmann and Milek 2018, 562).

2.6.4 Attempts at Stress Management: Successful or Unsuccessful

Stressors occur in all people, even if the intensity and frequency of stress or even trauma diverge. However, there are large interindividual divergences in stress management strategies between healthy clients and various groups of clients with mental disorders. Based on the psychoendocrinological perspective, most subjective stress is processed through homeostatic regulation. This means that following a stressor, there is an activation of the physiological system, which is counter-regulated as a result of stress processing. As a result, this physiological system also returns to baseline (cf. Ehlert 2011, 34 f.). How the body responds to recurring stress situations depends, among other things, on the results of coping attempts. This has been researched using parachutists, fears and depression, and noise in the workplace (cf. Birbaumer and Schmidt 2018, 150).

> "During the first confrontations with the negative event, there is a significant increase in pituitary-adrenal cortex and adrenal medulla activity (…), as well as corresponding peripheral-autonomic physiological processes. Heart rate, skin resistance, blood pressure, muscle activity, peripheral glucocorticoids, peripheral adrenaline, noradrenaline, growth hormone, endorphins, and ACTH increase, (the) skin resistance decreases, testosterone and insulin are inhibited" (Birbaumer and Schmidt 2018, 150).

With increasing experience or increasingly successful coping behavior (for example, experienced parachutist), the intensity of activation during the stress event changes. The intensity decreases and subjectively shifts to positive areas, leading to "joy in danger," which in turn is associated with an increase in testosterone (cf. ibid., 150 f.). What if the coping attempt or coping behavior was not successful? If, for example, the level of stress is too high and/or the duration of the stress is too long, the various physiological systems regulate themselves to counteract the overload. This means that, in the case of a high hormone release, there is a significant down-regulation of the associated receptors. Conversely, if there is a hormone deficiency, the receptors are "up-regulated" (cf. Ehlert 2011, 35). However, if the stress persists or new avoidance attempts occur, some autonomic and hormonal reactions remain elevated even during rest periods. This results in, for example, immunosuppression (reduced T-lymphocyte cell activity) as well as organ damage (often due to persistent corticosteroid activity) and a number of other diseases, which were previously also referred to as psychosomatic (cf. Birbaumer and Schmidt 2018, 151). From a psychosomatic perspective, people who suffer from psychosomatic disorders are often considered difficult patients because they have nothing to say about the social and psychological backgrounds of their disorder, as these patients often seem to have marginal access to their emotions and find it difficult to build a connection to their emotional states and life circumstances. This phenomenon is also found in depressive patients, anxiety patients, or family members who do not understand why the daughter suffers from anorexia. Nevertheless, there are also psychosomatic patients who can very well perceive and describe their emotions. These often suffer from disorders that occur situation-specifically or disorders that developed immediately after a specific life event. So, when do problems in perceiving the psychological and psychosocial backgrounds develop? These difficulties arise particularly when the disorder or symptoms develop slowly and are based on long-standing life events and attitudes. The symptoms develop as a result of prolonged overload and chronic stress (cf. Meiss 2009, 548). What happens now from a psychoneuroendocrinological perspective as a result of an unsuccessful stress coping attempt? Here, it is first relevant to differentiate between active coping ("active coping") and passive coping ("passive coping") in coping attempts. Active coping ("active coping") is referred to when the (unsuccessful) coping attempt is more somatic-muscular oriented (fight-flight reaction). In this case, after punished or unsuccessful coping attempts, damage predominantly occurs in the cardiovascular system (affecting the heart and vascular system) and diseases in the muscle and support apparatus (such as chronic muscle pain). In passive coping ("passive coping"), coping is more through passivity and withdrawal; the organ damage is predominantly in the influence area of corticosteroids. These are the intestinal systems (meaning: affecting the intestines) and the immune system (for example, duodenal ulcers or asthma). In summary, this means that the consequences of stress depend on individual coping. Active coping with stress and direct confrontation with the stress leads to a reduced stress response. In the case of repeated punished or unsuccessful coping attempts, illness is the result (cf. Birbaumer and Schmidt 2018, 151). What happens now when the feeling of helplessness manifests? Learned helplessness is seen as a consequence of prolonged unsuccessful coping with stress. A so-called learned helplessness or learned uncontrollability arises. It should be noted that learned helplessness leads to motor as well as cognitive-associative disorders. This means that motor deficits such as immobility or movement stereotypes as well as associative deficits such as no avoidance learning for a certain period or performance decline in learning and concentration tasks can occur (cf. ibid., 149 f.).

> "The negative consequences of learned helplessness are strongest when previously successful avoidance behavior is suddenly punished, i.e., has negative consequences" (Birbaumer and Schmidt 2018, 150).

2.6.5 Stress and the Brain: From Homeostasis to Allostasis

The term homeostasis comes from the Greek "homoios" (= same) and "stasis" (steady state). Homeostasis describes a process that aims to ensure that the internal state remains constant. This can be, for example, the regulation of body temperature or water balance. Homeostasis is comparable to a thermostat that is connected to both an air conditioner and a heater. When the temperature rises, the air conditioner automatically turns on (cf. Fredrickson et al. 2007, 466 f.). Homeostasis is thus the tendency of an organism to maintain a balanced and constant internal state. This system compensates for ongoing changes in the external environment that could otherwise harm the internal state (cf. Chamary 2016, 136). These physiological adaptations of the organism can be understood as physiological efforts, which are associated with physiological costs, according to Ehlert. McEwen (1998) referred to these physiological costs as a shift in homeostasis, called "allostasis" ("allostatic load"). The severity of the allostatic load depends on many factors (cf. Ehlert 2011, 35). Birbaumer and Schmidt note that long-term stress without successful coping leads to the collapse of homeostatic counter-regulations. This, in turn, results in allostasis (Greek for imbalance) and disease (cf. Birbaumer and Schmidt 2018, 151). The extent of allostasis ("allostatic load") depends on many factors, such as the quality of the stressors themselves, as well as individual prior experiences, genetic predispositions, and the person's psychosocial stress-coping competence (cf. Ehlert 2011, 35). Additionally, the hypothalamic-pituitary-adrenal system is of relevance. As previously shown, the activity of the hypothalamic-pituitary-adrenal system is determined by the frequency, duration, and intensity of stress stimuli, as well as by subjective evaluation (attribution) and individual coping behavior. Like Ehlert, Birbaumer and Schmidt also mention the importance of the person's genetic vulnerability and the cognitive experiences already encountered with stress. Moreover, the circadian periodicity influences the effects. The focus in this complex interplay is the brain. In the brain, the hypothalamic CRF system acts anxiogenic, immunosuppressive, and excitatory. As a negative feedback stimulus, glucocorticoids cause the limitation and counter-regulation of the hyperactivity of this system, although this counter-regulation system fails during prolonged or repeated stress. This failure, however, is caused by learning processes. The disruption of homeostasis, also referred to as allostasis, and the long-term consequences of stress and the transition to disease are also called allostatic load. Memory, sleep, stress evaluation, and stress coping are intertwined in the brain, which is evident in their hormonal commonalities. The processes behind these behavioral categories determine whether the organism becomes ill or not (cf. Birbaumer and Schmidt 2018, 151). The interplay of environmental demands and individual competencies in coping with stress and trauma is thus complex, and there is evidence that various physiological systems are involved in these adaptations (cf. Ehlert 2011, 35).

2.6.6 Stress and Neurochemical Imbalance

The temporary assumptions are that

> "(…) the relative balance of catecholaminergic and serotonergic stimulation, which determines CRH production, decides whether hypothalamic-pituitary-adrenal axis activity habituates (gets used to) or sensitizes (escalates) with repeated stress" (Birbaumer and Schmidt 2018, 153).

The decline in CRH stimulation and the stress response, as observed in extreme social stress and status loss, leads to apathy. If the serotonin system is also depleted, it can lead to excessive violence and/or suicide. The balance of catecholaminergic and serotonergic influence on CRH production is important here, as it limits the sensitivity of the adrenal cortex axis to repeated stress (cf. Birbaumer and Schmidt 2018, 153 f.).

2.6.7 Stress, Norepinephrine, Cell Loss, and PTSD

Stress that cannot be controlled prolongs peripheral and central catecholamine synthesis. With repeated and prolonged stress, tyrosine (the precursor of catecholamines) is increasingly produced in the nuclei of the sympathetic nervous system and in the locus coeruleus. This increases selective attention to stress stimuli on the one hand and excitability in the hippocampus on the other (cf. Birbaumer and Schmidt 2018, 151 f.). This leads to the "(…) implicit imprinting of emotional stimuli" (ibid., 152) being enhanced. The same happens in the amygdala. The increased avoidance tendency (whereby traumatic situations are better imprinted) generates anxiety, symptoms of depression, and post-traumatic stress disorder (PTSD). Animal experiments have shown that after extreme and prolonged stress, the end state is a depletion of norepinephrine stores in the brain. However, this was always preceded by an increase in norepinephrine production (cf. Birbaumer and Schmidt 2018, 152).

Noradrenaline (NA)

To better understand this, the following section will delve into noradrenaline in connection with psychoneuroendocrinology. Noradrenaline, like dopamine, is a catecholamine. NA is related to adrenaline but differs by the absence of a methyl group. The absence of this methyl group results in a different effect. Noradrenaline is synthesized from dopamine, specifically by dopamine-β-hydroxylase. It is released either as a hormone by the adrenal medulla into the blood or as a neuromodulator in the brain. Noradrenergic cells respond to novelty. This means they are activated as soon as an event appears relevant to the brain for temporary or future behavior. This occurs regardless of whether the event is perceived as positive or negative. In the target areas of noradrenergic neurons, such as the hippocampus and cortex, NA binds to various receptor types, and the signal-to-noise ratio is enhanced. This means it amplifies the activity of those cells involved in processing novel and significant stimuli and reduces the activity of nerve cells not involved in stimulus processing. Noradrenergic cells respond to the significant stimulus with what is known as phasic activation. Phasic activation promotes focused attention, allowing for an optimal response to the stimulus (cf. Roth and Strüber 2021, 130). However, this is only possible in a state of relaxed alertness and not in moments of stress or fatigue. This is because the phasic stimulus response can only be effective if the tonic baseline arousal is neither too low (fatigue) nor too high (stress). Additionally, other substances are involved. For example, corticotropin-releasing factor (CRF) increases tonic activity in stressful situations, putting the body on alert. When the stress or strain ends, endogenous opioids bind to their receptors in the locus coeruleus, shifting the activity pattern to low tonic activity and a relaxed baseline activity. Depending on the extent of NA release, NA binds to various receptor types, which can have contrasting effects on brain activity. Adequate NA release, without stress and strain, allows humans to map and maintain their behavioral goals in working memory. The individual does not feel threatened and can act flexibly and purposefully. However, if the situation is associated with stress, the high concentrations of NA bind to less sensitive receptors such as the alpha-1 receptor (cf. Roth and Strüber 2021, 130 f.). This stress-based shift in brain activity leads to a deactivation of the dorsolateral prefrontal cortex. In contrast, activity in the amygdala or striatum is increased (Arnsten et al. 2015, cited in Roth and Strüber 2021, 131 f.). This, in turn, means that the person can process the situation with less cognitive flexibility and their attention is rigidly focused on the stress stimulus. Additionally, the person falls back on habitual behavioral strategies, sometimes associated with a fight-or-flight response. Thoughts are shut down, which often leads to the proverbial "headless" behavior under excessive stress. The various activity patterns of noradrenergic cells can thus best adapt behavior to the temporary demands of the environment. How does the previously mentioned PTSD (post-traumatic stress disorder) develop? As already mentioned, NA promotes the storage of memories of frightening situations and is thus also involved in preparing for future dangers. However, in life-threatening events, based on massive impacts of NA on the amygdala, there can be an over-consolidation of traumatic memories or a long-lasting storage of memories in the brain, characteristic of PTSD (cf. Roth and Strüber 2021, 132). The end state, which results in the complete depletion of the NA store, also implies reversible or permanent atrophy with cell loss in the hippocampus. The same has been observed in the amygdala and prefrontal cortex in melancholic depression. In humans, this could be accompanied by amnesia (loss of explicit memory storage) and apathetic syndromes. Desensitization, also known as immunization, can also occur (cf. Birbaumer and Schmidt 2018, 152).

> "Desensitization (or also called immunization) of the organism through slow and increasingly intensive and repeated confrontation with stress stimuli and the possibility of coping limits the allostatic deviation of the adrenal-pituitary axis" (ibid.).

Birbaumer and Schmidt also mention the significant influence of genetics here. Because in connection with genetic vulnerability, extreme stress stimuli, due to noradrenaline release, can lead to increased emotional imprinting and cell loss in the hippocampus. This is referred to as post-traumatic stress disorder (PTSD) (cf. Birbaumer and Schmidt 2018, 152). As already mentioned, it is about the balance of catecholaminergic and serotonergic stimulation. After having described the catecholamine noradrenaline in detail, the following will discuss serotonin in this context. PTSD will be discussed in more detail in Sect. 2.7.

2.6.8 Stress, Serotonin, and Psychological Functions

Much has already been written in this book about the importance of serotonin and the relevance of the serotonin system. Here, once again, the enormous relevance of serotonin for our physical and mental health is presented.

Serotonin (5-hydroxytryptamine, 5-HT) is of great relevance for various physiological systems of our body, such as the gastrointestinal tract or the circulatory system. However, the serotonin formed there cannot cross the blood-brain barrier. To trigger effects in the brain, serotonin is produced in the raphe nuclei from the amino acid tryptophan, which is ingested with food. Felt, uncontrollable stress stimulates the activity of these cells, leading to increased serotonin secretion (cf. Roth and Strüber 2021, 122 f.). Within the serotonin system, activation can then lead to opposing effects. In the case of extreme and prolonged stressors, the serotonin of the dorsal raphe nucleus, by activating the so-called 5-HT_2 receptors, induces anxiety in the amygdala, neocortex, and hippocampus. However, if the serotonin of the median raphe nucleus stimulates the 5-HT_{1A} receptors in the hippocampus, this has a rather "therapeutic" effect on stress disorders. Previously learned emotional connections are dissolved, and forgetting is enabled (cf. Birbaumer and Schmidt 2018, 153).

1) **Serotonin and psychological functions**
It is important to note that serotonin influences a variety of psychological functions. Serotonin affects mood, emotions, sleep, memory, appetite, and temperature regulation. Above all, serotonin influences the emotions of anxiety and fear (cf. Roth and Strüber 2021, 123 f.).

> "Circulating glucocorticoids in chronic stress increase the 5-HT synthesis rate specifically for the 5-HT_2 system and inhibit the 5-HT_1 receptors, reinforcing the vicious cycle of anxiety/stress and improved imprinting of the stress situation" (Birbaumer and Schmidt 2018, 153).

This is the reason why one can never consider the total amount of serotonin, but primarily the synthesis rates of the receptors (cf. ibid.). The effects of serotonin secretion depend on which receptors are active in which brain region. Depending on the receptor type, anxiety is then either reduced or increased (cf. Holmes 2008, cited in Roth and Strüber 2021, 124). It is generally assumed that serotonin in the amygdala promotes anticipatory anxiety but inhibits a panic reaction. It is believed that serotonin is generally relevant for the inhibition of behavior. For example, reduced serotonergic transmission causes some people to have great difficulty adopting a waiting or passive attitude. In this respect, serotonin could be seen as a counterpart to dopamine (cf. Daw et al. 2002, cited in Roth and Strüber 2021, 125). If the serotonin system in the central nervous system is underactivated, this is associated with increased suicidality, hostility, as well as an increase in the risk of heart attack and violence (cf. Birbaumer and Schmidt 2018, 153). In stressful situations, however, it is important to be flexible and control the stress with an active coping strategy, such as a fight or flight reaction. In this situation, tonic dopamine secretion is then increased. However, if stressors are unavoidable or uncontrollable, it is sometimes better to react passively, like an animal that plays dead. A person is then "paralyzed with fear" or immobilized based on fear and/or pain. In situations like these, tonic dopamine secretion is reduced, and serotonin release is increased in many areas of the forebrain. This results in so-called behavioral inhibition (cf. Roth and Strüber 2021, 126).

2) **Serotonin and the influence of genes and experiences**
Diverse genetic variants have great relevance for the personal development of the serotonin system. The most well-known are various gene variants ("polymorphisms") for the serotonin transporter. The serotonin transporter removes serotonin from the synaptic cleft after its effect. Depending on how the gene is expressed, serotonin can act longer or shorter in the synaptic cleft (cf. Roth and Strüber 2021, 126). The S-allele, for example, leads to reduced serotonin reuptake and a prolonged effect of serotonin. The L-allele variant, on the other hand, is associated with a lower effect of serotonin in the synaptic cleft (cf. Canli and Lesch 2007, cited in Roth and Strüber 2021, 127). According to current studies, this polymorphism is relevant for personality development as well as the risk of developing mental disorders. The S-allele is thus associated with anxiety-related personality traits, an increased amygdala response to threatening stimuli, increased stress sensitivity, irritability, and a tendency to depression. However, it is discussed whether this is only the case if this genetic variant is accompanied by early or significant stress experiences, meaning only if a gene-environment interaction occurs. Polymorphisms of other components of the serotonin system can also affect and modulate the serotonergic influence on the psyche. The promoter region of the gene for the 5-HT_{1A} receptor, for example, can be present in various variants. This variant causes a tendency towards excessive anxiety and depression. But it is also important to mention here that not only individual genes modulate the development and function of the serotonin system, but also experiences. For example, early abused children who already suffer from depression show higher serotonergic activity than children who did not experience abuse. In adults, however, who experienced early abuse, serotonergic activity is reduced (cf. Roth and Strüber 2021, 127 f.). Whether early traumatic experiences promote the development of mental disorders or lead to a change in the serotonin system depends on the gene-environment interaction. Compared to the L/L genotype (one L-allele from the mother and one from the father), people with an S-variant of the gene are more likely to have depression and tendencies towards suicide if they were exposed to significant stress, such as experiencing abuse in the first decade of life (cf. Caspi et al. 2003, cited in Roth and Strüber 2021, 129). Similarly, the experience of a less sensitive mother can have more severe consequences for children with at least one S-allele than for children with the L/L genotype. Depending on which genotype one has, it influences whether and how certain experiences affect one. Prenatal influences are also important here. For example, if the mother has severe anxiety in the last trimester, children with 2 S-alleles are much more anxious and tend to depressive symptoms, whereas in children with the L/L genotype, under the same conditions, aggressive behavior is promoted (cf. Roth and Strüber 2021, 129). Also relevant for the development of behavioral disorders based on early experiences is a polymorphism of the gene for monoamine oxidase A (MAO-A). People with a certain variant of this enzyme, which is relevant for the breakdown and resynthesis of

serotonin, have an increased tendency to develop violent criminality or antisocial personality disorder in adulthood (cf. Caspi et al. 2002, 2006, cited in Roth and Strüber 2021, 129). Additionally, they show an increased amygdala response to emotional stimuli and a lower involvement of prefrontal regions. In serious criminals, this could explain the frequently found increased sense of threat, which then manifests in reactive violence (cf. Roth and Strüber 2021, 129 f.). Now that serotonin has also been examined from the psychoneuroendocrinological and genetic perspectives, it is still important to address endogenous opioids. When endogenous opioids are released, as well as the effects of genetic influences and experiences, will be explained in the following.

2.6.9 Stress, Endogenous Opioids, and the Influence on Emotions and Behavior

The following will illustrate the relationship between endogenous opioids, emotions, and behavior. It will be explained what effects endogenous opioids have in connection with stress on human behavior. Among other things, attachment and pain insensitivity will be discussed.

1) **Opioids and Stress Analgesia (Pain Insensitivity)**
As previously stated, neurotransmitters influence the activity of the ACTH-adrenal cortex system. The secreted ACTH stress hormone also functions as a precursor to the endogenous opioids β-endorphin, α-endorphin, γ-endorphin, and Met-enkephalin. This means that opioids are also released during stress, which in turn can lead to stress analgesia (insensitivity to pain). The reason for stress analgesia is the release of ACTH and β-endorphin during stress. Insensitivity to pain is observed in accident victims (cf. Birbaumer and Schmidt 2018, 154). The body's own opioids are neuropeptides that have an opiate-like effect. In the case of insensitivity to pain, the neurons in the spinal cord are active. Pain processing is impaired because the activation of the responsible brain centers is reduced, thereby directly reducing pain. However, this pain-inhibiting effect is not only focused on physical pain but also affects emotional pain, such as in cases of exclusion and social rejection (cf. Roth and Strüber 2021, 135). By binding to μ-receptors, opioids promote a person's sense of well-being in their social environment. Furthermore, studies show that looking at a photo of one's partner has a pain-relieving effect (cf. Hsu et al. 2013, cited in Roth and Strüber 2021, 135 f.).

2) **Opioids and the Reward System**
Additionally, opioids play a significant role in the reward system. Dopamine mediates the pursuit ("wanting") of reward, while endogenous opioids are responsible for the hedonic experience in the brain, i.e., the liking ("liking"). However, this only occurs when the corresponding receptors bind in "(…) specific areas of the nucleus accumbens or the ventral pallidum" (Roth and Strüber 2021, 136). In other areas of the nucleus

accumbens, opioids promote motive-driven behavior or the pursuit of rewards (cf. Berridge and Kringelbach 2013, cited in Roth and Strüber 2021, 136).

3) **Opioids and Social Interactions**

The μ-receptors in the nucleus accumbens are also involved in the rewarding effect of social interactions. For social interactions to appear attractive to the individual, these receptors are stimulated by, for example, β-endorphin. Personality disorders, social behavior disorders, autism, or schizophrenia seem to be based on a dysfunction of the μ-receptor. Additionally, sadness could also be related to a lower binding of opioids to μ-receptors. The basis of negative emotions thus seems to lie in a deactivation of the μ-opioid system. However, activation of these receptors can have positive emotional effects. When opioids bind to these receptors, they can dampen stressful stimuli. Fear in threatening situations, as well as anxiety reactions, such as in the separation of mother and child, can thus be suppressed (cf. Roth and Strüber 2021, 136). Jaak Panksepp developed the so-called "brain opioid theory of social attachment." This theory assumes that opioids are a significant basis for both the maintenance and formation of social bonds. When opioids are secreted in the context of social bonds, they can convey a rewarding effect of social belonging and the associated sense of well-being (cf. Nelson and Panksepp 1998, cited in Roth and Strüber 2021, 137). It is also assumed that, based on individual predispositions, low opioid secretion increases the need for social closeness, thereby motivating the individual to seek more social contacts, whereas high opioid activity can reduce social needs (cf. Roth and Strüber 2021, 137).

4) **Opioids and Bonding**

Opioids are also the basis for mammals preferring their own mother over other mothers. If an infant or toddler is separated from its mother for too long and cries or calls for her, the reunion of the two leads to a positive emotional state and increased "affiliative" behaviors such as vocal and physical caresses and clinging. Animal studies have shown that when the receptors were blocked, the animal sought comfort from another mother. However, the bonding-promoting effect is not limited to mother and child but also plays a significant role in partner bonding. This was demonstrated in monogamous voles. The μ-receptors in the dorsal striatum of the females were blocked, which led them to mate just as frequently with unfamiliar partners as with the known partner. This means that a higher receptor density could be significantly involved in our social bonding behavior. However, studies with Homo sapiens are still pending (cf. Roth and Strüber 2021, 137 f.).

5) **Endogenous Opioids and the Influence of Genes and Experiences**

Genetic polymorphisms can influence the individual functioning of the opioid system. This is evident for the polymorphism of the gene for the μ-receptor. Carriers of the G allele exhibit different characteristics compared to carriers of two A alleles. The G allele occurs more frequently in women than in men. It is especially widespread in the Asian region. Individuals with this allele react, compared to other people, not only particularly sensitively to physical pain but also more sensitively to social rejection. Fundamentally, they are more interested in social interactions than people with other gene variants, and they also tend to avoidant attachment behavior less frequently. However, they more often exhibit anxious attachment behavior, as they desire close contact but simultaneously fear being hurt (cf. Roth and Strüber 2021, 138 f.). In the gene-environment interaction, the individual opioid system influences the effect of environmental experiences. For example, it can be seen that carriers of the G allele, compared to the A/A genotype, react to terrible childhood experiences with lower agreeableness, a greater tendency to anger and hostility, as well as other negative manifestations of social traits (cf. Carver et al. 2016, cited in Roth and Strüber 2021, 139).

2.6.10 Stress and Pathophysiological Consequences

> "Psychological and physiological causal factors of stress-related diseases are so closely intertwined that they are usually neither conceptually nor experimentally separable" (Birbaumer and Schmidt 2018, 154).

1) **Psyche—Soma, a False Dichotomy**
Birbaumer and Schmidt (2018) clearly hold the view that a clear separation between purely somatic and psychosomatic diseases, as advocated by so-called psychosomatic medicine, can neither be empirically nor theoretically maintained. In mental disorders such as depression, patients exhibit massive hormonal-physiological changes, which, when frequently repeated, have lasting pathophysiological consequences. Psychosomatic disorders such as chronic pain conditions, stomach and duodenal ulcers, essential hypertension, and many other diseases develop from complex structures of endogenous rhythm disturbances, molecular genetic changes, and stress events. The boundaries between body physiology and environmental influence are often not discernible. Likewise, "purely" organic disorders or diseases such as some heart diseases, forms of epilepsy, type 2 diabetes mellitus, and immune deficiency diseases have psychological triggers. Here, too, a strict separation between organic and psychological can often not be made. Epileptic seizures, for example, are mostly triggered by sudden changes in the level of arousal (up or down). These rapid changes in arousal are often dependent on social environmental stimuli or rapidly changing emotional changes. Thus, Birbaumer and Schmidt (2018) state that physiological and psychological causal factors of stress-related diseases are so closely intertwined that they are usually neither experimentally nor conceptually separable. The following summarizes some of the pathophysiological consequences of chronic stress and helplessness known to date (cf. Birbaumer and Schmidt 2018, 154).

Stress-induced stress reactions can, for example, suppress immune reactivity, increase muscle tension, suppress digestion, and inhibit growth and reproductive function. In addition, many diverse pathophysiological effects can result from prolonged stress, such as back, facial, and headaches, migraines, some forms of epilepsy, psychogenic dwarfism, loss of libido, infertility, anovulation, and impotence. Diabetes, reduced resistance to a variety of diseases, accelerated aging of cognitive functions and memory, ulcers, and more (cf. Birbaumer and Schmidt 2018, 155). A well-known example of the relationship between stress and disease is stomach ulcers. Although it is now known that stomach and duodenal ulcers can be co-caused by Helicobacter pylori (bacteria), the stress-weakened immune system of the stomach lining and the inhibition of prostaglandin synthesis cause an increase in acid sensitivity. This, in turn, facilitates the colonization of the bacteria. This situation is similar in many so-called psychosomatic diseases. A psychological-emotional stimulus increases the risk of a physical illness or a physically induced pathological change. This psychological-emotional stimulus inhibits or activates a brain region, which then changes the internal environment of an organ system via the autonomic nervous system. An example of this is a lesion of the medial nucleus of the amygdala. This lesion promotes stress-induced stomach ulcers, whereas the administration of high doses of a dopamine agonist into the brain reduces them (cf. ibid., 154).

2) **Stress, Aging, and the Hippocampus**

In animal experiments, it was found that the administration of high doses of glucocorticoids over a longer period leads to the destruction of hippocampal neurons. Destruction of the hippocampus results in the impairment of explicit short-term memory, thereby preventing the storage of new context-related (explicit) information. Stress stimuli that were stored earlier, however, cannot be forgotten. In elderly people, an increase in serum glucocorticoids is generally observed. This is sometimes associated with a reduction in core sleep (the first deep sleep phase). This increase also parallels memory defects in old age. The feedback regulation of the hypothalamic-pituitary-adrenal axis weakens with age. This, in turn, means that the hormonal response to stress stimuli persists longer. Additionally, elevated glucocorticoid levels accelerate the aging of memory because hippocampal neurons are destroyed more rapidly (this particularly affects the CA3 region). The situation is further dramatized because the hippocampus has an inhibitory influence on CRH secretion, which in turn affects ACTH release. If the CA3 region of the hippocampus is partially destroyed, an increase in CRH and ACTH follows, as well as a further increase in glucocorticoids (cf. Birbaumer and Schmidt 2018, 154 f.). This creates "(…) a vicious circle of aging → stress increase → and memory loss" (ibid., 155). In animal experiments, this vicious circle could be prevented. The animals were well-treated during their childhood and adolescent development and were only gradually introduced to or confronted with stress. Thus, they were immunized and showed no memory disorders or loss of hippocampal cells in old age. This can be associated with some people who can maintain their mental productivity into old age, and others who, after significant life events such as war, concentration camps, and torture, exhibit permanent memory disorders and accelerated aging (cf. Birbaumer and Schmidt 2018, 155).

The influences of glucocorticoids, particularly cortisol, and the extent to which genetics and experiences play a role in this will be explained and demonstrated in the following.

2.6.11 Stress, Cortisol, and Mental Disorders

The basic knowledge about cortisol was already presented in Chap. 1. Now I will go into more detail about its significance for the psyche and behavior. Furthermore, it will be shown what role genes and early experiences play in connection with cortisol. Cortisol is an important substance in the stress processing system. This means that the body responds to a threatening situation with a rapid stress response. This includes, in addition to the stimulation of the sympathetic nervous system, a secretion of norepinephrine and CRF, which enables the body to react within seconds. In a second, slower response, additional energies are activated, and the initial stress reaction is dampened again. This second reaction is mediated by cortisol, which is the end product of the HPA axis (hypothalamic-pituitary-adrenal axis). For cortisol to take effect, it must bind to one of its receptors. This is either a glucocorticoid receptor (GR) or a mineralocorticoid receptor (MR). Numerous studies have now shown that this hormone is significant for the influence of early experiences on the psyche, personality, and the development of mental disorders. Cortisol, like other neuromodulators, is capable of influencing the excitability of brain structures. For example, when it binds to MR, it can trigger an activation of the brain structure, and 1–2 hours later, when the genomic effect of the receptors sets in, it is normalized again. Thus, cortisol can, for example, first cause activation and then inhibition in the amygdala. However, brain areas such as the dorsolateral cortex are not affected like the amygdala: In an acute stress situation, cortisol initially reduces its activation during cognitive tasks, but a few hours later, it is enhanced (cf. Roth and Strüber 2021, 150 f.). This results in seeing things or problems differently after a longer period. Furthermore, it is important to mention that cortisol is released both basally (i.e., under resting conditions) and as part of a stress response. This particularly affects memory performance and behavior in stressful situations and mobilizes energy (cf. Roth and Strüber 2021, 151 ff.). Another significant function of cortisol is to inhibit the stress response driven by NA and the sympathetic nervous system. This is intended to prevent an overreaction of the body's response to an acute stress situation. Since cortisol, as already described, can have opposite effects depending on receptor occupancy, it also influences behavior differently in stressful situations (cf. Roth and Strüber 2021, 154). Initially, cortisol promotes a rapid response to direct stress stimuli. Anxiety and vigilance are promoted, but this comes at the cost of usual control. When the stress subsides, the allocation of resources is reversed (cf. Fernandez et al. 2014, 304). Thus, attention is directed to the threat, energy resources are activated, and often, rigid and unconsidered responses with practiced strategies occur (cf. Roth and Strüber 2021, 154). Only a few hours later, when the effect of delayed genomic cortisol sets in, the influence is reversed, and individual neural resources are directed towards flexible and goal-oriented behavior (cf. Roth and Strüber 2021, 154). The development of the respective receptors is individual in humans, meaning that depending on the individual ratio of receptor types, one effect of cortisol may predominate. It is assumed that in people who suffer from PTSD or have had to experience severe early childhood stress, the "calming" effect of cortisol is rather reduced (cf. Fernàndez et al. 2017, cited in Roth and Strüber 2021, 155). The HPA axis is particularly stimulated when pronounced physical and psychological resources are needed. These can be socially risky events such as a presentation in front of an audience, family conflicts, separation, or social rejection, in infants a temporary separation from the mother, in children, for example, parental conflicts and social rejection, more so than in physical challenges. Discussions with parents also lead to activation of the HPA axis in children, especially if they are anxious and the outcome of the discussion is unpredictable. In general, it should be noted that unpredictable and uncontrollable events lead to significant cortisol responses. Even positive unpredictable events, such as the anticipation the day before Christmas, can lead to stimulation of the HPA axis. The cortisol system develops very early and is characterized by the so-called "stress hyporesponsive period" (SHRP). This means that in the first years of life, both the cortisol stress response and the resting cortisol level are dramatically reduced. This SHRP is maintained by parental care, which achieves a dampening of cortisol secretion (cf. Roth and Strüber 2021, 155). This seems to be based on the release of oxytocin, which is secreted during caring interaction with parents, especially with a caring mother, and thus has an inhibitory effect on the cortisol system (cf. Roth et al. 2014, cited in Roth and Strüber 2021, 156). However, stressors that involve a loss of social contacts or parental care can trigger a stress response in children (cf. Roth and Strüber 2021, 156).

1) **Cortisol and the Influence of Genes and Experiences**

Here, the influence of genes and experiences plays a particularly significant role. Certain gene variants of the stress system are associated with reduced or increased cortisol secretion. This means that the risk for stress-related disorders is either lower or higher, which, for example, decreases or increases the risk of developing PTSD (cf. Roth and Strüber 2021, 156). In this context, the CRF-R1 receptor is a significant polymorphism. This influences the regulation of CRF production and consequently also the production of ACTH and cortisol. This gene variant increases the risk of developing depression after early childhood trauma (cf. Binder et al. 2008, 190). Similarly, polymorphisms of the gene for the GR (glucocorticoid receptor) can represent a vulnerability factor for stress-related (psychiatric) disorders and thus increase the risk of developing PTSD and depression (cf. Entringer et al. 2008, 179). Furthermore, the gene for the MR receptor type exists in various variants. This influences both the extent of basal and stress-related cortisol secretion. Additionally, the polymorphism of the FKBP5 gene, which in turn encodes the FK506-binding protein 5, is significant for stress- and trauma-related disorders. This protein acts, among other things, as an inhibitor of the GR binding capacity for cortisol and is thus a functional antagonist of the GR. The risk allele variant therefore increases the risk of developing post-traumatic stress disorder based on negative early childhood experiences. The results of this study show that there is a potential interaction between genes and childhood environment concerning PTSD in adulthood (cf. Binder et al. 2008, 1291). It has long been proven that early childhood experiences have a significant influence on the development of our cortisol system or the HPA axis. Through epigenetic mechanisms, the early extent of cortisol secretion seems to shape how many receptors for cortisol are formed in the long term. Through the feedback mechanism, their individual function is determined by the extent of long-term cortisol secretion (cf. Roth and Strüber 2021, 157).

2) **Prenatal Epigenetic Imprinting of the Cortisol System**

The epigenetic imprinting of the cortisol system begins prenatally (before birth). If, for example, hypercortisolism (overactivity of the cortisol system) occurs in the mother during pregnancy, based on extreme stress experiences or psychological disorders (cf. Roth and Strüber 2021, 157), "(…) then this influences the development of the fetal stress processing system" (ibid.). The maternal and fetal blood circulations are connected via the placenta and the umbilical cord. Glucocorticoids can cross the placental barrier, with normally only about 3/10 of the maternal cortisol passing through. This intercepts acute increases in cortisol concentration in the maternal blood, which is essential for normal fetal development of the stress processing system, as the fetus is much more sensitive to cortisol. However, animal experiments have shown that a chronic increase in cortisol levels in the blood plasma and brain of the pregnant woman leads to the placenta allowing a dramatically higher amount of cortisol to pass through the placenta (cf. Roth and Strüber 2021, 157 f.). This can sustainably damage the development of the fetal stress axis. Additionally, the CRF and oxytocin receptors, which are located in the placenta, are influenced in a long-term effect (cf. Binder et al. 2015, cited in Roth and Strüber 2021, 158). Besides stress during pregnancy, trauma experienced by the mother in childhood or adolescence can also be effective. Trauma, especially in early childhood, leads to either hypocortisolism or hypercortisolism depending on the severity of the stress (cf. Roth et al. 2014, cited in Roth and Strüber 2021, 158). This effect can persist into pregnancy and then lead to a similar effect as if the trauma had occurred during pregnancy. This can mean that the child is negatively affected even though the pregnancy appears "unremarkable." Thus, trauma can be passed on to the next generation and even to the subsequent one. Prenatal effects on the development of the child's cortisol system, based on the maternal cortisol balance, can influence both the child's temperament and the risk of developing behavioral disorders and affective diseases. However, the consequences of prenatal stress can be mitigated by secure postnatal attachment (cf. Roth and Strüber 2021, 158).

3) **Postnatal Imprinting of the Cortisol System**

Postnatal (post-birth) stress can also have long-term effects on the function of the cortisol system. This can influence the child's emotional as well as cognitive development and lead to a change in the risk for, for example, aggressive behavior or depression. The mother-child bond and maternal care have great relevance in the prenatal influence on the child's stress system. Tests have shown that securely attached children do not respond with cortisol secretion during the SHRP despite high stress stimuli, whereas children with a disorganized or insecure-ambivalent attachment often show an increase in cortisol release. This occurs especially when these children already have a rather reserved or anxious temperament. It is assumed here that this early activity of the cortisol system can "program" its functioning in the long term (cf. Roth and Strüber 2021, 158 f.).

4) **Early Childhood Trauma and the Cortisol System**

In early childhood trauma, the cortisol system is significantly and long-term altered. If children suffer from neglect, abuse, or maternal withdrawal, this affects both basal and stress-induced cortisol release. Pronounced underfunctions are the result here (cf. Roth and Strüber 2021, 159). "This underfunction is often accompanied by helplessness" (ibid.). This means that the children accept their situation or accept that they cannot change anything, whereupon they shut down their emotions. However, their perception of stress is not shut down; it seems rather the opposite. Abused women, for example, who have not processed their trauma, experience stress most intensely but show the lowest cortisol response (cf. Roth and Strüber 2021, 159). If, on the other hand, they have processed their trauma, for example through psychotherapy, and have an organized attachment representation, stress is perceived intensely, but the cortisol response hardly diverges from that of non-abused women. They may even be able to process stress better (cf. Dimitrova et al. 2009, 924). Experiences during the first years of life can thus influence the stress system in the long term. A large study found that the severity of early negative experiences is particularly relevant for the development of the cortisol system (cf. Roth and Strüber 2021, 159 ff.). Severe and prolonged abuse and maltreatment, especially when it came from close persons, have a more severe impact, particularly on the lower basal morning cortisol concentration. Since these subjects grew up in a positive environment after their early childhood, it can be assumed that these are indeed long-term effects of early childhood abuse (cf. Roth et al. 2014, cited in Roth and Strüber 2021, 161). This was also studied in children who were confronted with war for a long time. Children with war experiences responded to the experimental stress situation with an increased cortisol response. They tended to seek security and protection from their mothers. Other children who had to experience war, on the other hand, showed an underfunction of the cortisol system. For these children, not only was withdrawal behavior and the tendency to want to comfort themselves characteristic, but also the development of

PTSD (cf. Eidelman-Rothman et al. 2013, 943). This noticeable change in cortisol function can apparently develop as early as the second year of life. Basal morning cortisol release begins to decrease in early abused children as early as 19 months of age (cf. Roth and Strüber 2021, 161 f.). However, it has been clearly shown that children who had early active interventions showed cortisol secretion that did not differ from non-abused children, even after the interventions had already ended for a year. The results of this study particularly underscore the value of psychosocial interventions. In early childhood abuse, such normalization of biological regulatory processes can be achieved (cf. Cicchetti et al. 2011b, 789). Likewise, an early therapeutic program conducted in foster families can normalize the cortisol secretion of early abused children. It is important to convey to the children that they are allowed to express feelings such as anger and to be able to influence their own environment (cf. Nienstedt and Westermann 2007, cited in Roth and Strüber 2021, 163). This experience could then be the basis for a normalization of cortisol release (cf. Roth and Strüber 2021, 163). However, sensitive periods must be considered. If early neglected children are placed in foster families within the first two years of life, the function of the stress system is often normalized. A later move to a foster family is less likely to result in normalization. Obvious intervention effects were only observed in children who were placed in foster families before the 24th or 18th month of life. This clearly shows a sensitive period in humans, during which it can be assumed that the environment changes the development of the stress response system (cf. Fox et al. 2015, 5637). However, if there remains a lower cortisol secretion, this has significant implications for mental health. It also affects the body and how it responds to later trauma (cf. Roth and Strüber 2021, 163).

5) **Later Chronic Stress and the Cortisol System**

Later chronic stress also leads to a change in the cortisol system. In particular, chronic stress that is not controllable is a significant risk factor for some neuropsychiatric disorders. The mechanisms are complex and multifactorial (cf. Hall et al. 2015, 174). Initially, it seems as if chronic stress produces hyperfunction. However, when a state of exhaustion is reached and the affected individual can no longer cope with environmental stress, the cortisol system can switch to hypofunction. Studies show that most states of deepest exhaustion indicate hypofunction of the HPA axis. The changes in cortisol balance caused by early or later chronic stress have significant effects on the brain (cf. Roth and Strüber 2021, 163). The excitation of nerve cells is affected, as is the formation of synapses and their stabilization. Additionally, the formation of new nerve cells is impaired and how they develop in brain structures. Furthermore, the activity of nerve cells and how well they are connected are influenced (cf. Hall et al. 2015, cited in Roth and Strüber 2021, 163 f.).

> "Through modulation of these processes, stress experiences can significantly promote the development of mental disorders" (Roth and Strüber 2021, 164).

As elaborated in detail in this chapter, cortisol is of enormous relevance to our well-being, our behavior, and our mental health. The specific mental disorders for which the cortisol system is particularly relevant are discussed in Sect. 2.7.

In the following, I would like to present some results from recent studies by the Biological Stress Research Group to illustrate possible gender differences in psychosocial stress.

2.6.12 Neurobiological Gender Differences in Psychosocial Stress

Before delving deeper into mental disorders in connection with psychoneuroendocrinology, some results from recent studies by the Biological Stress Research Group will be presented to address the question of possible gender differences in psychosocial stress. It is important to note here that this article always refers to gender in the sense of biological sex. The focus is always on the biological gender differences between men and women.

Although it has long been known that the two biological sexes differ in psychological and endocrine stress responses and in the prevalence of stress-related disorders, there is still little knowledge about gender-specific differences in stress regulation in the brain. A magnetic resonance imaging study examined the changes in cortisol levels under the influence of psychosocial stress. In both sexes, stress exposure led to significant increases in cortisol levels, but men showed higher levels than women. The different stress-related responses were particularly found in the striatolimbic area. The higher increases were associated with deactivation in women, whereas they were associated with activation in men. Thus, various stress responses were found in an identical brain structure. No gender-specific differences were found in terms of affect or heart rate. Generally, it is assumed that there are no detectable divergences in stress response between men and women, and if there are, they are only partially attributable to biological sex. However, it is suggested that future studies consider sociocultural gender. Even though the two biological sexes differ in their general stress reactivity and in the prevalence of certain stress-related disorders, the result of this study is that there is no clear neuroanatomically distinguishable typically "female" or typically "male" stress response. However, the data provide indications (cf. Bärtl et al. 2021, 972–984),

> "(…) that considering complex interactions and quantitative variables such as individual cortisol increases is a more suitable approach to elucidate gender-specific differences in central stress regulation" (ibid., 984).

2.7 Mental Disorders, Psychoneuroendocrinology, and Gene-Environment Factors

As repeatedly stated in this book, there are connections between the endocrine system, genetic-epigenetic factors, and mental disorders as well as personality disorders. This section of the book now provides a brief insight into some mental disorders and personality disorders and shows the connection of the disorders with both genetic and environmental experiences as well as endocrine influences. It is important to emphasize here that the explanations and presentations of the various mental disorders are merely intended to provide an overview or insight into the disorders to make the connections with psychoneuroendocrinology understandable.

The psyche of a person does not always develop as it should. Based on a certain genetic-epigenetic makeup as well as early childhood or later stressors, these factors can lead to suboptimal development of the psyche and impair a person's well-being. It should be mentioned at the outset that genes and experiences determine synaptic connections, which in turn determine where and in what quantity neuromodulators are secreted and the corresponding receptors are formed. This affects whether a person is depressed or happy, courageous and willing to take risks, or reacts to certain external and internal stimuli with unbearable fear, whether a person is empathetic and helpful to others, or rather exploits and abuses other people. If a mental illness or behavioral disorder has developed, it is often associated with pronounced and individual suffering. Certain mental illnesses and personality disorders can occur in mild, moderate, or severe forms, and certain symptoms can be more or less pronounced. In addition, comorbidities are often present, where a person develops more than one illness. However, before I go into more detail about the respective illnesses and show how negative experiences lead to impairments in psychological development, it is important to note that not all people react to negative early childhood experiences or stressors with a mental illness or problematic development of the psyche. There are people who seem to be resilient, which in turn is due to certain genes. These specific genes mitigate the risk of mental illness, just as there are certain genes that increase the risk of developing certain mental illnesses. Moreover, substitute relationships with good bonding and care for early neglected or abused children can have a positive effect. The decisive factor in the mentioned resilient individuals is (cf. Roth and Strüber 2021, 285 ff.)

> "(…) additional adjustments in their brain function that allow them to effectively compensate for subliminal psychiatric symptoms" (ibid., 286).

The following provides an insight into some mental illnesses and personality disorders, and psychoneuroendocrinological findings related to them are presented. As already mentioned, only brief overviews of the various disorders and mental illnesses are given here.

2.7.1 Post-Traumatic Stress Disorder (PTSD)

Post-traumatic stress disorder (PTSD) has already been frequently mentioned in this book. Here, it is now explained in more detail what PTSD (or "post-traumatic stress disorder") is, what causes and symptoms this illness has, and how PTSD is related to hormones, genes, and experience.

PTSD is linked to the experience of fear but differs from other anxiety disorders because an exceptionally stressful life event or continuous trauma occurred before the onset of PTSD. This can involve an immediate traumatic experience that the person had to endure themselves, such as acute life-threatening situations, serious injuries, sexual violence, or secondary traumatizations (witnessing traumatic experiences of others). A few weeks to months after the experienced trauma, the characteristic symptoms of PTSD appear (cf. Roth and Strüber 2021, 313). The three main symptom groups of PTSD are intrusion, avoidance, and hyperarousal. These can each manifest in the form of various individual symptoms (cf. Dittmar 2013, 43).

Intrusive Re-experiencing

> "Intrusions are unwanted recurring and distressing memories or memory fragments" (Dittmar 2013, 43).

Intrusions often do not just appear as mere recollections but as an unwanted re-living of the traumatic event or a re-experiencing of individual aspects of the event with all sensory qualities and affects. This feels to the affected individuals as if the event is happening again in the present. The most well-known intrusions are the so-called flashbacks, which are characterized by sudden onset and very detailed memories. The affected person feels as if they are experiencing the traumatic event again, and depending on the severity of the flashback, they may completely lose touch with the present and not know what is happening. This is a dissociative state that can last for seconds, hours, or even days. Intrusions can occur in the form of images, smells, sounds, taste sensations, as well as bodily perceptions. It is also common to experience a subjectively perceived state of being overwhelmed. Additionally, intrusions can also appear as diffuse feelings of fear, helplessness, or inability to act, without visual or audible memory fragments. They are triggered by key stimuli, known as triggers, that have an association with the traumatic event. Triggers can be similar situations, objects, scents, sounds, or words, as well as anniversaries or media reports or films (cf. Dittmar 2013, 43 f.).

Avoidance Behavior and Emotional Numbing

Since memories of the experienced trauma are associated with extremely strong emotions, those affected try with all their might to avoid those overwhelming and distressing thoughts and emotions. The affected individuals often try not to think about the experienced events, which usually fails. Additionally, people, situations, objects, or places associated with the trauma are avoided. This shutting off of memories leads to dissociative states such as partial amnesias, which are characterized by a blurred memory of the experienced events. This self-induced form of avoidance is an attempt at coping, which, however, can lead to the symptoms of PTSD persisting longer. These avoidance strategies can include attempts to stop thoughts as well as complete social withdrawal, where the affected individuals can no longer leave the house. Numbing (emotional numbness) also falls into the symptom category of avoidance. This implies any symptoms associated with the inability to experience and express positive emotions. This means, for example, a reduction in interest in participating in everyday life or activities that brought joy before the traumatic event; there is a minimized range of affect with the sensation of limited future prospects. The trauma has massively damaged the emotional life of the affected individuals (cf. Dittmar 2013, 45 f.).

Hyperarousal

Based on the traumatic experience, the arousal threshold of the autonomic nervous system decreases. Stressors affect the affected individuals both earlier and more sustainably. Even stressors that could be easily compensated before the event now trigger stronger arousal. The autonomic nervous system is in a constant state of alert, which implies that even the smallest stressors lead to strong startle responses or irritability and impair sleep behavior (falling asleep and staying asleep). Hyperarousal is fundamentally a very useful reaction of the organism to dangerous situations, intended to serve as a survival aid by perceiving threatening stimuli earlier and faster. However, after a trauma, the ability to distinguish between a real danger and a state of safety is often lost. This can lead to neutral stimuli being associated with the traumatic experience and the affected individuals interpreting them as dangerous (cf. Dittmar 2013, 46).

Other Post-Traumatic Disorders

The spectrum of post-traumatic disorders also includes acute stress disorder, complex post-traumatic stress disorder, and developmental trauma disorder. Additionally, other post-traumatic diagnoses include persistent personality changes and post-traumatic embitterment disorders. There are divergences between the temporal criteria and the increased dissociative symptomatology. Furthermore, the occurrence of acute stress disorder is not a determining factor for later long-term consequences. This means that the occurrence of acute stress disorder cannot be used to infer later post-traumatic stress disorder. There are also divergences in the severity of symptoms, which can be similar to those of borderline personality disorder. Symptom constellations can occur that, for example, imply disturbances in affect regulation, dissociative tendencies, disturbances in self-perception, disturbances in sexuality and relationship formation, somatization disorders and physical illnesses, interpersonal disturbances, revictimization tendencies, as well as changes in the meaning system (complex post-traumatic stress disorder).

In developmental trauma disorder, for example, neurobiological and developmental psychological explanatory models are combined, which are considered an advancement of the complex PTSD concept. In other post-traumatic diagnoses such as persistent personality change after extreme stress or post-traumatic embitterment disorder, the research situation still seems unclear or the demarcation debates rather contradictory (cf. Dittmar 2013, 47–52).

In summary, it should be noted that the symptoms in PTSD patients lead to impairment of life, fear and startle responses, anger and a negative mood, increased irritability and aggressiveness, guilt or shame, as well as difficulties in experiencing emotions such as happiness, love, and satisfaction. Depression and suicidal thoughts are not uncommon in PTSD patients, where it is important to mention that people's reactions to the same severely stressful events diverge. One-third of people show no symptoms of psychotrauma, another third recover from the symptoms after a few months, while one-third suffer from the consequences of these events for several years or even decades. This is related to the resilience and vulnerability, genetic makeup, as well as the individual histories of the affected individuals. Furthermore, the symptoms can also appear later, based on memories as well as temporary experienced stress or re-experienced traumatic events, or even be intensified. In older individuals, this can particularly be related to a deterioration in health and cognitive abilities as well as social isolation (cf. Roth and Strüber 2021, 314).

Neurobiological Changes and Psychoneuroendocrinological Findings in PTSD

An overfunction of the amygdala seems to be responsible for the increased anxiety as well as the continuity and intensity of traumatic memories. This increased amygdala activity occurs both under resting conditions and in response to specific triggers and anxious faces. Compared to anxiety disorders and depression, it is observed that in PTSD, particularly the vmPFC (ventromedial prefrontal cortex) shows generally reduced activity. This area of the brain is responsible for capturing the emotional significance of the situation and linking it with previous or prior experiences. The deactivation of the vmPFC can be related to the feeling of inner emptiness that is characteristic of PTSD. The typical symptomatology of overwhelming intrusions is due to a suddenly driven strong activity of the amygdala (cf. Roth and Strüber 2021, 315). Additionally, significant changes in the stress system are observed. Individuals suffering from PTSD show both a lower morning cortisol release and a lower cortisol response when confronted with stress compared to healthy individuals. These changes occur particularly in connection with early childhood trauma (cf. Buxbaum et al. 2013, 1–14). It is interesting to mention here that individuals who develop PTSD after a specific event show reduced cortisol release immediately after the traumatic event, along with a higher heart rate compared to individuals who do not develop PTSD. From this, it can be concluded that, based on an early childhood traumatic experience, reduced cortisol release influences how the body responds to later traumas and whether the risk of developing PTSD is increased (cf. Roth and Strüber 2021, 316). People with PTSD thus show a reduced cortisol level, but the CRF release in the "rapid stress response" is increased. A normal function of the stress system includes that a rapid stress response (CRF, catecholamines, autonomic nervous system) is moderated by cortisol release, thus preventing an overshoot. However, if cortisol release is reduced based on previous stress experiences, cortisol cannot perform this task in a recurring traumatic situation. This leads to an overshoot of the rapid stress response. Prolonged physiological arousal can, in turn, promote the development of PTSD (cf. Noll et al. 2010, 405–417). Based on these findings, a preventive measure against this disorder could be derived. If a single high dose of hydrocortisone (100–140 mg) is administered within 6 hours after a traumatic event, such as a car accident, the core symptoms of acute stress and subsequent development of PTSD could be mitigated (cf. Roth and Strüber 2021, 316). PTSD has also been linked to adult neurogenesis, which could be related to a period of overfunction preceding trauma-induced cortisol underfunction. For example, abuse or neglect during childhood initially leads to cortisol overfunction, and only after a period does cortisol underfunction develop (cf. Noll et al. 2010, 165–175). Psychologically, this is due to the child's resignation when the child gives up resistance. If chronic stress occurs later, it is also initially accompanied by hyperactive cortisol function, which, however, shifts to underfunction when a state of exhaustion is reached. Adult neurogenesis is necessary for distinguishing new experiences from stored memories, and it is assumed that a reduction can lead to the generalization of similar events. For example, a traumatized soldier seeing a campfire may, based on the feature similarities, trigger a recall of war memories and any emotions experienced at that time, such as physical arousal and fear. A healthy person, however, stores this experience as a separate and safely associated event (cf. Roth and Strüber 2021, 317).

The Influence of Genes and Environment on the Development of PTSD

Various genotypes can either mitigate or increase the risk of developing PTSD. An increased risk exists, for example, for individuals who have had both early negative childhood experiences and later traumatic experiences, especially if they also possess 1 or 2 S-alleles of the serotonin transporter gene. The definition of the cause of PTSD development is based on environmental events. Additionally, as previously mentioned, early experiences such as early childhood trauma determine the influence of later traumatic experiences or increase the risk of developing PTSD. Social support, on the other hand, can have a protective effect and thus reduce the risk of PTSD. Another important aspect is the intergenerational transmission of PTSD susceptibility. Particularly, offspring of mothers with PTSD already show reduced cortisol concentration in the first year of life compared to children of healthy mothers. This, in turn, increases the risk of developing their own PTSD, which proves that an increased risk of PTSD susceptibility is passed on to descendants (cf. Roth 2016, cited in Roth and Strüber 2021, 317 f.).

2.7.2 Depression

Depressive illnesses are among the most severe and important medical conditions worldwide. In their various forms, they affect up to 20% of the population. In this process, thinking, emotions, the body, and social relationships are impaired. This means that the entire life or every area of life is thus influenced by this illness. Nevertheless, depression is often not recognized or inadequately treated. This causes a loss of quality of life, both for those affected and for their relatives. In recent years, it has also been recognized that depression is a chronic stress-related illness, which is why it is also referred to as stress depression. This, in turn, means that it is a risk factor for the occurrence of other serious common diseases, such as stroke, heart attack, osteoporosis, diabetes, and dementia. An untreated depression can therefore shorten life expectancy, yet on average only 10% of those affected are adequately and appropriately treated. A scientifically based therapy that leads to complete healing is important because patients with residual symptoms suffer a relapse in 80% of cases. In maintenance therapy to prevent relapses, patients are accompanied for at least another 6 months after the symptoms of the illness have subsided. The more frequently depressive phases have already occurred and the more severe they were, the more imperative long-term therapy is, which means that it goes beyond the period of maintenance therapy (cf. Keck 2017, 8 f.). Furthermore, it is important to mention that, in terms of biological sex, women are twice as likely to suffer from depression as men. This is partly explained by the fact that the symptoms of depression in men are often not recognized as such. It should also be mentioned that depression can occur at any age, meaning: from childhood to old age. In 15-20% of cases, a chronic course can develop if treatment is inadequate or does not take place. In 50-75% of cases, at least a second episode follows, and with each further period of illness, the risk of another increases, which is why careful therapy is all the more important. Worldwide, depression is among the 5 most common diseases, which are associated with increased mortality, a high degree of disability, and chronic psychosocial impairment. According to calculations by the WHO (World Health Organization), depression will continue to increase by 2030 and will be the disease in industrialized nations that requires the most financial resources, ahead of heart disease (cf. ibid., 14).

Symptoms and (Special) Forms of Depression

In general, it can be stated that people with depressive episodes suffer from a depressed mood as well as a reduction in drive and activity. They find it difficult to enjoy anything, to show interest, or to concentrate on something. Those affected often suffer from sleep disorders, have feelings of guilt, low self-esteem, and little self-confidence. Depending on the severity of the illness, suicidal thoughts or actions may occur. Changes in opposite directions are also possible, such as insomnia and increased need for sleep, psychomotor agitation and slowing down, decreased or increased appetite, and thus significant weight loss or weight gain. Regarding the forms of depression, it can already be mentioned here that depressive episodes are classified as an affective disorder, which also includes bipolar disorder, in which depressive episodes alternate with manic episodes, i.e., an elevated mood with increased drive. If the disorder is characterized by repeated depressive episodes, it is referred to as recurrent depressive disorder. If the episodes are less severe but persistently occur and lead to considerable subjective suffering, this is called dysthymia. Dysthymia can occur before a depressive episode, follow it, or occur without severe depressive episodes (cf. Roth and Strüber 2021, 287).

Depressive episodes can thus occur in the context of so-called uni- or bipolar disorders. This means: If only depressive episodes occur, it is called unipolar depression, but if manic episodes (e.g., unrestrained drive, elevated mood, lack of need for sleep, grandiose ideas, or shopping sprees) also occur at different times, it is called bipolar affective disorder. However, unipolar depression can also develop into a bipolar disorder with manic phases over time. It is important to mention that depression can exhibit a variety of symptoms as well as various degrees of severity, typical complaints, and considerable individual variations (cf. Keck 2017, 15).

"Criteria of Depression by the World Health Organization (ICD-10)

- Depressed mood
- Loss of interest and/or joylessness, even in otherwise pleasant events
- Reduced drive, lack of energy, increased fatigue, exhaustion (burnout)
- Anxiety, inner restlessness
- Reduced ability to concentrate and pay attention
- Lack of self-confidence and self-esteem, feelings of worthlessness
- Severe uncertainty in making decisions
- Ruminating thoughts, tendency to brood
- Negative future perspectives, hopelessness, pessimism
- Severe guilt feelings, self-reproach
- Persistent sleep disturbances
- Reduced appetite, weight loss
- Loss of libido, that is, decreased interest in sexuality
- Deep despair, thoughts of death, suicidal thoughts, suicidal actions

These symptoms must be present for at least two weeks" (Keck 2017, 16). It should be noted here that there has been an ICD-11 since 2022, and thus a new version of the International Classification of Diseases has come into force. However, although it has been in force since early January 2022, it is not yet used in the German-speaking area, as the ICD-11 must first be translated and modified. Additionally, it must be integrated into the existing structures in the country. How long it will take until the ICD-11 can be used in the German-speaking area is still unclear (cf. Mocker 2022, n.p.).

In addition, depressive disorders often occur together with anxiety disorders, obsessive-compulsive disorders, substance abuse, and borderline personality disorder. Furthermore, different subtypes of depressive disorders are distinguished. Here, for example, it is significant whether the depression is accompanied by anxiety or is associated with psychotic symptoms (cf. Roth and Strüber 2021, 288). The earlier terms such as "endogenous depression," "neurotic depression," and "reactive depression" are considered outdated, as earlier concepts of origin have been refuted by current research (cf. Keck 2017, 20). Among the various subtypes is, for example, a depression with melancholic features, which is characterized by melancholy and, in particular, the loss of pleasure in almost all activities. The affected individuals are sullen, hopeless, desperate, and feel guilty in an inappropriate way. They feel helpless, worthless, and suffer from a self-focused anxiety (cf. Roth and Strüber 2021, 288). Additionally, a pronounced morning low, joylessness, weight loss, and loss of libido and interest are characteristic of melancholic depression (cf. Keck 2017, 20). This form of depression is particularly common among patients who suffer from severe depressive episodes and are thus often in inpatient treatment (cf. Roth and Strüber 2021, 288). However, depression can also manifest differently. This means that the depression manifests differently than previously mentioned, that is, not with dejection or sadness, but with irritability, aggressiveness, anger, and increased alcohol consumption. Sometimes, excessive exercise is also reported, and the affected individuals feel stressed and burned out. It is important to mention that men are more frequently affected by this type of symptoms than women (cf. Keck 2017, 20). Another form of depression is the "atypical depression." Despite the term "atypical," it is estimated that 15–50% of depressive patients exhibit symptoms like these. Here, the patients are indeed able to feel joy or be cheered up. Typical features include a feeling of inner emptiness, increased appetite and corresponding weight gain, and an increased need for sleep. The symptoms worsen throughout the day, and the affected individuals feel a "leaden" paralysis in their limbs. They also show an enormous sensitivity to rejection, which often leads to social and professional impairments. This form of depression often begins during school years, has a more chronic than episodic course, and occurs more frequently in women than in men. Individuals affected by these features have also more frequently experienced depression with abuse, neglect, and depressive disorders in their childhood than others (cf. Roth and Strüber 2021, 288 f.). Additionally, certain special forms of depression can be distinguished based on particularly striking symptoms. One of the most significant is the "larvated depression" or "masked depression." Here, physical symptoms, organ complaints, and vegetative disorders are in the foreground. This masked or larvated depression is spoken of when the physical complaints are so prominent that the mental complaints are difficult to recognize (cf. Keck 2017, 20 f.). An increasingly common form of depression is the so-called**Burn-out syndrome.**This form is an exhaustion depression or its precursor, which arises particularly based on prolonged occupational stress. Women are often additionally burdened by the stresses of household and family, whereby it should be mentioned that pure household management also corresponds to occupational stress. Typical features here are energy loss, reduced performance, cynicism, and indifference, as well as a reluctance, despite previously often long-term above-average performance and extremely high commitment. After the long-term accumulation of stress, often only a relatively minor trigger is needed to bring about the onset of the illness. Symptoms also often include unclear physical complaints such as sweating, headaches, dizziness, muscle pain, and gastrointestinal problems. Sleep disturbances are also frequently observed as a symptom. The increase in this state of exhaustion is attributed to the changed working conditions, such as constant availability via mobile phone and/or email, as well as increasing pressure but lack of recognition. New demands are placed on health, which requires the proper handling of occupational stress (cf. Keck 2017, 22). If a depression or mood episode occurs about 4 weeks after the birth of a child, it is referred to as **"postpartum depression."** Typical features here are increased neglect or disinterest in the child's needs or the mother's fear of being alone with the child (cf. Roth and Strüber 2021, 289). Postpartum depression occurs in 10–15% of women. It should be mentioned that the postpartum phase is characterized by pronounced and rapid hormonal changes. During the first 48 hours after delivery, a significant drop in the hormones progesterone, estrogen, cortisol, and thyroxine is observed. Why these hormonal changes lead to such an illness in some women is still unclear (cf. Keck 2017, 23). It is important to mention that these episodes should be differentiated from the baby blues (so-called "crying days"), which are observed in up to 70% of all women in the first 10 days after birth (cf. Roth and Strüber 2021, 289). Typically, the baby blues do not begin before the 3rd day and last a few hours to days. The baby blues have no disease value (cf. Keck 2017, 23). Another special form is the so-called **male depression ("male depression")**. This form of depression in its various manifestations is often overlooked. Increased risk and addictive behavior, irritability and aggressiveness, dangerous sports, and risky behavior in traffic are symptoms that occur here. Additionally, social withdrawal, lack of utilization of help options, and failure to seek medical help are more common than in women. This form of depression is often recognized only after a long history of suffering (cf. Keck 2017, 24). Depression in older age, from about 65 years, is referred to as **"age-related depression."** Depressive disorders do not occur more frequently in older age; there are even indications that they occur somewhat less frequently in younger seniors between 65 and 75 years. However, in older patients, depression often goes unnoticed and thus remains untreated for years. For people with age-related depression, there is a high risk of chronicity and the need for care. Older patients increasingly complain about other physical illnesses but are more likely to conceal depressive symptoms. Therefore, various physical symptoms are at the forefront in older patients, and it should be mentioned that unclear pain is often an expression of an underlying depression. It should also be mentioned that age-related depression can arise or be favored by malnutrition and inadequate fluid intake. Regular physical activity and a generally active lifestyle, even in old age, are also considered proven protective factors. Especially in older age, persistent or inadequately treated cognitive impairments are a risk factor for later developing dementia, making therapy particularly important. In general, it should be noted that depression doubles the risk of developing Parkinson's disease or Alzheimer's dementia (cf. Keck 2017, 22 f.). It should also be mentioned that, even if older people do not have a tendency to suicide, untreated depression can very quickly lead to life-threatening conditions due to withdrawal to bed, loss of appetite, and low fluid intake. It is also now very well documented that the course of many diseases, such as diabetes or the condition after a heart attack, is extremely negatively influenced if untreated depression is present in the patients (cf. ibid., 26). Furthermore, the so-called **seasonal depression (winter depression)** should be mentioned, as dark and foggy winter days can worsen the mood. In individual cases, this can lead to a severe or even life-threatening illness. The cause is the seasonally reduced light exposure through the eyes, which leads to a lack of electrical stimulation and, in susceptible individuals, to a disruption of brain metabolism. This, in turn, leads to the development of depression (cf. Keck 2017, 24).

Depression as a Stress-Related Illness: Changes in Stress Hormone Regulation
Before I delve into the neurobiological changes and psychoneuroendocrinological findings of depression in more detail, I would like to explain the connection between stress and depression. As mentioned several times, any confrontation with internal or external stressors triggers a meaningful stress response. The body and brain respond to any challenge for change with stress. Everyday stress is diverse and can exist both in professional performance demands as well as in leisure time. Likewise, an acceleration of daily life, an increasing flood of information, and relationship conflicts can lead to stress. If a stressful episode is only of short duration, healthy people can indeed perceive it as beneficial or stimulating. The stress response usually ends quickly. However, if it is chronic stress, the stress response does not come to rest, leading to increased concentrations of stress hormones in the brain and promoting the development of depression, which is why it is also called stress depression. A predisposition for this can be genetically determined or based on early childhood experiences such as abuse or neglect. The gene-environment factors will be discussed in more detail later. In general, it should be noted that it is not the stress itself but the negative individual evaluation and processing of stress or stressful events, such as professional problems, job loss, death, family conflicts, or moving, etc., that is disease-promoting (cf. Keck 2017, 30 f.). Prolonged stress thus harms health. This chronic stress is often accompanied by a feeling of loss of control. In certain brain regions, such as the limbic system, which is responsible for our emotion regulation, there is an overactivity of the amygdala, which is of enormous importance for the regulation of our feelings. This leads to a pathological, permanent activation of the stress hormone system (hypothalamic-pituitary-adrenal axis) on the hormonal level. Thus, the brain loses control over the stress hormone system. In depression, this hormonal change and shifts in the regulation of the stress hormone system are best documented. The majority of patients show an increased blood concentration of stress hormones. In addition to the hypothalamic-pituitary-adrenal axis, another stress system is affected, as depressive patients also show dysregulation of the autonomic nervous system. An increase in sympathetic activity leads to an increased release of adrenaline. A permanent overactivation of the stress hormone systems can ultimately lead to further changes in metabolic regulation, which can result in additional pathophysiological diseases. In the case of depression, it becomes particularly clear how mental and physical illnesses strongly influence

each other. Mental illnesses are based on a neurobiological disease process in the brain, with depression in most cases being based on a dysregulation of the stress hormone system. Furthermore, Keck notes here that thus every mental illness is “psychosomatic” and requires a holistic, comprehensive treatment (cf. Keck 2017, 30–34).

In the following, the psychoneuroendocrinological findings and neurobiological changes in depression will be explained in more detail.

Neurobiological Changes and Psychoneuroendocrinological Findings in Depression
Changes in both the structure and function of various brain areas as well as neurochemical abnormalities have been found in depressive patients. Additionally, it has been shown in recent years that so-called “adult neurogenesis” (i.e., the formation of new nerve cells in adulthood) is significantly altered in depressed individuals. For example, in brain areas, the ventromedial prefrontal cortex (vmPFC) shows altered activity in connection with depression. The vmPFC is part of the brain’s resting state network. An activated vmPFC ensures that attention is directed to internal processes such as self-reflective thoughts and autobiographical memories. However, when a person is engaged in specific tasks, this brain area is deactivated, which in turn allows for focusing on new stimuli and pursuing behavioral goals. Depression, especially severe cases, is characterized by overactivity in the vmPFC, even under resting conditions (cf. Buchheim et al. 2012, cited in Roth and Strüber 2021, 290). In contrast, dorsolateral areas of the PFC, which are involved in planning and executing actions, show reduced activity. People with depression often show a tendency towards pronounced introspection and self-reflection and an increased self-focus (cf. Böker et al. 2009, 2617–2627). Particularly those affected by melancholic depression seem to be affected by an overfunction of the limbic brain areas. The amygdala, which is responsible for threat detection, is also more active in depressive patients. This overfunction could lead to the affected individuals attributing a threatening content to actually neutral stimuli and overvaluing negative stimuli. This could also explain the extraordinarily high comorbidity of depression and anxiety disorders (cf. Roth and Strüber 2021, 290 f.). Furthermore, other studies of patients indicate damage to the hippocampus. It has been shown that the longer the depressive illness lasts, the more pronounced the reduced hippocampal volume is. It is suspected that the prolonged high cortisol release in the affected individuals leads to damage to the hippocampal cells. This, in turn, can prevent the hippocampus from inhibiting cortisol release as it normally would. A vicious cycle is created, as hippocampal damage and increased cortisol release reinforce each other (cf. Ravnkilde and Videbech2004, 1957–1966). There is a theory of reduced monoamine supply related to decreased activity of various neuromodulatory systems, which is associated with various symptoms of depressive disorders. The reduced motivation or general lack of interest (anhedonia) could be due to disturbances in the dopaminergic system, while anxiety and negative mood are more likely related to disturbances in the noradrenergic and serotonergic systems. Numerous changes in components of monoaminergic systems have been demonstrated in depression. These changes affect, among other things, proteins responsible for the synthesis of these

components, as well as transport molecules and individual receptors. However, the results of studies are controversially discussed. For example, the formation of the serotonergic 5-HT1A receptor has been found to be upregulated in some depressed individuals and downregulated in others (cf. Roth and Strüber 2021, 292 f.). The so-called serotonin transporter, which removes serotonin from the synaptic cleft and transports it back into the presynaptic cells, is of particular importance for the treatment of depressive disorders. Therefore, so-called selective serotonin reuptake inhibitors (SSRIs) are used in pharmacological treatments. They block the serotonin transporter, reducing reuptake, thereby increasing the serotonin concentration in the synaptic cleft. With a delay of a few weeks, they have an antidepressant effect. Recent studies suggest that the increased serotonin concentration after administration of SSRIs activates various processes. For example, increased oxytocin release or the promotion of adult neurogenesis in various parts of the brain should be mentioned here. However, it should also be mentioned that there are various arguments against the monoamine hypothesis of depression (cf. Roth and Strüber 2021, 293 f.). For example, monoaminergic psychopharmaceuticals have a positive and long-lasting effect in only about one-third of patients. Moreover, an experimental withdrawal of serotonin causes a slight mood deterioration in depressed people and those at increased risk for this disorder, but healthy people do not react to it. Therefore, it is assumed, according to Hasler (2010), that a monoamine deficit is a secondary, "downstream" effect of other primary changes (cf. Hasler 2010, 155–161). A primary effect could be the alteration of the stress system. Depression is often accompanied by increased function of the HPA axis. The significant substances here are CRF, ACTH, and cortisol, with an overfunction of the stress system particularly affecting melancholic and psychotic depression. If cortisol release is increased, this could be the cause of various other changes in the brains of depressed individuals (cf. Roth and Strüber 2021, 294). Additionally, depression, especially in women, seems to be associated with reduced oxytocin concentration in the blood (cf. Carson et al. 2014, 30–36). However, it should be mentioned that not all studies come to the same conclusion. One possibility is that the form of depression plays a role here, as well as the question of whether psychopharmaceuticals were taken before the survey, as SSRIs stimulate serotonin receptors, which in turn leads to the release of oxytocin (cf. Roth and Strüber 2021, 294 f.). The significance of vasopressin for mood and behavior has already been explained in more detail, but it should now be noted that the vasopressin system is also altered in affective disorders such as depression and anxiety disorders. Depression and anxiety disorders are associated with excessive vasopressin function. This is particularly observed in patients with melancholic depression and patients with a suicide attempt. These individuals exhibit significantly increased synthesis and release of vasopressin. Since vasopressin can stimulate the stress axis, the increased vasopressin function may also be involved in the development of elevated cortisol levels (hypercortisolism). In depressed patients, this mechanism seems to be more pronounced than in healthy individuals. Likewise, endogenous opioids, which are associated with pleasure and joy and have a pain-inhibiting effect, are dysregulated in depressive disorders. This explains the high comorbidity of depression and pain disorders. Furthermore, dysregulation of the acetylcholine system, which is associated with nicotinic receptors, could explain why smoking is much more common among depressed patients than among healthy people, and quitting the addiction is accompanied by an increase in depressive symptoms (cf. Roth and Strüber 2021, 295 f.). Finally, the importance of adult neurogenesis should be mentioned once again. The formation of new nerve cells in the brain is also of particular importance in adulthood and occurs primarily in the hippocampus. However, depressive disorders are associated with a significant reduction in neurogenesis in the hippocampus. These deficits in neurogenesis can not only lead to a smaller hippocampal volume but also manifest in the difficulty depressed patients have in integrating new positive experiences into neural circuits and storing them as memories (cf. Roth and Strüber 2021, 296 f.). It is now believed that neurogenesis or the formation of new nerve cells has enormous significance for both mood and behavior of the individual (cf. Blackshaw and Lee 2012, 615–621). Additionally, stress should be mentioned once again, which is of enormous importance for the relationship between depression and neurogenesis, as experiencing stress leads to increased release of stress hormones, which inhibit neurogenesis and thus promote the development of depression (cf. Roth and Strüber2021, 298). Ultimately, it should be noted here that depression is a common psychiatric disorder associated with significant suffering, mortality, morbidity, and costs. Despite numerous treatment methods for severe depression, many affected individuals do not respond to traditional antidepressants, which is why more effective treatments for depression are needed. Targeting specific hormone systems is a concept-based approach that has already proven promising in treating this disorder. A number of hormones and hormone-manipulating compounds have been evaluated as monotherapies and as adjunct treatments. Some promising results have been shown in the search for new effective therapies for severe depression (cf. Aftab et al. 2020, Et al. 686–705). The significance of genes or predisposition and environmental factors for the development of depression will be explained below.

The Influence of Genes and Environment on the Development of Depression
Based on inheritance studies, it has been shown that individual genetic-epigenetic makeup plays an enormous role in the development of depression. First-degree relatives of a person with depression have a 2- to 4-fold increased risk of also developing depression compared to people without relatives with depression. This is especially true if it is an early-onset depression or a depression with recurrent episodes (cf. Roth and Strüber 2021, 298 f.). A connection between genetic factors and a depressive disorder is now undisputed (cf. Mattheisen 2018, 1). For example, the University Hospital of Würzburg, in a study led by Prof. Dr. Mattheisen, identified 44 gene loci associated with severe depression. Findings like these can serve as a foundation for even more efficient treatments for depression. "A gene locus refers to the exact location of a specific gene or genetic marker on a chromosome" (ibid.). Of these 44 identified gene loci, 30 were

described for the first time, and 14 had been discovered earlier. The result of this study clearly shows that individuals who combine a higher number of genetic risk factors also have an increased risk of developing depression. It is important to mention that many other (environmental) factors also play a role, but the findings of genetic correlations can open the door to exploring the biological causes of depression (cf. Mattheisen 2018, 1). Various gene variants have thus been associated with depression. The previously mentioned polymorphism of the serotonin transporter gene is one of them. For example, it is assumed that the S-variant of the gene promotes the development of depression, especially when this gene variant coincides with early or severe stress experiences, leading to a gene-environment interaction. The polymorphism affecting the gene for the 5-HT_{1A} receptor is also worth mentioning. This receptor can, on the one hand, act on the serotonergic cells themselves, leading to inhibition of serotonin release, and on the other hand, it occurs as a postsynaptic 5-HT_{1A} receptor or heteroreceptor on the target cells of serotonergic neurons. The gene for the 5-HT_{1A} receptor can exist in various alleles (cf. Roth and Strüber 2021, 298 f.). "The G-allele leads to increased expression of the 5-HT_{1A}autoreceptors, while the expression of the postsynaptic 5-HT_{1A}receptor is reduced" (ibid., 299). This results in less serotonin being released and the inhibitory and calming effect of serotonin in the target areas not being adequately effective. The target areas then tend to be overactive. Additionally, due to the complicated feedback loops, similar to a vicious cycle, the reduced serotonin release is maintained in the long term. The G-allele is found more frequently in affected individuals (cf. Roth and Strüber 2021, 299).

> "It is assumed that the reduced serotonin release observed in depression and the increased activity of the vmPFC in some patients are due to the presence of the G-allele" (ibid.).

Gene variants, such as those of the oxytocin receptor, also increase the risk of a depressive disorder (cf. Roth and Strüber 2021, 299).

Since, as already mentioned, medications and therapies are not effective for all patients, the need for research is still great. However, with related research efforts, it is possible to develop tools for the treatment of severe depression. Through these findings, for example, better predictions of therapy success are possible, and in the field of pharmacogenetics, these findings open up the possibility of predicting the response to therapies with antidepressants (cf. Mattheisen 2018, 1 f.). However, it should also be mentioned here that, in addition to genetic-epigenetic factors, environmental factors also have enormous significance. For example, early negative childhood experiences such as disturbances in mother-child interaction, physical and sexual abuse, experiencing natural disasters, or the loss of parents can promote the development of depression in adolescence and adulthood. In particular, disturbances in interpersonal relationships during childhood and adolescence have been shown to significantly increase the risk of developing depression. Additionally, the risk increases both through parental neglect and through maternal overprotection, and in children who experience their parents as unloving and highly controlling (cf. Benecke 2014, cited in Roth and Strüber 2021, 300). However, the permissive parental upbringing style (a highly tolerant, minimally controlling, and boundary-setting upbringing style) is more closely associated with depression than, for example, instability experienced in childhood and lack of continuity regarding primary caregivers. In contrast, individuals not affected by depression most frequently experienced an authoritative upbringing style, characterized on the one hand by control and authority and on the other hand by a loving response to the child's concerns and needs. Therefore, loving responsiveness is particularly important for healthy psychological development. But not only experiences in childhood can contribute to the development of depression; later environmental conditions can also increase the risk of developing depression. Here, for example, the death of a loved one, rape, divorce, prolonged unemployment, a low level of education, a chronically low income, and above all, the lack of trustworthy personal relationships should be mentioned. The presence of close relationships, on the other hand, can be noted as a protective factor against the development of depression. In the development of depression based on negative experiences, gene-environment interactions are usually to be expected. Early stress experiences can trigger epigenetic changes, which in turn lead to genes no longer being expressed (not "translated" into proteins) to the normal extent. Additionally, it should be mentioned in this context that these epigenetic changes can be passed on to the next generation. In contrast to gene variants that promote depression, those variants that convey resilience to stress should also be mentioned. In individuals with such a genetic makeup, experiencing early childhood stress has no negative impact on mental health but, in the best case, promotes the development of a strong personality (cf. Roth and Strüber 2021, 300 ff.).

Yoshimura notes that a possible path to depression could lead through experiencing significant and unavoidable stress during early childhood. This experience causes an increased release of cortisol and thereby an altered formation of cortisol receptors. This, in turn, can affect feedback regulation and result in a long-term increased release of cortisol. This can have further effects on the brain and psyche. This includes, on the one hand, an inhibition of neurogenesis, which can result in a reduced volume of the hippocampus and basal ganglia as well as possibly a reduced ability to adapt behavior to current circumstances. On the other hand, the increased release of cortisol can impair the formation of 5-HT_{1A} receptors and thereby cause a reduced inhibitory effect of serotonin on the limbic cortex areas. An increased tendency to persistently focus on one's own emotional state could be the result (cf. Yoshimura et al. 2017, 610–614). The reduced ability to change behavior and to leave the emotional state can form the basis for the development of a depressive episode (cf. Roth and Strüber 2021, 305).

In summary, it should be noted here that, in addition to the individual genetic-epigenetic makeup of people, stress experiences promote the development of depression. This involves uncontrollable or unavoidable stress. Since depressive disorders are based on such heterogeneity, a comprehensive model of action is not available. Ultimately, it is important to note that not all forms of depression are equally affected by all changes, and neurobiological changes not discussed here may also play a role (cf. Roth and Strüber 2021, 302).

2.7.3 Anxiety Disorders

Having anxiety disorders means experiencing states of excessive fear or anxiety (cf. Roth and Strüber 2021, 306). According to ICD-10, anxiety disorders are divided into 2 groups: phobic disorders (phobia), consisting of agoraphobia (without or with panic disorder), social phobias, and specific (isolated) phobias, and other anxiety disorders, which include the following types: panic disorder (episodic paroxysmal anxiety), mixed anxiety and depressive disorder, generalized anxiety disorder, and mixed other anxiety disorder (cf. Morschitzky 2000, 34 f.). In phobic disorders, the emotions are related to specific environmental situations, whereas in panic disorders or generalized anxiety, the anxiety itself is the focus (cf. Roth and Strüber 2021, 306).

Phobic Disorders

Phobic disorders describe an unfounded, exaggerated, and above all, persistent fear of objects, activities, people, or situations. The patients perceive the fear as uncontrollable, and even though they are aware of the groundlessness of their fears, they still avoid the triggers. There are various forms of phobias. They are divided into three main groups: agoraphobia, social phobias, and specific phobias (for example, acrophobia = fear of heights or arachnophobia = fear of spiders), whereby it must be mentioned that in DSM-5, agoraphobia is categorized as a separate disorder. The term phobia is a generic term, as the individual diverse phobic fears are not understood as independent disorders. They are integrated into the three main groups (cf. Schäffler 2022, n.p.). In phobic disorders, the fear is triggered by (mainly harmless) situations such as social situations, the use of means of transport, the prospect of a ride in an elevator, or the encounter with even a small spider (cf. Roth and Strüber 2021, 306).

- **Social Phobia**

> Social phobia is the "second most common anxiety disorder with a lifetime prevalence of 8–10%" (Schäffler 2022, n.p.).

Social phobia, also referred to as social anxiety disorder, is a common and severe illness that usually begins in adolescence. In addition to the performance pressure associated with the illness, many patients suffer from comorbidity with addiction disorders. Furthermore, the illness is associated with an increased suicide rate (cf. Bandelow and Wedekind 2014, n.p.).

> "Characteristic of social phobia is the exaggerated and unrealistic fear of being negatively evaluated by other people" (Bandelow and Wedekind 2014, n.p.).

Patients often report significant self-doubt and insecurities regarding social interactions, especially with strangers. Like other anxiety disorders, social phobia can also trigger psychosomatic symptoms such as irritable bowel syndrome, flushing, sweating, tachycardia, nausea, and urinary urgency. The symptoms can intensify to the point of panic attacks and, in extreme cases, lead to complete social isolation. Many affected individuals suffer from addiction problems and depressive symptoms, possibly in connection with suicidal thoughts. This illness can thus massively impair patients in both their social and professional habits (cf. Roth and Strüber 2021, 306). Various forms of cognitive behavioral therapy (CBT) have proven effective in treatment or have been shown to be effective in studies. In pharmacological therapy, serotonin reuptake inhibitors (SSRIs) and selective serotonin-norepinephrine reuptake inhibitors (SNRIs) are recommended (cf. Bandelow and Wedekind 2014, n.p.).

- **Agoraphobia**

Agoraphobia is the most common anxiety disorder with a lifetime prevalence of about 5% (cf. Schäffler 2022, n.p.).

It is the anxiety disorder that occurs when affected individuals are in a public or crowded place—places where a quick escape, especially without help, is difficult (cf. Balaram and Marwaha 2023, n.p.). There is a fear of leaving the house alone, being in crowds, being in public places, or using public transportation (cf. Roth and Strüber 2021, 307). This illness is characterized by the fact that affected individuals experience panic attacks in the mentioned situations or that panic-like symptoms occur. Agoraphobics therefore strive to avoid such crowded places or situations (cf. Balaram and Marwaha 2023, n.p.). Therefore, after some time, affected individuals increasingly tend to avoid public life, which is why they rarely leave their homes (cf. Spektrum Lexikon der Neurowissenschaft 2000f, n.p.). Agoraphobia is considered an independent diagnosis, which can occur independently of other diagnoses such as generalized anxiety disorder. However, to meet the criteria for the diagnosis, affected individuals must not only fear public places but also avoid these situations. Additionally, the criteria must be present for longer than 6 months (cf. Balaram and Marwaha 2023, n.p.). Commonly described symptoms include, for example, palpitations, sweating, tightness, shortness of breath, trembling, dizziness, nausea, and weakness. The symptoms can begin harmlessly and, due to the increasingly perceived threat and rising fear, the complaints intensify. Genes play a significant role in the development of this anxiety disorder. It is assumed that the illness is almost 50% hereditary (cf. Spektrum – Psychische Störungen 2014a, n.p.).

- **Panic Disorders**

Panic disorders consist of the repeated occurrence of spontaneous and unexpected panic attacks (cf. Morschitzky 2000, 34 f.). However, the anxiety here is not related to a specific environmental situation, but rather there are recurring severe and unpredictable attacks. Such an attack is characterized by intense and nameless fear (cf. Roth and Strüber 2021, 307). These recurring and unexpected panic attacks are to be described as sudden and intense surges of fear with symptoms such as shortness of breath, palpitations, nausea, dizziness, chest pain, and fear of death (cf. Balaram and Marwaha 2023, n.p.). Panic attacks can also be associated with other psychological and physical disorders, such as thyroid dysfunctions or depression. Likewise, heart diseases can cause the mentioned symptoms (cf. Spektrum – Psychische Störungen 2014b, n.p.).

> "Around two to three percent of all Germans suffer from a panic disorder at least once in their lives, with or without agoraphobia, and around six percent experience a panic attack at least once in their lives. Women are about twice as likely to be affected as men" (ibid.).

If the disorder is not treated, it lasts for over 7 years in 80% of those affected. Between the panic attacks, there can be long symptom-free phases, as they vary depending on stress and strain. The concern of those affected about another panic attack contributes to the chronicity of the disorder. Increasingly frequent panic attacks can lead to social withdrawal. There is a tendency to stay in one's own home as a safe environment. The guiding principle of action is a constant fear that something bad might happen. This often leads to the "fear of fear." This social withdrawal can ultimately lead to agoraphobia (cf. Spektrum – Psychische Störungen 2014b, n.p.).

- **Generalized Anxiety Disorder**

Generalized anxiety disorder (GAD) is considered a common and serious condition, where the worries of those affected, which relate to real dangers, are the focus. However, both the risk of occurrence and the negative consequences are greatly overestimated (cf. Bandelow et al. 2013, n.p.). GAD is often accompanied by restlessness, irritability, nervousness, difficulty concentrating, muscle tension, easy fatigability, and sleep disturbances. Even everyday life circumstances such as household management, health, being late for an appointment, and concern for family members, professional responsibility, and income cause excessive worries. Patients find it difficult to control these worries; the worries also distract them from current activities that actually require their attention (cf. Roth and Strüber 2021, 307 f.). The worries can quickly generalize to numerous areas. Consequently, a behavior of reassurance and avoidance emerges, which is why activities or trips considered dangerous are postponed or avoided. The fears then lead to typical physical expressions of anxiety (cf. Bandelow et al. 2013, n.p.).

"Diagnosis of generalized anxiety disorder according to ICD-10:

- Tension, worry, and fears related to everyday events and problems for at least six months, with the following findings:
  - vegetative symptoms such as increased heart rate, sweating, tremor, or dry mouth
  - symptoms in the chest or abdomen (breathing difficulties, feeling of tightness, chest pain, abdominal discomfort)

- psychological symptoms (dizziness, derealization, fear of losing control, fear of dying)
- general symptoms (hot flashes or chills, paresthesia)
- symptoms of tension (muscle tension, restlessness, lump in the throat)
- other nonspecific symptoms (exaggerated startle response, difficulty concentrating, irritability, sleep disturbances)" (Bandelow et al. 2013, n.p.).

In terms of differential diagnosis, neurological diseases, internal medical conditions, and other psychological disorders, particularly anxiety disorders, must also be delineated. In individuals with GAD, there is a comorbidity with depression of 40–67%. If, in addition to feelings of anxiety, symptoms such as suicidal ideation, diurnal variations, feelings of guilt, etc., are also present, it must be checked whether depression is the primary condition. Regarding treatment, various forms of cognitive behavioral therapy (CBT) have proven effective in supervised studies. The focus here is on psychoeducation, various cognitive strategies, exposure, emotion regulation (e.g., muscle relaxation techniques), and problem-solving techniques (cf. Bandelow et al. 2013, n.p.). As with other anxiety disorders, traumatic life experiences, faulty conditioning, neurobiological dysfunctions, and genetic influences are discussed as causes. Twin studies have found a moderate hereditary factor, which is, however, less pronounced than in other anxiety disorders such as panic disorder. Neurobiological changes associated with GAD include disturbances in the serotonin system, the adrenergic system, or GABA binding. Abnormalities were also found in the amygdala, the dorsomedial prefrontal cortex, and other areas (cf. ibid.).

Neurobiological Changes and Psychoneuroendocrinological Insights in Anxiety Disorders

> "Etiology, symptomatology, and course of anxiety disorders are to be explained as multicausal" (Ehlert 2006, n.p.).

Neurobiologically, it is clear that the amygdala represents the central structure for the experience of fear and anxiety. As already described, it is responsible, with specialized neural networks, for recognizing potentially threatening environmental stimuli and aligning behavior accordingly. If an environmental stimulus is associated with danger based on a previously established fear conditioning, the basolateral amygdala receives information about the perceived stimuli. From the central nucleus of the amygdala, the hypothalamus and brainstem are activated, where the actual affective and vegetative fear reaction is then triggered. Symptoms such as rising blood pressure, palpitations, and sweaty hands are typical here (cf. Roth and Strüber 2021, 308), although it should be mentioned that the amygdala does not merely react to fear or fear-associated stimuli but also to other emotionally arousing, surprising, and significant, yet positively connoted stimuli. Likewise, the medial prefrontal cortex, including the anterior cingulate cortex, is significant in the context of fear conditioning. It is active in learning fear, through observation as well as in response to emotional stimuli. The insular cortex is stimulated by negative stimuli such as sadness and is then active. These structures are also activated by emotions, stimuli, and information from other people (for example, through photographs of emotional faces). In connection with anxiety disorders, these mentioned brain structures are often overly active. However, differences can be observed in anxiety disorders. For example, in social phobia, increased amygdala activity is noticeable, which occurs, for instance, when speaking in public. An overfunction of limbic cortical areas has also been measured. The ventral striatum, which includes the nucleus accumbens, is less active in social phobia when one has to speak in public. In panic disorder, overfunction in the limbic brain areas and particularly in the amygdala, thalamus, and periaqueductal gray (PAG) is observed. In generalized anxiety disorder (GAD), however, the state of knowledge is not as clear. There are indications of both increased amygdala activity and increased activity of the limbic medial cortex and the lateral prefrontal cortex. Furthermore, in GAD, there is a reduced hypothalamus volume (cf. Roth and Strüber 2021, 308 f.). As already mentioned, anxiety disorders can only be explained as multicausal. A partial aspect of psychobiological explanatory approaches is endocrine abnormalities, through which certain subtypes of pathological anxiety can be characterized. In particular, the HPA axis and the sympathoadrenomedullary system are associated with emotion regulation and pathological anxiety. Both hormone systems are of enormous importance in adapting to individual stress situations and thus sustainably influence the psychobiological adaptation to anxiety-inducing situations, according to Ehlert. Endocrine dysregulations of the HPA axis and the sympathoadrenomedullary system therefore play a significant role in various subtypes of anxiety disorders in connection with genetic findings (cf. Ehlert 2006, 165–175). A dysregulation of the serotonergic system is, for example, characteristic not only of depression but also of anxiety disorders. This leads to both diseases exhibiting numerous overlapping symptoms. However, not all forms of anxiety disorder are equally affected by the dysregulation of the serotonergic system. Particularly, patients with social phobia, panic disorders, and people with PTSD suffer from serotonergic underfunction (cf. Roth and Strüber 2021, 310). Regarding oxytocin, the plasma concentration in people with social phobia seems to differ little compared to healthy individuals, but the administration of oxytocin (OXY) appears to have a positive effect on brain function in anxiety patients. However, OXY cannot yet be used as a therapeutic agent in the treatment of anxiety disorders, as animal models show that chronic administration of OXY can also have the opposite effect and thus increase anxiety (cf. Neumann et al. 2014, 225–236). Additionally, a reduced availability of serotonin and norepinephrine has been identified as a risk factor for panic disorders (cf. Domschke et al. 2017, n.p.).

The Influence of Genes and Environment on the Development of Anxiety Disorders
Only 30% of patients suffering from anxiety disorders respond inadequately or not at all to pharmacotherapeutic and psychotherapeutic interventions. In light of this therapy

resistance rate, research efforts are aimed at identifying risk markers for the pathogenesis of anxiety disorders as well as for non-response to therapeutic interventions. The following findings are intended to promote effective preventive measures as well as individualized and innovative therapeutic approaches. Genetic and epigenetic markers are of importance here (cf. Domschke 2014, 1263–1268).

Anxiety disorders are favored by temperament traits, particularly neuroticism and inhibited behavior. This finding suggests that genes and very early experiences play a significant role in the later development of anxiety disorders (cf. Roth and Strüber 2021, 311). Family studies show that first-degree relatives of panic patients have an approximately 3- to 5-fold increased risk of illness compared to the general population. Heritability is also evident in generalized anxiety disorders and specific phobias (cf. Domschke et al. 2017, n.p.).

> "(…) the proportion of genetic factors in the development of a disorder is up to 48 percent for panic disorder, heritability rates for generalized anxiety disorder and specific phobias are around 30 percent, for social phobia 51 percent, for blood-injection phobia 59 percent, and for agoraphobia 67 percent, with the remaining variance explained by individual environmental factors such as life events" (Domschke et al. 2017, n.p.).

Furthermore, anxiety disorders and depression may have common genetic foundations, with the individual clinical picture being shaped by the respective environmental conditions. For example, the S-allele of the serotonin transporter polymorphism is associated not only with depression but also with GAD, social phobia, general anxiety, and on the neurobiological side with increased amygdala activity (cf. Roth and Strüber 2021, 312). Regarding environmental factors, risk-increasing environmental factors include critical life events shortly before the onset of the disorder, such as deaths, separations/divorces, illnesses/injuries, or financial problems, as well as stressful life events during childhood, such as emotional and/or physical abuse, sexual violence, and emotional and/or physical neglect (cf. Domschke and Schiele 2017, n.p.). Early separation from parents and parental overprotection are also among the involved environmental risks (cf. Roth and Strüber 2021, 312). In addition to the S-allele, the T-risk allele of the neuropeptide S receptor gene *(*NPSR1*)* also appears to be associated with stressful childhood experiences. They are also associated with recently experienced traumatic events, which also increase the risk of heightened anxiety sensitivity and thus the risk of anxiety disorders (cf. Domschke and Schiele 2017, n.p.), with panic disorders being more strongly associated with early abuse, and factors such as parental separation, lack of parental warmth, or parental overprotection seeming to favor agoraphobia. A specific phobia is usually preceded by a traumatic encounter with the feared stimulus. Agoraphobia can also result from an assault. The months before the first panic attack were usually marked by stressful situations such as deaths in the family, interpersonal stress, or illnesses (cf. Roth and Strüber 2021, 312 f.).

The pathogenesis of anxiety disorders is thus clearly multifactorial and involves complex interactions between psychological mechanisms, biological factors, and environmental influences (cf. Domschke and Schiele 2017, n.p.). However, based on (epi)genetic findings and psychoneuroendocrinological insights, individually tailored and targeted therapeutic interventions can lead to faster treatment success and a significant reduction in the suffering time of patients (cf. Domschke et al. 2017, n.p.).

2.7.4 Obsessive-Compulsive Disorder

Obsessive-compulsive disorders are referred to as conditions characterized by obsessive thoughts and/or compulsive actions. Obsessive ideas are understood as actions and impulses to act, against whose occurrence the affected individuals struggle in vain. However, compulsive phenomena belong to one's own self, yet they are mostly experienced as nonsensical and threatening. Obsessive symptoms can also occur in connection with other mental illnesses (cf. Laszig and Rieg 2004, 418). The diagnosis of an obsessive-compulsive disorder is made when the compulsions are distressing and time-consuming or severely restrict the patients in professional and social areas. When obsessive thoughts are predominant, this is often referred to as obsessive rumination. In this case, it happens that the affected individuals weigh the pros and cons of alternatives in a distressing endless loop but cannot make everyday decisions in life. Additionally, exaggerated fears of, for example, infection with disease or fire can dominate the thoughts. Compulsive actions and rituals are often characterized by exaggerated orderliness, cleanliness, and control behavior. Examples of this include washing hands after every touch, checking six times whether the stove is really turned off, and arranging certain objects symmetrically repeatedly to avert possible threats. Such compulsive actions have the background of reducing the anxiety that accompanies the obsessive thoughts. Moreover, many patients with an obsessive-compulsive disorder exhibit maladaptive beliefs, such as an exaggerated sense of responsibility, a tendency to overestimate dangers, perfectionism, and strong risk aversion (cf. Roth and Strüber 2021, 318 f.). The course of obsessive-compulsive disorders is often described as chronic. The symptoms of the condition can fluctuate significantly. The obsessive symptoms can also change over time, with it being important to mention that the complaints increase under general stress exposure. Long-term studies show that 83% of patients showed some form of improvement in symptoms and social functioning within 40 years, but only 20% of patients achieved complete remission. Additionally, it seems that an initially intermittent course is associated with a better prognosis than a chronic course from the beginning. Particularly in men, where the onset of the condition occurs before the age of 20, there is a higher risk of unfavorable courses. A low social status also worsens the prognosis (cf. Kathmann et al. 2022, 2). A major problem of this condition is the high tendency towards suicide. Up to 50% of those affected experience suicidal thoughts at some point, and a quarter attempt suicide. The risk of suicide is particularly high when there is comorbidity with a depressive disorder. Within obsessive-compulsive disorder, a distinction is made between obsessive-compulsive disorder (OCD) and obsessive-compulsive personality disorder (anankastic personality disorder, "obsessive-compulsive personality disorder"). Obsessive-compulsive personality disorder is not characterized by compulsive actions or thoughts; rather, the entire personality is marked by exaggerated conscientiousness, doubt, constant checking, perfectionism, caution, rigidity, and stubbornness. Unwanted, persistent thoughts can occur but are not as severe as in obsessive-compulsive disorder (cf. Roth and Strüber 2021, 319). Additionally, obsessive-compulsive disorders can often occur in childhood and adolescence. The disorder's symptomatology impairs their quality of life, yet the condition is often recognized late (cf. Jans et al. 2011, n.p.).

According to ICD-10 (Jans et al. 2011, n.p.), the following symptoms are crucial for both adults and children and adolescents:

- Compulsions must be recognizable to the patient as their own thoughts or impulses.
- At least one of these compulsions is resisted.
- The obsessive symptoms are not experienced as relaxing in themselves.
- The compulsions repeat in an unpleasant manner, and the patients are significantly impaired.

The treatment of obsessive-compulsive disorders must be specific and as early as possible to avoid chronicity. According to the guidelines for obsessive-compulsive disorders, the first-choice therapy is particularly cognitive behavioral therapy (CBT) with exposure and response management. Pharmacotherapy with serotonin reuptake inhibitors is only recommended if CBT does not work adequately, is not available, is rejected by the affected individuals, or the disorder is so severe that CBT with exposure is not feasible. Despite evidence-based treatment options, the treatment usually does not lead to complete remission but only to an improvement, whereby it must be mentioned that the proportion of treatment-resistant chronic courses is very high. Comorbidities such as PTSD or severe personality disorders also play a significant role here. Currently, the influence of the COVID-19 pandemic must also be mentioned, as many affected individuals suffer from contamination fears, which are associated with exaggerated cleaning rituals and frequent hand washing and disinfecting. After the first lockdown, 394 British patients with obsessive-compulsive disorders were surveyed about the consequences of the pandemic for the disorder. Of these, 72% reported that their obsessive-compulsive symptoms definitely increased during the pandemic. Particularly those affected with washing compulsions reacted with an increase in symptoms. Additionally, the patients felt more like experts in advising others on infection prophylaxis but reported receiving negative feedback from others for this. The negative effects of the pandemic were also evident not only in patients with obsessive-compulsive disorders but also in patients suffering from depression, anxiety disorders, or eating disorders (cf. Favreau et al. 2021, 27–31).

Neurobiological Changes and Psychoneuroendocrinological Insights in Obsessive-Compulsive Disorders

Neurobiologically, the dorsal and ventral loops of the basal ganglia seem to be particularly affected in obsessive-compulsive disorders. This means that the feedback pathways originating from the cortex via the striatum, pallidum, and thalamus are affected. Especially the ventral loop shows changes. These mentioned structures are more active in people with obsessive-compulsive disorders both at rest and when symptoms occur. It appears that individual symptoms are each tied to a pattern of changes. For example, patients suffering from washing compulsions have, in addition to changes in prefrontal regions, a reduced volume of gray matter in the basal ganglia. In contrast, those affected by control compulsions have a reduced volume of white and gray matter in the lower inner temporal lobe. The amygdala and hippocampus are located here (cf. Graybiel and Rauch 2000, 343–347). It is important to mention here that the functions of the ventral loop include "unlocking" certain situation-appropriate actions while simultaneously suppressing inappropriate action alternatives (cf. Roth and Strüber 2021, 320). The loops are involved in building motor and cognitive habits. In obsessive-compulsive disorders, errors seem to occur here, as the disorder prevents constantly repetitive, habitual compulsive actions and thoughts from being suppressed when they are inappropriate (cf. Graybiel and Rauch 2000, 343–347). Additionally, Roth notes that considering the calming function of serotonin and the motivating function of dopamine, it is plausible that this disorder is also associated with altered function of these two systems. A reduced function of a specific class of serotonin receptors in various areas of the prefrontal cortex has been found, as well as indications of increased dopaminergic function in the striatum. This could also contribute to the inability of these patients to resist inappropriate action impulses. Furthermore, some findings support the assumption that serotonergic and dopaminergic excitation processing is faulty in obsessive-compulsive disorders. For example, treatment with serotonin reuptake inhibitors can be successful (cf. Roth and Strüber 2021, 321). The oxytocin system also seems to be linked or involved in this disorder, as the gene for the oxytocin receptor is increasingly methylated in affected individuals. The more pronounced the obsessive-compulsive disorder, the more strongly this gene is methylated (cf. Cappi et al. 2016, 79).

The Influence of Genes and Environment on the Development of Obsessive-Compulsive Disorders

Obsessive-compulsive disorders, like anxiety disorders, are also associated with temperament traits such as neuroticism and behavioral inhibition. It has been shown that adults suffering from an obsessive-compulsive disorder tended to exhibit anxious, withdrawn behavior and negative emotionality in childhood and were more socially isolated than other children. First-degree relatives of affected individuals have a twofold increased risk of developing this disorder as well. However, if the obsessive-compulsive disorder already appeared in close relatives during childhood or adolescence, the risk is increased tenfold. Twin studies indicate that not only the experiences with compulsive parents play a role, but genetic factors also contribute, as identical twins show a greater concordance in the development of compulsions than fraternal twins. Both certain variants of the serotonin transporter gene and genetic variants of other components of the serotonergic and dopaminergic systems can increase the risk of developing this disorder. However, it should be mentioned that the contribution of individual genetic variants is only minor, and only the cumulative effect of various genes leads to an increased disease risk. Physical or sexual abuse in childhood increases the risk of developing an obsessive-compulsive disorder, and traumatic or highly stressful experiences in childhood also lead to an increased risk of developing this disorder. Physical abuse, for example, is associated with a sevenfold increased likelihood. The attachment status can also be of enormous importance, as adolescents with an obsessive-compulsive disorder predominantly exhibit an insecure-avoidant status (cf. Roth and Strüber 2021, 321 f.).

2.7.5 Borderline Personality Disorder

> "A personality disorder is present when the inner experience or behavior deviates long-term from societal norms starting from adolescence or early adulthood and leads to significant problems in social behavior and partnerships" (Roth and Strüber 2021, 322).

Even though personality and behavioral disorders are different diagnoses and exhibit clear differences, there are still similar behavior patterns, particularly concerning lifestyle and the relationship to oneself and others (cf. ibid.). Marsha Linehan first provided scientific evidence of the effectiveness of dialectical behavior therapy (DBT) in 1991 and, based on her own experiences, declared borderline personality disorder (BPD) as a profound disorder of emotion regulation. Therefore, DBT also focused on improving skills in stress tolerance and emotion regulation. This groundbreaking approach significantly contributed to the foundation of neurobiological research (cf. Bohus 2019, 3). BPD is an emotionally unstable personality disorder of the borderline type (cf. Roth and Strüber 2021, 323). BPD (or "border personality disorder," BPD) is characterized by extreme sensitivity to perceived interpersonal slights, an unstable sense of self, intense and fleeting emotionality, and impulsive behavior, which is often self-destructive. Most patients experience symptomatic remission over time. The remission rate can be accelerated by evidence-based psychosocial treatments. Despite the gradually decreasing crisis susceptibility and the reduction of self-injurious behavior, the natural course usually leaves lasting severe social impairments associated with depression or self-injurious behavior. Therefore, it is of enormous importance in therapies to address issues of interpersonal relationships and unstable identity. However, it is important to mention that patients with BPD are often not correctly diagnosed, which in turn leads to inadequate pharmacological interventions that are rarely successful (cf. Gunderson et al. 2018, n.p.).

The diagnostic criteria according to DSM-5, which were adopted by ICD-11, are as follows:

A. "A persistent pattern of inner experience and behavior that markedly deviates from the expectations of the individual's culture. This pattern is manifested in at least two of the following areas:

   1. Cognition (i.e., ways of perceiving and interpreting self, other people, and events).

   .

   2. Affectivity (i.e., the range, intensity, lability, and appropriateness of emotional response).
   3. Interpersonal functioning.
   4. Impulse control.
   5. The enduring pattern is inflexible and pervasive across a broad range of personal and social situations.

B. The enduring pattern leads to clinically significant distress or impairment in social, occupational, or other important areas of functioning.
C. The pattern is stable and of long duration, and its onset can be traced back at least to adolescence or early adulthood.
D. The enduring pattern is not better explained as a manifestation or consequence of another mental disorder.
E. The enduring pattern is not attributable to the physiological effects of a substance (e.g., a drug of abuse, a medication) or another medical condition (e.g., head trauma)" (Bohus 2019, 4).

In a second step, the subtype is specified:

"A pervasive pattern of instability in interpersonal relationships, self-image, and affects, and marked impulsivity. The onset is in early adulthood and the pattern is present in a variety of contexts. At least five of the following criteria must be met:

1. Frantic efforts to avoid real or imagined abandonment. (Note: Do not include suicidal or self-mutilating behavior covered in Criterion 5.)
2. A pattern of unstable and intense interpersonal relationships characterized by alternating between extremes of idealization and devaluation.
3. Identity disturbance: markedly and persistently unstable self-image or sense of self.
4. Impulsivity in at least two areas that are potentially self-damaging (e.g., spending, sex, substance abuse, reckless driving, binge eating). (Note: Do not include suicidal or self-mutilating behavior covered in Criterion 5.)
5. Recurrent suicidal behavior, gestures, or threats, or self-mutilating behavior.
6. Affective instability due to a marked reactivity of mood (e.g., intense episodic dysphoria, irritability, or anxiety usually lasting a few hours and only rarely more than a few days).
7. Chronic feelings of emptiness.
8. Inappropriate, intense anger or difficulty controlling anger (e.g., frequent displays of temper, constant anger, recurrent physical fights).

9. Transient, stress-related paranoid ideation or severe dissociative symptoms" (Bohus 2019, 5).

In summary, it should be noted here that affected individuals are constantly internally tense and have great difficulty regulating their emotions. The subjective level of suffering is extremely high, and their relationships with their partners are often intense and at the same time unstable. However, they have a great fear of being abandoned and being alone. Additionally, they tend to alternately idealize and devalue their partners (cf. Roth and Strüber 2021, 323). BPD patients are attributed with a great need for attention, with some achieving this through clothing and others through positive means such as art, music, or acting. They have a reduced tolerance for frustration and are unable to delay gratification, which is why affected individuals often prematurely terminate their schooling or vocational training (cf. Bandelow et al. 2010, 623–636). BPD is found in approximately 1.7% of the general population and in 15–28% of patients in psychiatric clinics (cf. Gunderson et al. 2018, n.p.). The disorder is associated with pronounced psychosocial impairments. There is also a significant suicide rate of up to 10% among those affected. Furthermore, BPD has a high comorbidity with other disorders such as depression, PTSD, social phobias, obsessive-compulsive disorders, drug addiction, and other mental disorders and behavioral disturbances (cf. Bohus et al. 2004, 453–461). The symptoms usually decrease with increasing age, yet a tendency towards impulsivity and intense, unstable relationships remains. BPD is particularly diagnosed in women (cf. Bader et al. 2013, cited in Roth and Strüber 2021, 324).

Neurobiological Changes and Psychoneuroendocrinological Insights in Borderline Personality Disorder

In BPD, imaging studies show a reduced volume of the hippocampus, amygdala, as well as the orbitofrontal and anterior cingulate cortex, which can be up to a quarter of the normal volume. A reduced volume of the hippocampus is also seen in other disorders such as PTSD, but a reduction in the amygdala and limbic cortical areas is relatively specific to BPD. However, it should be noted that in adolescents with newly diagnosed BPD, no volume reduction of the hippocampus and amygdala is found, which means that this reduction only occurs in the course of the disease. The volume of the right orbitofrontal cortex, however, is already reduced in adolescents. When confronted with emotional stimuli, the activity of the amygdala is increased in people with BPD. The difficulties in controlling emotions and impulses seem to stem from changes in brain activity in the ventromedial, prefrontal, and orbitofrontal cortex areas as well as the hippocampus (cf. Bader et al. 2013, cited in Roth and Strüber 2021, 324 f.). Additionally, BPD is associated with malfunctions of various neuromodulatory systems, such as the serotonergic and dopaminergic systems, as well as the opioid, oxytocin, and vasopressin systems. In affected women, reduced oxytocin concentrations in blood plasma can also be found, and it should be mentioned that the OXY level in cerebrospinal fluid, urine, or plasma is demonstrably negatively correlated with childhood trauma (plasma oxytocin especially with abuse and emotional neglect), aggressive behavior, and suicide attempts. Thus, it is assumed that the oxytocin system plays an outstanding role in BPD, as BPD is characterized by (para)suicidal behavior and aggressiveness and is closely related to traumatic experiences in childhood (cf. Bertsch et al. 2013, 424–429). Furthermore, reduced OXY release can impair the recognition of social cues, the assessment of others' emotional states, the building of trust, and the ability to form close bonds. Additionally, increased vasopressin concentration can lead to increased irritability and aggression in interpersonal interactions (cf. Roth and Strüber 2021, 326). In addition to the dysfunctions of several neurotransmitter systems, including serotonergic and dopaminergic systems, the sensitivity of opioid receptors and the availability of opioids are also mentioned as part of the pathophysiology of BPD (cf. Bandelow et al. 2018, n.p.).

> "The alarming symptoms and self-destructive behaviors of affected patients can be explained by uncontrollable and unconscious attempts to stimulate their endogenous opioid system (EOS) and the dopaminergic reward system, regardless of the possible harmful consequences" (Bandelow et al. 2018, n.p.).

The frantic efforts to avoid abandonment, frequent and risky sexual contacts, as well as attention-seeking behavior, can also be explained by the fact that the EOS (opioid system) mediates the rewarding effect of human bonding. Anhedonia and the feeling of emptiness can also be expressions of reduced EOS activity. Additionally, affected individuals tend to abuse substances that target μ-opioid receptors (cf. ibid.).

> "Self-injury, food restriction, aggressive behavior, and sensation seeking can be interpreted as desperate attempts to artificially put the body into survival mode to mobilize the last reserves of the EOS" (Bandelow et al. 2018, n.p.).

The assumption that self-injurious behavior leads to increased opioid release and the effect on particularly sensitive opioid receptors explains the fact that the injuries are hardly perceived as painful and that rather a sense of well-being up to euphoria is triggered (cf. Roth and Strüber 2021, 327).

The Influence of Genes and Environment on the Development of Borderline Personality Disorder

The previously mentioned neurobiological changes in BPD patients can be both genetically determined, a direct consequence of early emotional trauma, and an effect of increased activity in stress-associated neurobiological systems (cf. Bandelow et al. 2018, n.p.). The fact that people whose first-degree relatives have BPD have a fivefold increased risk of developing this disorder themselves compared to the general population points to a significant genetic-epigenetic basis for this condition (cf. Roth and Strüber 2021, 327). According to a large twin study, 69% of the variance is based on genetic factors, although it is not yet clear why patients with such an increased genetic risk for BPD also seem to have an increased risk for traumatic events in childhood. However, these factors are obviously interconnected. If parents of BPD patients also had symptoms of this disorder, there is a higher likelihood of their limited parenting skills. This can be based on drug abuse, frequent absence (due to hospital stays), unfavorable social and family environmental conditions, as well as a tendency towards sexual deviations (cf. Bandelow et al. 2018, n.p.). Since the oxytocin and opioid systems are dysregulated in affected individuals, it is suspected that polymorphisms in these two systems are involved in the development of BPD (cf. Roth and Strüber 2021, 328).

In addition to the significant genetic predisposition, environmental influence is also substantial for the development of BPD. It is evident that BPD patients very often experienced sexual abuse or other traumatic events in early childhood, namely in 74% of all cases. Among healthy individuals, this rate is 6%, yet it is also significantly higher compared to individuals with other mental disorders. Mental illnesses of family members, especially those with depression, anxiety disorders, and suicide, as well as parental separation and parents with less caring parenting methods, also favor the development of BPD. Only 6% of borderline patients do not report such negative experiences (cf. Bandelow et al. 2005, 169–179). Early negative attachment experiences also influence the development of BPD. This can be either a disorganized or an insecure-ambivalent attachment disorder. The disorganized attachment experience is particularly significant, as it is characterized by contradictory tendencies of approach and withdrawal, which is also characteristic of BPD. Additionally, 80% of all children of mothers with BPD develop a disorganized attachment disorder, which in turn increases the risk that the child will develop borderline disorder. Whether the child develops a disorganized attachment through the relationship with a traumatized mother and is thus predisposed to BPD depends, however, on the child's disposition (cf. Roth and Strüber 2021, 328 f.).

2.7.6 Antisocial Personality Disorder and Psychopathy

First, it should be mentioned that antisocial personality disorder (ASPD) is referred to as dissocial personality disorder in the ICD-10 classification system. However, since many of the studies presented here are based on the American DSM-5 classification system, the term antisocial personality disorder (ASPD) is used (cf. Roth and Strüber 2021, 330).

Patients with APS regularly disregard and violate the rights of other people. This is particularly evident in illegal behavior, lying and cheating for their own advantage or pleasure, lack of planning ahead, impulsivity, irritability, and aggressiveness. Similarly, disregard for their own safety and the safety of others, irresponsible behavior, for example at work, and especially a lack of remorse are frequently observed. Instead, the affected individuals react with indifference and rationalize their actions. To make this diagnosis, 3 of the mentioned characteristics must appear from the age of 15 (cf. Spektrum – Psychische Störungen 2014, n.p.). This is because individuals who develop APS in adulthood already stand out before the age of 15 due to a conduct disorder. They often show aggression towards people and animals as children, are deceitful, steal, destroy others' property, or disregard the normal rules of coexistence. Typical impairments of emotional functions are observed in people with APS. They not only tend to blame others but also offer explanations such as: "He deserved it." Additionally, patients have an exaggerated and arrogant self-assessment, are overly argumentative, conceited, and self-confident. Some of them have a superficial charm and impress others with their eloquence and verbosity (cf. Roth and Strüber 2021, 329 f.). Psychopathy is considered a severe, special form of APS, and in addition to the already mentioned characteristics, the affected individuals exhibit a pronounced lack of fear and empathy. Psychopaths are not distinguishable from their fellow humans at first glance, as they usually present themselves as extremely charming and eloquent, but are also considered assertive and in need of recognition. They are highly adaptable, but they lie and cheat others without hesitation (cf. Spektrum – Psychische Störungen 2014, n.p.). Regarding the aggressiveness of their actions, there are significant differences between patients with psychopathy and those affected by APS. Aggressive behavior can be impulsive-reactive, meaning the aggression is an unplanned, very emotional reaction based on the subjective perception of a threat or provocation. This is often followed by superficial remorse. In contrast, instrumental aggression, which characterizes psychopaths, is planned, unemotional, and "cold," serving to gain power, status, drugs, or other goals (cf. Lück et al. 2008, 93–121). Therefore, not every person with APS is also a psychopath. Studies on prisoners have shown that 70–80% of inmates meet the criteria for APS, but only a third of these inmates can be classified as psychopathic. Additionally, APS is particularly found in men and often co-occurs with other mental disorders such as depression, anxiety disorders, substance abuse, gambling addiction, and a general impulse control disorder (cf. Roth and Strüber 2021, 331). Regarding evidence-based therapy strategies and successful psychological interventions, there is definitely a need for further research and discussion for both APS and psychopathy. Fiedler, for example, reports on multimodal approaches to psychotherapy for dissocial subjects, where therapy optimism has proven to be a significant factor for treatment success. Similarly, there are reports from the USA on the possibilities of pharmacotherapy for impulsive aggression in the context of psychopathy (cf. Habermeyer and Saß 2018, 183–185). However, there is very limited evidence on psychological interventions for adults with APS. According to studies, no intervention has been reported to provide convincing evidence for a change in antisocial behavior (cf. Cheung et al. 2020, n.p.).

Neurobiological Changes and Psychoneuroendocrinological Insights in Antisocial Personality Disorder and Psychopathy

Neurobiological changes can already be detected during childhood or adolescent development in people with APS, which, among other things, impair learning from experiences (cf. Roth and Strüber 2021, 332). In healthy individuals, the brain is able to use information about the negative consequences of one's actions for future behavioral orientation. For example, if a punishment is worse than expected, this leads to reduced activity in the striatum, which in turn is an important signal for a corresponding behavioral change. In adolescents with a conduct disorder, however, this does not function in the same way. The malfunction of the striatum as well as the vmPFC (ventromedial prefrontal cortex) and the anterior insular cortex seems to be associated with reduced abilities in these adolescents to link certain actions or stimuli with punishment. The reduced empathetic response to the distress of others is primarily based on a reduced responsiveness of the amygdala to distress signals. The deficits in decision-making and reinforcement learning, on the other hand, reflect a dysfunction in the vmPFC and the striatum. It can already be mentioned here that both genetic and prenatal factors contribute to the abnormal development of these neural systems (cf. Blair 2013, 786–799). Lesion studies by Anderson (1999) demonstrated that early childhood damage to ventromedial and frontopolar areas leads to social-moral deficits and psychopathy-like behavior (cf. Roth and Strüber 2021, 333).

Psychopathy can be clearly distinguished from other forms of APS by means of neurobiological findings, whereby these divergences, as already mentioned, can be observed early (during childhood or adolescence). The impairment of processing information about punishment affects, for example, both adolescents with psychopathic traits and adolescents with a reactive-aggressive behavior disorder. However, if this deficit occurs in combination with a reduced sensitivity of the amygdala, it explains the emotionless and punishment-resistant behavior of highly criminal juvenile offenders with psychopathic traits. An APS with psychopathic traits is already evident in adolescence through a reduced response of the amygdala or through compassionless and emotionless behavior. In the context of this disorder, emotional processing generally appears to be flattened. Adults who suffer from an APS with psychopathic traits often show reduced physical arousal in response to emotional stimuli. This indicates an emotional underfunction (cf. Roth and Strüber 2009, 587–609).

A clear connection exists between psychopathy and a reduced cortisol level (cf. Roth and Strüber 2009, 587–609).

> "Both callous-unemotional behavior and aggressive tendencies are accompanied by a cortisol underfunction under resting conditions as well as under stress" (ibid., 333).

A cortisol underfunction can already be detected in 10-year-old boys who stand out due to increased aggressiveness. It is important to note here that only the boys whose aggressive behavior is not emotional respond to a stressful situation with a lower cortisol release. Children whose aggressiveness is associated with great fear, on the other hand, show a much higher cortisol response than non-aggressive children (cf. Roth and Strüber 2021, 333 f.). Unlike in depression, where, as already described, a cortisol overfunction leads to changes and symptoms, in psychopaths, it is exactly the opposite.

> "A cortisol underfunction leads to a chronic underfunction of the vmPFC and the associated emotional and moral deficits through an increased formation of serotonergic 5-HT1A receptors" (Roth et al. 2014, cited in Roth and Strüber 2021, 334).

In addition, neuromodulators such as dopamine are associated with the development of psychopathy. Psychopaths are characterized by an increased sensitivity of the dopamine system, which would explain the abnormal reward sensitivity and high risk-taking. These results also suggest that this is the reason for impulsive-antisocial behavior and substance abuse in psychopathy (cf. Buckholtz et al. 2010, 419 ff.). The sex hormone testosterone also plays a role, as it promotes aggressive actions as well as motivated and reward-oriented behavior. Testosterone is capable of activating the dopaminergic system and thus enhancing reward sensitivity. The testosterone-cortisol ratio also seems to form the basis for particularly violent aggression and lack of empathy in psychopathy. In addition, both factors, i.e., a high testosterone level and a low cortisol level, reduce communication between the amygdala and the vmPFC and thus presumably also the transmission of emotional information to the differentiated processing cerebral cortex (cf. Roth and Strüber 2021, 334 f.). It is also clear that a dysregulation of the oxytocin system is responsible for the typical impaired abilities of psychopaths, as the recognition of others' emotions, empathy, and the formation of social bonds are influenced by OXY (cf. Chen et al. 2013, 83). It is already evident in children and adolescents with psychopathic traits that they exhibit increased methylation and reduced formation of oxytocin receptors. This suggests that even high amounts of this neuropeptide are unlikely to have an effect on them. These children and adolescents also have low oxytocin levels in their blood. Thus, the reduced oxytocin production and the reduced formation of oxytocin receptors are indeed related to the characteristics of psychopathy (cf. Dadds et al. 2014, 33–40).

In contrast to psychopathy, antisocial personality disorder with reactive aggression (the second, reactive-impulsive form of antisocial behavior disorder) is already accompanied by increased amygdala activity in youth. Here, the amygdala reacts particularly sensitively to signals of threat and provocation. This sensitivity could form the basis for the tendency towards reactive-aggressive behavior (cf. Roth and Strüber 2021, 335 f.). Adolescents with a reactive-impulsive APS seem to have both an increased sensitivity of the "threat circuit" and a reduced regulation of the limbic cortical areas. The increased activity of the amygdala also increases the risk that these adolescents will later develop affective disorders such as depression or anxiety disorders (cf. Blair 2013, 786–799). Adults with a reactive-impulsive APS also respond to fearful or angry faces with high arousal, increased amygdala activation, and reduced involvement of limbic cortical areas. Regarding neuromodulators, a low serotonin turnover is particularly in focus for impulsive aggressive behaviors, whereby it must be noted that the influence of serotonin on aggressive behavior depends on the individual tendency towards aggression. For serotonin does not inhibit aggressive behavior per se, but impulsivity, meaning the willingness to give in to impulses. In individuals with an APS, however, the reduced serotonin release can be responsible for reactive and impulsive aggression (cf. Roth and Strüber 2021, 336 f.).

The Influence of Genes and Environment on the Development of Antisocial Personality Disorder and Psychopathy

Genetic approaches have definitely improved the understanding of the neurobiological foundations of social behavior and cognition, as well as the epigenetic mechanisms that regulate genetic function and expression without changes to the DNA sequence and are of enormous importance for mental disorders or socio-behavioral phenotypes (cf. Chen et al. 2013, 83).

> "The epigenetic modification of genes involved in oxytocin signaling could be part of the mechanisms that mediate the long-term influence of early negative experiences on social behavior outcomes" (ibid.).

In the development of APS, based on adoption studies, both genetic and environmental factors are involved, as both adopted children and biological children of adults with APS show an increased risk of developing this mental disorder themselves. Since children adopted by parents with APS also show an increased risk of developing it, environmental influence is to be mentioned as a contributing factor. When the biological children of parents with APS are adopted, they still resemble their biological parents more, which in turn suggests a genetic influence or speaks for the genetic factor (cf. Roth and Strüber 2021, 337). Various gene variants are associated with the development of an antisocial disorder. A genome-wide association study also suggests a robust and replicable connection of genetic variants with APS (cf. Rautiainen et al. 2016, 883). Nevertheless, early negative experiences such as abuse, neglect, and inconsistent or unpredictable parental behavior also increase the risk of a later disorder (cf. Roth and Strüber 2021, 337).

> "Furthermore, the degree of maternal unavailability during childhood predicts the extent of antisocial traits occurring 20 years later" (ibid.).

The connection between disorder and experiences is based on the influence on brain development. For example, the worse the early experiences of neglect as well as physical and sexual abuse were, the more pronounced is a reduced volume of the anterior cingulate cortex in individuals with APS. Within psychopathy, a distinction is made between primary psychopaths with an innate disorder of social-affective behavior and secondary psychopaths, in whom the disorder is based on early negative experiences. The characteristic lack of empathy in psychopaths seems to be more strongly influenced genetically than the behavior of patients with a reactive type of APS. This influence is already visible at the age of 7 years. Genes can influence the development of brain structures associated with psychopathy, such as reduced sensitivity, particularly of the amygdala and the vmPFC (cf. Glenn 2011, cited in Roth and Strüber 2021, 337 f.). The L-allele of the serotonin transporter gene is capable of producing such an effect. Actually, the L-allele is attributed a positive influence on resilience, as it protects against developing depressive symptoms after a strong stress confrontation. However, the L-allele is not as harmless as thought, as carriers of two L-alleles have an amygdala that reacts less to negative emotional stimuli. Similarly, parallels between the L/L genotype and psychopathic traits appear during stress activity. Prenatal stress, for example, leads to increased aggression only in children with two L-alleles. Adolescents with this genotype tend to lack empathy and exhibit narcissism in a low socioeconomic status, whereas this is not the case in people with, for example, an S-allele (cf. Glenn 2011, 612–620). This could be the reason why it is so difficult or even impossible to change the psychopathic character traits of emotional and empathy deficits. Accordingly, parental educational measures and psychosocial interventions to reduce those psychopathic symptoms are far less effective than, for example, in children and adolescents with other behavioral disorders. It is suspected that particularly fearlessness and insensitivity to punishment make their socialization and upbringing difficult (cf. Blair 2013, 786–799). However, a secure and strong attachment can protect these emotionally deficient children and adolescents. Because if parents manage to maintain high empathy despite the children's emotional deficits and build a secure attachment, this can lead the children to accept parental values and intentions and further develop a social conscience (cf. Aksan and Kochanska 2006, 1587–1617). However, if the children's emotional deficits are not compensated for by correspondingly positive early experiences, for example, due to abuse, emotional unavailability of the parents, or early separation from the parents, this increases the risk of developing APS. In contrast to psychopathy, APS, which is associated with reactive aggression and violence, has been primarily linked to a mutation of the enzyme monoamine oxidase A (MAO-A). It is important to note that MAO-A contributes to the breakdown of monoamines such as serotonin, dopamine, and norepinephrine. Thus, a deficit in enzyme function leads to an excess of these substances in the brain (cf. Roth and Strüber 2021, 339 f.). According to Buckholtz and Meyer-Lindenberg (2008), individuals with the MAO-A-L variant, which leads to low production of this enzyme, exhibit a reduced volume of the amygdala, hippocampus, and anterior cingulate cortex. Furthermore, carriers of this variant show heightened amygdala activity and increased activity of the insular cortex and reduced activation of the orbitofrontal and anterior cingulate cortex under emotional stress (cf. Buckholtz and Meyer-Lindenberg 2008, 120–129). This, in turn, leads to an increased tendency towards aggressive behavior. However, a gene-environment interaction plays a significant role here. Children with the MAO-A-L genotype have a greater risk of developing a conduct disorder, violent behavior, or even an antisocial personality due to early traumatic experiences, compared to children with a highly active MAO-A genotype (cf. Caspi et al. 2002, 851–854). The effect of this genotype on early childhood serotonin concentration is of particular importance. As mentioned earlier, serotonin has a significant influence on brain development. Therefore, if there is an excess of serotonin in the brain during early childhood development due to the MAO-A-L variant, this could destabilize a circuit between the amygdala and limbic cortical areas responsible for social evaluations and emotion regulation. Increased sensitivity to threats, reduced control over emotions, and an enhanced fear memory would be the result (cf. Buckholtz and Meyer-Lindenberg 2008, 120–129). A destabilized connection between the amygdala and limbic cortical areas, combined with abuse, neglect, persistent insecurity, inadequate role models, unpredictable threats, and inconsistent reinforcement of prosocial behavior, leads to a massively increased risk of overt aggression and impulsive violence (cf. Roth and Strüber 2021, 342).

2.7.7 Conclusion

In this section, mental illnesses were outlined, in which it becomes clear that dysregulated substances and brain areas are very likely associated with the symptoms of the illnesses. Psychoneuroendocrinological, neurobiological, as well as genetic-epigenetic findings bring new knowledge that could be used for individual therapies. The findings recorded here further show that genes and epigenetic factors always predispose to the development of mental illnesses. Here, the influence of systems that impair brain development, such as the serotonergic system, is particularly important. Equally significant for the development of mental disorders are prenatal and early childhood experiences, which also negatively influence the development of systems such as the oxytocin or cortisol system. Traumatic experiences, as well as early attachment disorders, should also be mentioned here. Roth and Ryba (2019) state this as follows: Disorders or impairments of the psyche are caused by temporary or persistent disturbances in the interaction of the 6 psychoneuronal basic systems. These are partly genetically-epigenetically or by negative environmental factors or even by both (cf. Roth and Ryba 2019, 146). Therefore, the following will present and explain the 6 psychoneuronal basic systems and their relationship to our behavior.

2.8 The 6 Psychoneuronal Basic Systems According to Roth and Strüber

In this section of this book, the 6 psychoneuronal basic systems, as described by Roth and Strüber (2021), are presented. It is a neurobiological model that provides an overall picture of some significant psychoneuroendocrinological findings and explains how certain endocrine substances influence our behavior, our psyche, and also our personality. It is once again made clear how enormously important hormones are for humans and their behavior. Additionally, it is shown how the findings of the psychoneuronal basic systems can be implemented in psychosocial and psychotherapeutic practice.

2.8.1 Stress Processing System

For the psyche, behavior, and personality of a person, it is relevant how he or she deals with stress, how resilient he/she is, that is, how pronounced his/her stress resistance is. This implies the individual's competence to deal with negative, threatening things, how quickly it recognizes the danger and can activate the stress system in the brain and body and subsequently dampen the excitement again. Physical as well as psychological stresses and challenges are to be managed by the stress processing system. The interaction of many substances enables the brain and body to adapt to their environment. This allows the person, for example, to be alert, to run away, or to seek protection from parents. If a stressful situation is perceived, this information is forwarded to the hypothalamus, the amygdala, the hippocampus, and other brain structures. The sympathetic nervous system is activated, and CRF production occurs in the hypothalamus and amygdala. CRF is crucial for a rapid stress response. Exploratory behavior is inhibited, alertness is increased, and at higher doses, CRF has a fear-inducing effect, which in turn leads to withdrawal. Additionally, it acts in the locus coeruleus, leading to increased release of norepinephrine in several brain areas (for example, in the amygdala, hippocampus, and ventromedial prefrontal cortex). This leads to increased alertness and also promotes emotional learning. If the stress persists, the rapid stress reaction is followed by the activation of the HPA axis. This is triggered by CRF and the subsequent release of ACTH in the pituitary gland. ACTH, in turn, leads to the synthesis and release of cortisol into the bloodstream in the following minutes. This initially promotes adequate stress processing and dampens the stress reaction over time through negative feedback. There are specific receptor types for a variety of substances. They respond differently to various concentrations of the substances and also have opposing effects on brain activities. The individually different receptor formation affects how quickly the body "ramps up" and how quickly the brain activity returns to a flexible resting mode (cf. Roth and Strüber 2021, 164 f.). Furthermore, the connection between genes and experiences influences the individual function of the stress processing system. As already mentioned, a genetic predisposition or a predisposition shaped during pregnancy of the stress processing system can be mitigated by positive bonding experiences in early childhood or exacerbated by negative or traumatic childhood experiences. This results in increased or decreased stress tolerance. Additionally, an individual's stress behavior can be transmitted to offspring in various ways:

- through inheritance, purely genetic,
- epigenetically, that is, through mechanisms determining gene expression,
- through prenatal, physical, and neural influences of the expectant mother
- as well as through care and interaction with the children in early childhood (cf. Roth and Strüber 2021, 166).

Mahlmann notes that, based on the stress processing system described here, it is important in psychosocial and psychotherapeutic practice to explain to clients the goal of dealing with distress. This means conveying to them how to handle unpleasant, overwhelming, or threatening stress (distress) or obstacles and difficulties. It is important to learn which strategies the clients have already had success or failure with and what would be within their capabilities. Practical exercises should be offered that are resource-oriented, implement ratio and emotion, and link motives of avoidance and approach. It is crucial to make clients understand that the stress processing system is a firmly anchored system that does not merely conform to the norms of the psychosocial counselor or psychotherapist. This also applies if the clients are additionally treated with psychopharmacological therapy (cf. Mahlmann 2020, n.p.).

2.8.2 Internal Calming System

Closely connected to the stress processing system is the internal calming system. Following a stressful situation, or when a situation requires "suppressed" stress, it is important to be able to quickly switch back to rest mode. The return to rest mode works, among other things, through the released cortisol, which dampens the initial stress reaction with a slight delay. In the body, this is realized by activating the parasympathetic nervous system. The internal calming system is considered the counterpart of the sympathetic nervous system, which is responsible for fight and flight reactions. A return to rest mode involves the prefrontal cortex becoming increasingly active and the amygdala, which is particularly sensitive to threats, being deactivated. There are substances that can support the shift to rest mode, such as oxytocin, which is released in social interaction situations, as well as the neuromodulator serotonin, which thereby brings about an internal calming system (cf. Roth and Strüber 2021, 166 f.). Through certain receptor types of serotonin (primarily the 5-HT_{1A} receptor), it is determined how active the brain structures of the upper limbic level are. This means that it is determined how pronounced an individual's tendency is to brood or dwell on their memories. Through the inhibitory 5-HT_{1A} receptors, this activity is dampened, and everything calms down again ("Everything is fine—don't get upset!"). Thus, serotonin is of enormous relevance for the suppression of action impulses ("Better do nothing than something wrong!"). If the inhibition via these receptors does not work well, this can contribute to the development of depressive disorders (cf. Hahn et al. 2012, cited in Roth and Strüber 2021, 167). Of enormous importance here is the interaction of serotonin with the stress system, as cortisol in high concentrations reduces the formation of 5-HT_{1A}receptors of the serotonin system. This leads to the "soothing" of the emotional brain areas being only limitedly possible. A poor or even harmful interaction of the stress system with the serotonin system is especially found when genetic burdens of the serotonin system meet prenatal or early postnatal negative environmental influences (cf. Roth and Strüber 2021, 167). These include, for example, emotional or physical stress of the pregnant woman or mother, neglect, abuse or mistreatment of the infant or toddler, as well as a mental disorder of the mother. These circumstances have a strong negative impact on the further psychological development of the child. When people have a serotonin deficiency, they experience the world as more threatening and are constantly worried. This leads to depression in both biological sexes, as well as reactive physical violence in men and more often to feelings of guilt and suicidal tendencies in women. In general, a serotonin deficiency can cause the following psychological disorders and emotional impairments (cf. Roth and Strüber 2021, 167 f.): "Depression, anxiety, risk aversion, reactive aggression, and impulsivity" (ibid., 168).

Applied to psychosocial and psychotherapeutic practice, this means, for example, addressing the following questions: How do clients regulate themselves? How do they control intense feelings, aggressiveness, and impulsivity? To what extent do clients perceive the world as threatening, are they willing to take risks, and also to fail? To what extent can clients be calm or regain calmness? The stress system and the self-calming system influence each other. The more active the stress system, the less controlled the self-calming system is. This means for practice that the resilience, resilience, and stability of the clients come into focus. Thus, Mahlmann recommends the same psychotherapeutic attitude and work that also apply to the stress processing system (cf. Mahlmann 2020, n.p.).

2.8.3 Internal Evaluation and Reward System

All our actions are determined by motives and reasons. These can be unconscious, conscious, or preconscious-intuitive. The universal principle on which all these motives are based is to strive for what is pleasant or appears advantageous, and to end or avoid what is disadvantageous or painful. This principle is determined on the one hand by innate drives and on the other hand by our own experiences in action and interaction with the world. This means that experiences and their consequences are evaluated in the "reward and punishment (pleasure-displeasure) memory." Subsequently, the resulting "reward and punishment expectations," which are generated when experiencing similar situations, are developed. The internal evaluation system is based on two subsystems. The first can be referred to as the actual reward system. It is associated with satisfaction, pleasure, and our hedonistic experiences and is based on the release of endogenous opioids. These act in the amygdala and thus generate unconscious reward experiences. This activity is then mapped in the orbitofrontal, ventromedial, and insular cortex, creating the conscious feeling of pleasure and satisfaction associated with receiving rewards. The second system is referred to as the reward expectation system. Here, dopamine is the mediating substance. It is based on the first system, builds upon it, and develops expectations from it. These follow the principle: What once led to a reward will be repeated, and those experiences that caused displeasure or pain should be avoided in the future. The dopaminergic neurons encode "the type, size, and probability of occurrence of an expected reward and the associated risk" (cf. Roth and Strüber 2021, 168 f.) under the influence of the amygdala and hippocampus (ibid., 169). Genes and epigenetic factors influence the extent to which we are guided by rewards. What we perceive as a reward and how expectant we are is individually different. Early childhood experiences and especially attachment experiences play a significant role here. It should also be mentioned that the influence of certain preferences on the opioid and dopamine system is stronger the earlier they are developed by the individual. Furthermore, they then have a stronger impact on the individual's personality. However, negative experiences in early childhood lead to an impaired opioid and dopamine system, which in turn leads to deficits in the reward and reward expectation system. When the reward system is impaired, the effect is that no sufficient feeling of reward or satisfaction follows actually rewarding events. This can lead to an increased urge or craving for reward (cf. Roth and Strüber 2021, 169). This may presumably predispose to drug addiction. If individuals have a deficit in the reward expectation system, motivational problems become apparent. This means that these people cannot associate enough reward expectations with their own actions. As a result, goals seem unattainable, unattractive, or require too much effort. This can lead to apathy and hopelessness, as observed in melancholic depression, for example. The problem also becomes apparent when rewards need to be delayed, as seen in children with ADHD. The affected individuals are well guided by immediate rewards, but because the anticipatory dopamine signal (which mediates reward expectation) is impaired, there is a reduced sensitivity to temporally delayed rewards. It is difficult for the children to keep this reward or its value in mind (cf. Roth and Strüber 2021, 170).

For psychosocial and psychotherapeutic practice, based on the reward system, the question of how much clients can be encouraged is significant. This does not only mean through conditioning experiences but also through experiences that lead to expectations. What drives the clients? What moves and activates the clients, and how do they respond to rewards and punishments (cf. Mahlmann 2020, n.p.)?

> "Important for psychotherapists here: The dopaminergic response is independent of the content of a confirmation. Even when a fear is confirmed, a reward occurs through increased dopamine release. For example, if a skeptical client does not receive help from the therapist from their perspective, they feel confirmed in their skepticism: 'I knew it, they can't help me either!' The fatal thing: Every confirmation is positive reinforcement—and this leads to repetition (in this case: an undesirable decision, expectation, behavior, action)" (ibid.).

2.8.4 Impulse Inhibition System

Equally significant for the ability to delay gratification is the so-called impulse inhibition system. Infants and toddlers generally do not accept delays; they want everything immediately. Impulse inhibition and the tolerance of delayed gratification are developed from the first year of life into adulthood, often representing a laborious process.

Impulsive actions are categorized into two types:

1) an uninhibited and unconsidered reaction to a stimulus, which can be, for example, an aggressive response to a threatening speech, and
2) the preference for an immediate reward instead of a delayed reward, such as preferring a sweet treat over the prospect of optimal body weight (cf. Roth and Strüber 2021, 170 f.).

Whether impulsive actions occur or not is primarily determined by the dopamine and serotonin systems. In stressful situations, where quick and impulsive actions (flight or fight) are important, dopamine release in the nucleus accumbens, the orbitofrontal and ventromedial prefrontal cortex, and the upper limbic level is increased. However, when restraint is needed in the situation, dopamine release is reduced, and serotonin release is increased in some areas of the forebrain, particularly in the orbitofrontal and ventromedial cortex. Serotonin signals to the body that it would be better not to react rather than to react incorrectly. However, a high testosterone level in men can counteract impulse inhibition (cf. ibid., 171).

Based on the impulse inhibition system, the leading question in psychosocial and psychotherapeutic practice for clients is to what extent they are able to actively control their impulses, how they deal with their impulses, and consequently, whether they are able to act in a socially accepted manner. High impulsivity also means high dopamine levels and is associated with personality traits such as extraversion and high risk-taking. Reactive impulsivity, on the other hand, means that affected clients live under constant distress and fear and find it challenging to distinguish between non-threatening and threatening situations. Low impulse control leads to the challenge of controlling or regulating one's impulses, which in turn can bring about negative moods and insecurity. Here too, it is important to work multidimensionally in psychosocial and psychotherapeutic contexts (cf. Mahlmann 2020, n.p.).

2.8.5 Attachment System

The attachment system develops in the first weeks after birth. This occurs when the infant begins to interact with the mother in various ways and smiles at her intentionally. The neuropeptide oxytocin (OXY) is of relevance here. It plays a role in the mother-child relationship, but also in pair bonding, sexual behavior, and trusting close social contacts. Oxytocin acts as a bonding hormone. An increased release of this hormone inhibits the stress system, and serotonin release is enhanced. Feelings such as fear are reduced by oxytocin. Additionally, oxytocin increases the ability to recognize social and emotional signals and supports social motivation (cf. Roth and Strüber 2021, 172). It has a positive effect on all kinds of social emotions and behaviors. Furthermore, it promotes trust and empathy towards parental behavior, pleasant social contacts, and much more. The stress-inhibiting effect is of particular importance for the child. During breastfeeding or familiar interactions, oxytocin is released and thus functions as physiological comfort. On the parents' side, OXY helps to perceive the behavior of the stressed child, such as shrill crying, not with aversion but with empathy for the child. Furthermore, OXY promotes the ability of parents to recognize and mirror the child's emotions through facial expressions. This supports the child's emotional development (cf. Strüber 2016, cited in Roth and Strüber 2021, 172). However, the release of OXY is not only tied to the parent-child relationship but is also released in other relationships with strong bonds, such as in partnerships or social interactions with friends. OXY promotes trusting and coordinated interactions (cf. Feldman 2017, cited in Roth and Strüber 2021, 172). Additionally, the OXY attachment system is closely linked to the reward and reward expectation system. Often, the effect of OXY is accompanied by the release of endogenous opioids, which, for example, convey the pleasant feeling during social contacts. This effect of the reward expectation system is noticeable when people look at their partners, their parents, or their child. Regions of this system, which have a high number of vasopressin and oxytocin receptors, are activated. Conversely, areas in the brain associated with negative emotions and more critical social evaluations are inhibited. Due to the effect of OXY on the dopaminergic cells of the reward expectation system and the release of opioids, the reward value of social contacts can be enhanced. An individual can thus be motivated to seek interaction with a bonding partner repeatedly. Although vasopressin has an effect on the stress system opposite to that of OXY, it still plays a significant role in the attachment system. Regarding the protection of the child, vasopressin enhances parental caregiving behavior (cf. Roth and Strüber 2021, 172 f.). There is also a strong influence of genetics and environmental factors on the attachment system. If both genetics and environmental factors are positive, one can expect stable attachment behavior in both adolescence and adulthood. However, if there are genetic-epigenetic predispositions affecting the oxytocin system combined with negative childhood experiences or early adolescence, this can lead to the promotion of attachment and personality disorders. If, however, one of the two factors is negatively predisposed and the other is positive, a balance can also occur. This means that secure attachment mitigates genetic-epigenetic predispositions, or a robust genetic-epigenetic makeup can be resilient to negative early childhood experiences (cf. ibid., 173).

Based on the findings about the attachment system, psychosocial and psychotherapeutic practice particularly addresses the questions of to what extent clients long for closeness, what prevents them from emotionally engaging with or approaching other people. Psychosocial and psychotherapeutic work can enable clients to engage with others more than before. This is done by addressing deep-seated motives, behaviors, and readiness and linking them with cognition (cf. Mahlmann 2020, n.p.).

> "Body/movement, mind/reason, and feeling/unconscious/fixed work most effectively together—and with an individually determined emphasis on utilization" (ibid.).

Additionally, the importance of the alliance between clients and counselors/therapists is mentioned in this system. A good alliance is indispensable for successful psychosocial and psychotherapeutic work (cf. Mahlmann 2020, n.p.).

2.8.6 System of Reality Sense and Risk Assessment

The focus here is on estimating a risk or the probability that a behavior will have negative consequences. If this system works well, the individual has a pronounced sense of reality and a good assessment of risk. If the individual has an increased willingness to take risks, it means that they ignore or underestimate possible negative consequences, whereby an increased willingness to take risks can be both impulsive and planned. For example, if someone sails across the ocean in a small sailboat despite turbulent weather, it is impulsive; if someone has been planning an Atlantic crossing for a long time, it is not impulsive, but still risky (cf. Nigg 2017, cited in Roth and Strüber 2021, 174). Like sensory and cognitive functions, the competence to realistically assess risks is associated with norepinephrine (NA) and acetylcholine. NA increases both general attention and focus, whereas acetylcholine enhances concentration and thus enables the targeted retrieval of memory contents. Ventral and medial prefrontal brain areas are then engaged in assessing risks and recognizing possible negative consequences of one's actions. It is therefore about the implementation of considered actions. This is again controlled by the impulse inhibition, reward expectation, and self-soothing systems. These three systems advise against risky and hasty actions. The development of the sense of reality and risk assessment begins around the age of 3. From then on, cognitive abilities gradually develop both in terms of attention and memory performance. The willingness to take risks increases during childhood, peaks in adolescence, and then decreases again. Evolutionary theorists assume that it was beneficial for the human species that adolescents have a high willingness to take risks. The path to adulthood is characterized by an increasingly reasonable and mature mind. The older adolescents get, the more they reflect on the possible consequences of their actions. However, this reflection does not necessarily lead to reasonable behavior full of understanding (cf. Roth and Strüber 2021, 174 f.). Famous studies have shown that, for example, patients with a damaged orbitofrontal cortex took great risks despite their better knowledge (cf. Anderson 1999, cited in Roth and Strüber 2021, 175).

In relation to this system, the cognitive-linguistic level plays a significant role, especially when it comes to formulating personal changes as a goal (cf. Mahlmann 2020, n.p.).

> "From a psychotherapeutic perspective, in addition to other methods, those that address reason and rationality, cognitive competencies, come into play with high weighting, in order to promote understanding processes as well as thinking abilities that are aimed at grasping realities and thinking about reasons for probabilities and possibilities of consequences, and justifying why one consequence is more likely than another and what that means for the personal field of action" (ibid.).

When this cognitive, intellectual work is linked with the emotional, affective level as well as intuition and the "gut feeling" (somatic markers), the effectiveness of psychosocial/psychotherapeutic work is increased (cf. Mahlmann 2020, n.p.).

> "The combination of emotive-cognitive work (reflection of feelings, affects), cognitive-emotive, cognitive-behavioral therapeutic intervention methods, including practical exercises, yields positive effects" (ibid.).

2.8.7 Psychoneuronal Systems and the 4-Level Model

The psychoneuronal systems presented here cut across the three limbic levels as well as the cognitive-linguistic level (cf. Roth and Strüber 2021, 175).

> "This means that all six systems, albeit to varying degrees, consist of components of the lower level, i.e., predominantly 'innate' reactions and temperament traits, the middle level of emotional conditioning, the upper level of socialization, and the level of cognitive-rational behavior" (Roth and Strüber 2021, 175).

Certain processes of the middle and upper limbic levels largely determine the attachment system. It is therefore shaped by early childhood experiences with the mother or other primary caregivers, later by social experiences with other family members as well as with peers in kindergarten and school. Our reality and risk perception system is based on our core personality on the one hand and on our experiences over time, which are predominantly processed at the upper limbic level as well as the cognitive-linguistic level. How well these systems are developed influences how capable we are of assessing certain consequences of our actions over a longer period (cf. Roth and Strüber 2021, 175 f.).

2.8.8 Conclusion: Psychoneuronal Basic Systems and the Psychosocial and Psychotherapeutic Practice

The findings on the psychoneuronal basic systems according to Roth and Strüber once again highlight the enormous importance of hormones for human behavior. When implementing these findings into psychosocial and psychotherapeutic practice, it is, however, of immense importance not to neglect the emotional level, not to overwhelm clients with cognitive knowledge, and especially to have a good alliance with the clients. Transferring these findings into practice entails multidimensional psychosocial/psychotherapeutic work. This work combines emotive-cognitive conversations, cognitive-behavioral interventions, and practical exercises. The integration of these findings with multidimensional psychosocial and psychotherapeutic work requires openness from psychosocial counselors/psychotherapists to a new approach as well as a diverse repertoire of tools/exercises that enable clients to achieve individual success. However, psychosocial counselors/psychotherapists and clients must be prepared for the fact that the path to success can be long and arduous. The neural networks involved in a problem cannot simply be "overwritten" in a short time. In a short time, one only experiences short-term successes, which soon cause clients to fall back into old patterns. Therefore, it is all the more important that clients become active themselves (exercises, homework, transfer tasks). There must be a phase in which clients practice/deepen better/adapted behaviors in everyday life. Ultimately, it is also of immense importance that psychosocial counselors/psychotherapists distinguish whether it is about lighter burdens and minor impairments or severe psychological disorders.

2.9 "Happiness Hormones" and the Importance of Precursors and Co-Factors

After the importance of the psychoneuronal basic systems has been explained, it is now important to elucidate the systemic connection between nutrition and hormones. This section will explain the relationship between nutrition and hormones and what can be done to balance or support hormone synthesis. As already explained in Chap. 1("Fundamentals of Endocrinology"), this science is closely related to water balance, appetite, and hunger—in short, our nutrition. It has also been repeatedly shown how individually perceived emotions or psychological well-being depend on several hormones and neurotransmitters. This connection between hormone levels and various emotions or psychological baseline mood is scientifically undisputed. These findings also provide the foundation for many psychotropic drugs and performance-enhancing medications. However, these medications are criticized for sometimes serious side effects. This section of the book aims to present alternatives to maintain and promote the natural hormone balance or the equilibrium of neurotransmitters (cf. Rotter 2021, 5).

As already noted several times in this book, there are neurotransmitters that trigger feelings of stress or anxiety, and others that trigger positive emotions, inner balance, calmness, and tranquility. To sufficiently form these neurotransmitters, some suggestions are given below. There are various causes for neurotransmitter deficiencies, which can be due to the insufficient availability of the necessary building blocks for synthesis or due to faulty regulation leading to neurotransmitter deficiencies. As already mentioned, various nutrients are considered so-called co-factors or precursor substances. A deficiency in these co-factors can have enormous effects on hormone synthesis and the formation of neurotransmitters (cf. ibid.).

The following will particularly focus on promoting the so-called "happiness hormones" serotonin, dopamine, and GABA, which are significantly involved in regulating our emotional balance. It will be shown how the body's own synthesis of these substances can be naturally modulated. The most important co-factors, effective adaptogens, and the importance of gut health will be examined. The effects and synthesis of serotonin, dopamine, and the neurotransmitter GABA will be explained. It is significant here which co-factors or precursor substances are needed for a healthy balance or synthesis of these neurotransmitters.

2.9.1 Serotonin and L-Tryptophan

A balanced amount of serotonin significantly contributes to our mental well-being or mental health and a balanced, positive basic mood. In addition to mood, serotonin also influences nerve signal transmission, social behavior, and the feeling of satiety. In the brain, serotonin acts as a neurotransmitter to excite our nerve cells. A lack of serotonin can be associated with low spirits and depressive moods, which is why the mechanism of action of many modern antidepressants is based on increasing the serotonin level in the synaptic cleft (cf. Blackwell et al. 2006, 325–338). Additionally, serotonin plays a role in the nervous system of the gut, the regulation of the cardiovascular system, the blood flow to skeletal muscles and organs, and blood pressure. If there is a serotonin deficiency, the following symptoms can occur (cf. Rotter 2021, 7):

- "Depression and anxiety
- inner restlessness and tension
- memory performance problems
- migraine and chronic headaches
- chronic muscle pain
- aggressive mood
- disturbances in the feeling of satiety
- sleep disorders (difficulty falling asleep and staying asleep)" (ibid.).

Serotonin must be produced by the body itself, with about 95% of serotonin being produced in the gut and only 5% in the brain. The essential amino acid L-tryptophan, which is ingested with food, is the natural precursor for the body's own serotonin synthesis. Tryptophan, in turn, is converted into serotonin via the intermediate stage 5-hydroxytryptophan (5-HTP) (cf. Blackwell et al. 2006, 325–338). However, the conversion steps are not only dependent on the extensive supply of the precursors but also require several co-factors. 1) For the conversion of L-tryptophan to 5-HTP, the body needs vitamins B_3 and B_6 as well as magnesium. 2) In the conversion step from 5-HTP to serotonin, vitamin $B_6$and zinc are needed. An adequate supply of co-factors is therefore indispensable for a functioning serotonin synthesis (cf. Rotter 2021, 7).

▶ **Tryptophan → 5-HTP → Serotonin**

Precursor: L-tryptophan to 5-HTP
Co-factor: vitamins B_3, B_6, magnesium, zinc

Another factor that must be considered is the tryptophan-degrading enzyme indoleamine 2,3-dioxygenase, or IDO for short. If the activity of this enzyme is increased by inflammatory cytokines, this can lead to the increased formation of N-formylkynurenine from tryptophan. Thus, tryptophan is no longer available for serotonin synthesis, and potentially neurotoxic substances can be formed from the kynurenine metabolism, which in turn can further exacerbate depressive symptoms. Administration of tryptophan can have negative effects here, which is why in these cases, 5-HTP should be given directly. There can be several reasons for a serotonin deficiency in the brain:

- an insufficient intake of tryptophan with food or inadequate absorption of this precursor substance into the brain,
- a lack of co-factors: if those vitamins and trace elements, which are indispensable for the individual synthesis steps, are not present in sufficient concentration,
- an increased indoleamine 2,3-dioxygenase (IDO) due to inflammatory diseases (cf. Bertrand et al. 2016, 56).

Tryptophan and 5-HTP

There are various preclinical and clinical studies that clearly demonstrate the positive effects of tryptophan as well as 5-HTP, but research on alternative treatment methods has significantly decreased in the last 20 years because the focus was on the development of modern antidepressants (cf. Blackwell et al. 2006, 325–338). However, it has been known for decades that people with depression often have a lowered tryptophan plasma level. An artificially induced serotonin deficiency, which was caused by the administration of a tryptophan-deficient diet, for example, leads to an acute deterioration in mood within hours. This is particularly true for people who have already experienced a depressive episode or have a familial disposition to depression, with it being noteworthy that women are more frequently affected than men (cf. Bertrand et al. 2016, 56). However, several studies demonstrate a contrary effect through the supplementation of tryptophan. Supplementation leads to a significant increase in positive emotions, positively influences memory, and leads to an improvement in resilience against negative moods and depressive episodes (cf. Kikuchi et al. 2020, 316–333). Likewise, supplementation of tryptophan resulted in prolonged sleep duration, improved sleep quality, and increased cognitive performance in the morning (cf. Bertrand et al. 2016, 56). It was already proven in 1998 that 5-HTP can effectively cross the blood-brain barrier and lead to an increase in serotonin in the central nervous system. The significant effect of 5-HTP on depression, insomnia, eating disorders, fibromyalgia, and chronic headaches has been demonstrated in various studies (cf. Blackwell et al. 2006, 325–338).

2.9.2 Dopamine and L-Tyrosine

After discussing serotonin, its precursor substances, and co-factors, the neurotransmitter dopamine will now be examined in more detail. Dopamine is associated with the "reward effect." This conveys positive feelings, which is why dopamine, like serotonin, is considered a "happiness hormone." Additionally, dopamine promotes energy, motivation, and drive. Dopamine fulfills important functions related to cognitive performance, memory, and information processing. Furthermore, dopamine is a precursor of the stimulating and drive-enhancing neurotransmitters norepinephrine and adrenaline. Dopamine is synthesized from the amino acid L-tyrosine, for which the co-factors vitamin $B_6$and zinc are required. Vitamin D is also considered a co-factor. Dopamine is particularly known for its role in Parkinson's disease. In this condition, the conversion of L-tyrosine to the intermediate stage L-Dopa is impaired (cf. Rotter 2021, 8).

▶ **L-Tyrosine → L-Dopa → Dopamine**

Starting material: L-tyrosine, co-factor: vitamin B_6, zinc, vitamin D

Based on several studies, it is proven that a change in dopamine metabolism is particularly based on increased stress. This includes, for example, post-traumatic stress disorders and addiction diseases (cf. Hernaus et al. 2015, 241–251). However, it should be mentioned that even in healthy people, the consumption of catecholamines (dopamine and norepinephrine) significantly increases in stressful situations. With decreasing dopamine levels in the brain, both cognitive performance and mood decrease. Here too, it is possible to stimulate dopamine production again by administering the starting substance L-tyrosine. Several studies demonstrate that the supplementation of tyrosine has a direct influence on both dopamine and norepinephrine concentrations in the brain (cf. Colzato et al. 2015, 50–57).

▶ **L-Tyrosine → L-Dopa → Dopamine → Norepinephrine → Adrenaline**

Apparently, tyrosine can achieve a correction of reduced memory performance and information processing, especially in physically or mentally challenging situations. Tyrosine also influences reduced mood. For these reasons, L-tyrosine is often used to restore stress resilience, for example, after burnout or in exceptionally stressful situations (cf. Rotter 2021, 9).

2.9.3 GABA and L-Glutamine

GABA can be described as the most significant inhibitory neurotransmitter, as it reduces nerve excitation and thus counteracts stress. The effect of GABA can therefore be described as relaxing, balancing, and sleep-promoting. To promote the body's own synthesis of GABA, the amino acid L-glutamine and the co-factor vitamin B_6 are needed (cf. Purves and Williams 2001, 681).

▶ **L-GLUTAMINE → GLUTAMATE → GABA**

Starting material: L-glutamine, co-factor: vitamin B_6
However, it is paradoxical that the most important excitatory, i.e., stimulating neurotransmitter glutamate is also formed from L-glutamine. If there is a vitamin B_6 deficiency, more glutamate and less GABA are produced. This disrupts the natural balance, leading to more excitation and less relaxation. In extreme cases and with particularly severe vitamin B_6deficiency, this can lead to seizures (cf. Arndt and Gressner 2019, cited in Rotter 2021, 9). More common health restrictions, however, include chronic stress, lack of ability to relax, and depression. It is now considered certain that a disturbance in the GABA-glutamate balance is of enormous relevance here (cf. Duman and Fogaça 2019, 87).

2.9.4 Co-Factors

As already mentioned, co-factors are needed for the body to form serotonin, dopamine, and GABA. These include vitamins (especially B vitamins) as well as certain minerals and trace elements (magnesium and zinc). The body necessarily requires these micronutrients as co-factors to carry out the corresponding synthesis steps. Therefore, it is of enormous importance not only to ensure the supply of building materials but also to pay attention to these co-factors to prevent a nutrient deficiency in this area (cf. Rotter 2021, 9). For example, vitamin B_6plays a significant role multiple times in brain metabolism. Vitamin $B_6$is a prerequisite for synthesizing 5-HTP in the brain, without which no serotonin can be formed. This also applies to the calming neurotransmitter GABA: In the case of a vitamin B_6 deficiency, synthesis gets stuck at the stimulating glutamate. Studies have shown that there is a correlation between the plasma level of vitamin B_6 and the severity of depression. Corresponding symptoms could be improved by administering vitamin B_6(cf. Aly and Engmann 2020, n.p.). Additionally, vitamin B_6, vitamin B_3, as well as zinc and magnesium, are necessarily required co-factors for the formation of serotonin, GABA, and dopamine. However, other vitamins, minerals, and trace elements also play a significant role. For example, vitamin D is needed for the conversion of L-tyrosine into dopamine. Vitamin B_1, B_9, and B_{12} are indirectly involved in neurotransmitter metabolism (cf. Kennedy 2016, 68).

2.9.5 Inflammations and Serotonin Metabolism

As already mentioned, reduced serotonin formation can also result from chronic inflammatory processes in the body. Inflammatory cytokines lead to IDO activity. This enzyme causes both a shift in the tryptophan/kynurenine ratio (in favor of kynurenines) and the formation of neurotoxic components from kynurenine metabolism (cf. Bertrand et al. 2016, 56). This metabolic shift increases susceptibility to depression. Additionally, neuropsychiatric disorders (such as schizophrenia and tic disorders) and inflammatory diseases like rheumatoid arthritis are promoted. Furthermore, the metabolic shift is associated with malignant diseases ("malignant" diseases that affect the entire organism as they progress) (cf. Rotter 2021, 11). Since chronic inflammations are one of the main factors for IDO activation, it is assumed that in some depressed individuals, a chronic inflammatory underlying disease is the cause of depression or at least strongly promotes it. The observed coincidence of depression with chronic inflammatory diseases such as rheumatoid arthritis, psoriasis, and chronic inflammatory bowel diseases also supports this. In these patients, symptoms improve with the administration of anti-inflammatory medications (cf. Havenaar 2011, 103–114). It is of enormous importance to mention here that supplementation with tryptophan can have negative consequences. This is because kynurenine metabolism is further fueled, but the formation of the urgently needed serotonin does not occur. Clients should therefore refrain from taking additional tryptophan and supplement with 5-HTP (5-hydroxytryptophan—the precursor of serotonin), as this substance is metabolized into serotonin independently of increased IDO activity. IDO enzyme activity can be determined with a simple laboratory test, regardless of a chronic inflammatory underlying disease (cf. Rotter 2021, 11).

2.9.6 Gut-Brain Axis: Healthy Gut—Healthy Mind

The interactions between the digestive tract and gut flora with brain function are of increasing scientific interest. The diverse interactions are described as bidirectional and are collectively referred to as the gut-brain axis (English: "gut-brain axis"). The connection between the brain, emotions, stress, and moods on our body system as well as our gastrointestinal function has already been explained in this book. In Germany, depending on the given criteria, between 5 and 10% of people are affected by the diagnosis of "irritable bowel syndrome" (cf. Arneth 2018, 446–452). A recent finding is that dysfunctions of the gastrointestinal tract also have a significant impact on brain functions, including stress resilience, cognitive performance, and mood. Connections to this are now being researched. Various approaches related to gut-brain communication or the messengers and neural structures are being discussed in science and research. For example, it is discussed that 95% of serotonin is produced in the gut. It is already known that prolonged stress leads to a change in the gut flora and the intestinal mucosa, which in turn results in reduced serotonin synthesis. Additionally, serotonin synthesis is suppressed by inflammatory mediators, interleukins, and interferons. These are produced, for example, in chronic intestinal problems and the so-called "silent inflammation" (cf. Dia et al. 2017, 3769–3787). These messengers directly inhibit the formation of 5-HTP, which is the blood-brain barrier-permeable intermediate product, resulting in a lack of serotonin. Likewise, disturbances of the gut flora and the intestinal mucosa can contribute to the development of a "leaky gut." This leads to toxins and food components entering the bloodstream, which are normally retained by an intact intestinal barrier. This not only has direct effects of toxins on the brain but also far-reaching consequences for all organs of the body and the immune system (cf. Tooley 2020, n.p.). These toxins in brain tissue disrupt the biochemical balance of the brain. This, in turn, has far-reaching consequences for both the mental and emotional stability of a person. The brain is generally particularly protected from such toxic substances, as only selected substances can cross the blood-brain barrier. Here too, researchers have been able to prove that the gut is involved in regulating this protective mechanism. Based on these findings, bacteria in the distal colon (rectum) produce substances that have a direct influence on the permeability of the blood-brain barrier (cf. Aigner et al. 2019, 1821–1827). It has also been found that the gut plays a role in the development of degenerative brain diseases such as Alzheimer's and dementia. In the meantime, researchers assume that the vagus nerve is the information mediator in this process. The vagus nerve is considered the longest cranial nerve and represents the neural connection between the brain and the gut in a bidirectional direction. There are indications that inflammatory processes in the gut, which are transmitted via the vagus nerve, can also lead to inflammatory and ultimately degenerative processes in the brain (cf. Amsterdam and Panossian 2016, 770–783 & Bravo et al. 2009, 397–401). Studies also show that in both healthy and mentally ill individuals, regulating the gut flora can improve both mental well-being and cognitive performance. When taking certain probiotics, the subjects showed a significant influence on various parameters such as the reduction of susceptibility to depression and a positive influence on attention (cf. Mattioli and Perfumi 2007, 37–43 & Amroyan et al. 2007, 343–348).

2.9.7 Conclusion

Stress, especially chronic stress, lack of sleep, and inflammation, particularly inflammatory bowel diseases, as well as mental concerns, can disrupt hormonal balance. This has a proven impact on certain physical changes in emotion-influencing hormones and neurotransmitters. This can result in mood swings, reduced concentration, and insomnia. The prescription for synthetic antidepressants is increasing annually; however, a functional neurotransmitter synthesis, for which the body needs the precursors and co-factors, is often sufficient (especially for mild to moderate symptoms). A lack of these precursors and co-factors leads to a halt in "happiness hormone synthesis." Both a healthy diet and a healthy gut are of enormous importance for mental health. To promote the body's own serotonin synthesis, for example, a systemic or interdisciplinary approach is needed, where all necessary precursors and co-factors are clarified (cf. Rotter 2021, 19).

2.10 Summary and Conclusion: Psychoneuroendocrinology

In summary, it should be noted at the end of this chapter that hormones not only influence our behavior, but they can also activate and control or direct it. They change our perception and also have an impact on our arousal thresholds. In particular, glucocorticoids and cortisol influence all human sensory systems. Additionally, the release of hormones usually occurs in circadian rhythms. This has significant effects on, for example, the growth of children as well as the human immune system. The connection between psychoneuroendocrinology and psychoneuroimmunology is particularly evident in relation to deep sleep stages and melatonin secretion. Cortisol is also produced in connection with sleep, leading to peak levels in the morning. Furthermore, the relationship between hormones and emotions was explained. Here, for example, the enormous importance of oxytocin for our social bonds, for the parent-child relationship, and the associated significance for the behavior and psyche of a child should be mentioned. Additionally, aggressive behavior and its connection with hormones were discussed. The result shows that male sex hormones are rather weakly positively correlated with aggression. However, it is clearly evident that not only do hormones influence our behavior, but our behavior can also influence our hormones. The enormous importance of stress for our health, our behavior, and our overall well-being was demonstrated. Stress can lead to depression, immune deficiency, and somatic disorders; extreme stress can lead to PTSD as well as loss of explicit memories and hippocampal degeneration. Additionally, the connection between genetics and PNE, as well as the connection between genetics and our psyche and behavior, is of enormous importance. It was demonstrated that modern PNE and thus also modern psychological and psychosocial fields of action are inextricably linked with behavioral genetics. The gene-environment interaction has an enormous impact on every individual, on our endocrine system, and thus on any scientific disciplines that deal with the human psyche. In this context, the influence of a pregnant woman's hormone secretions on the child's hormone secretions should also be mentioned. Hyper- or hypocortisolism during the perinatal phase can influence the development of the HPA axis and thus again promote mental disorders. Furthermore, human behavior and its psychosocial everyday life are controlled by 6 psychoneuronal systems, all of which are based on the effects of various hormones or endocrine systems. Ultimately, it should be noted that there is a connection between PNE and all disciplines or professions that work with people, whether in the medical, therapeutic, psychological, or psychosocial field. The relevance of these presented PNE findings for psychosocial and psychotherapeutic practice is therefore, in my opinion, undeniable, and openness to these interdisciplinary findings is thus an important aspect of modern, scientifically based, psychosocial counseling and psychotherapy.

Based on the findings presented here, an eclectic-integrative biopsychosocial coaching concept has emerged. Before this biopsychosocial coaching concept, the so-called "PNES Coaching," is presented and discussed, and the extent to which psychoneuroendocrinological findings are helpful in psychosocial and psychotherapeutic practice is examined, the following chapter will delve into psychosocial and psychotherapeutic methods or interventions and school-specific orientations, explain the concept of eclecticism, and further explore the biopsychosocial approach. Additionally, the importance of biopsychosocial diagnostics will be explained, and both methods from psychosocial fields of action and psychotherapeutic approaches and orientations will be presented and discussed. It will be shown which forms of psychotherapy have proven to be successful from a neuroscientific perspective and which approaches are compatible with "PNES Coaching." The goal is to provide a foundation on approaches, orientations, biopsychosocial diagnostics, methods, training, and interdisciplinarity to demonstrate suitable tools for the eclectic-integrative, biopsychosocial coaching concept "PNES Coaching."

References

Abbruzzese, Elvira (2011): Chronobiologie des Hormon- und des Immunsystems. In: Ehlert, Ulrike/von Känel, Roland (Hrsg.) (2011): Psychoendokrinologie und Psychoimmunologie. Berlin/Heidelberg: Springer-Verlag GmbH. 129–149.

Abney, Mark/Ober, Carole/Pan, Lin/Weiss, Lauren (2006): The sex-specific genetic architecture of quantitative traits in humans. Nat Genet 38(2): 218–222.

Aftab, Erwarte/Dwyer, Jennifer/Kalin, Ned H./McDonald, William M./Nemeroff, Charles B./Radhakrishnan, Rajiv/Rodriguez, Carolyn I./Widge, Alik/Zimmermann, Linda (2020): Hormonal treatments for major depressive disorder: State of the art. British Journal of Psychiatry. 177(8): 686–705. https://pubmed.ncbi.nlm.nih.gov/32456504/ [11.10.2022].

Aigner, Christoph/Bagga, Deepika/Cecchetto, Cinzia/Fischmeister, Florian/Holzer, Peter/Reichert, Johanna u. a. (2019): Einfluss einer 4-wöchigen Verabreichung von Probiotika mit mehreren Stämmen auf die funktionelle Konnektivität im Ruhezustand bei gesunden Freiwilligen. In: Europäische Zeitschrift für Ernährung. 58(5): 1821–1827.

Aksan, Nazan/Kochanska, Grazyna (2006): Children`s conscience and self-regulation. In: Journal of Personality 74(6): 1587–1617. https://pubmed.ncbi.nlm.nih.gov/17083659/ [22.10.2022].

Alleva, Enrico/Branchi, Igor/Champagne, Frances/Cirulli, Francesca/Curley, James/D`Andrea, Ivana (2013): Early interactions with mother and peers independently build adult social skills and shape BDNF and oxytocin receptor brain levels. In: Psychoneuroendocrinology 38(4): 522–532.

Aly, Janine/Engmann, Olivia (2020): Der Weg zum menschlichen Gehirn geht durch den Magen: Ernährungsfaktoren bei Major Depression. In: Front Neuroscience. 14: 582853. https://www.frontiersin.org/articles/10.3389/fnins.2020.582853/full [20.02.21].

Amroyan, E./Aslanyan, G./Darbinyan, V./Gabrielyan, E./Malmström, C./Panossian, Alexander (2007): Clinical trial of Rhodiola rosea L. extract SHR-5 in the treatment of mild to moderate depression. In: Nordic Journal of Psychiatry. 61(5): 343–348. http://www.tandfonline.com/doi/full/10.1080/08039480701643290 [26.05.2020].

Amsterdam, Jay/Panossian, Alexander (2016): Rhodiola rosea L. as a putative botanical antidepressant. In: Phytomedicine. 23(7): 770–783. https://linkinghub.elsevier.com/retrieve/pii/S0944711316000519 [26.05.2020].

Anderson, Steven/Bechara, Antoine/Damasio, Antonio/Damasio, Hanna/Tranel, Daniel (1999): Impairment of social and moral behavior related to early damage in human prefrontal cortex. In: Nature Neuroscience 2(11): 1032–1037.

Arndt, Thorsten/Gressner, Axel (2019) (Hrsg.): Lexikon der Medizinischen Laboratoriumsdiagnostik. Berlin, Heidelberg: Springer Medizin Verlag. In: http://link.springer.com/10.1007/978-3-662-48986-4 [20.02.2021].

Arneth, Borros (2018): Biochemische Signale der Darm-Hirn-Achse vom Gastrointestinaltrakt zum Zentralnervensystem: Darmdysbiose und veränderte Gehirnfunktion. In: Postgraduate Medical Journal. 94(1114): 446–452.

Arnsten, Amy/Connor, Daniel/Taylor, Fletcher/Raskind, Murray (2015): The effects of stress exposure on prefrontal cortex: Translating basic research into successful treatments for post-traumatic stress disorder. In: Neurobiology of Stress 1: 89–99.

Bader, Kerstin/Feiger, Bernd/Glauche, Volkmar/Jacob, Gitta A./Kaller, Christoph P./Kamphausen, Susanne/Klöppel, Stefan/Lieb, Klaus/Maier, Simon/Ohlendorf, Sabine/Schröder, Patricia/Silberschweig, David/Tebartz van Elst, Ludger/Tüscher, Oliver (2013): Mediale präfrontale Dysfunktion und verlängerte Amygdala-Reaktion während der instruierten Angstverarbeitung bei Borderline-Persönlichkeitsstörung. In: Das World Journal of Biological Psychiatry 14(4), 307–318. https://doi.org/10.3109/15622975.2012.665174.

Bahner, F. (1974): Klinik der Androgene. In: Androgene II und Antiandrogene. In: Handbuch der experimentellen Pharmakologie. Band 35/2. Berlin/Heidelberg: Springer Verlag. https://doi.org/10.1007/978-3-642-80859-3_5 [05.05.2023].

Bakermans-Kranenburg, Marian/van Ijzendoorn, Marinus (2006): Gene-envioronment interaction oft he dopamine D4 receptor (DRD4) and observed maternal insensitivity predicting externalizing behavior in preschoolers. In: Developmental Psychobiology 48(5): 406–409.

Balaram Kripa/Marwaha Raman (2023): Agoraphobia. In: StatPearls. Treasure Island (FL): StatPearls Publishing. PMID: 32119274. https://pubmed.ncbi.nlm.nih.gov/32119274/ [06.05.2023].

Bandelow, Borwin/Brooks, Andreas/Hajak, Göran/Krause, Johanna/Rüther, Eckart/Wedekind, Dirk (2005): Early traumatic life events, parental attitudes, familiy history, and birth risk factors in patients with borderline personality disorder and healthy controls. In: Psychiatry Research 134(2): 169–179.

Bandelow, Borwin/Falkai, Peter/Schmahl, Christian/Wedekind, Dirk (2010): Borderline personality disorder: A dysregulation oft he endogenous opioid system? In: Psychological Review 117(2): 623–636.

Bandelow, Borwin/Boerner, Reinhard/Kasper, Siegfried/Linden, Michael/Möller, Hans-Jürgen/Wittchen, Hans-Ulrich (2013): Generalisierte Angststörung: Diagnostik und Therapie. In: Deutsches Ärzteblatt 110(17): 300–310. https://www.aerzteblatt.de/archiv/137451/Generalisierte-Angststoerung [18.10.2022].

Bandelow, Borwin/Wedekind, Dirk (2014): Soziale Phobie. In: Nervenarzt 85. 635-647. https://doi.org/10.1007/s00115-013-3955-9 [05.05.2023].

Bandelow, Borwin/Falkai, Peter/Schmal, Christian/Wedekind, Dirk (2018): Borderline-Persönlichkeitsstörung: Eine Dysregulation des körpereigenen Opioidsystems? In: Psychologie-Blog: American Psychological Association. 117(2): 623–636. https://www.psycheblog.uk/2018/08/17/borderline-personality-disorder-a-dysregulation-of-the-endogenous-opioid-system/ [20.10.2022].

Bärtl, Christoph/Giglberger, Marina/Henze, Gina-Isabelle/Kirsch, Peter/Konzok, Julian/Kreuzpointner, Ludwig/Kudielka, Brigitte/Peter, Hanna/Streit, Fabian/Wüst, Stefan (2021): Geschlechtsspezifische Interaktion zwischen Cortisol und striato-limbischen Reaktionen auf psychosozialen Stress. In: Social Cognitive and Affective Neuroscience. 16(9): 972–984.

Beckrath-Wilking, Ulrike/Biberacher, Marlene/Volker, Dittmar/Wolf-Schmid, Regina (2013): Traumafachberatung, Traumatherapie und Traumapädagogik. Ein Handbuch für Psychotraumatologie im Beratenden, Therapeutischen und Pädagogischen Kontext. Paderborn: Junfermann Verlag.

Beckrath-Wilking, Ulrike/Biberacher, Marlene (2013): Einfluss von Bindungsfähigkeit und Bindungstraumata. In: Beckrath-Wilking, Ulrike/Biberacher, Marlene/Volker, Dittmar/Wolf-Schmid, Regina: Traumafachberatung, Traumatherapie und Traumapädagogik. Ein Handbuch für Psychotraumatologie im Beratenden, Therapeutischen und Pädagogischen Kontext. Paderborn: Junfermann Verlag. 94–99.

Belsky, Jay (1997): Variation in susceptibility to environmental influence: An evolutionary argument. In: Psychological Inquiry 8(3): 182–186.
Benecke, Cord (2014): Klinische Psychologie und Psychotherapie. Ein integratives Lehrbuch. Stuttgart: Kohlhammer Verlag.
Berner, Michael/Leiber, Christian/Wetterauer, Ulrich (2010): Testosteron und Psyche. In: Der Urologe. 49. Cham: Springer Nature Switzerland AG. 43–46. https://doi.org/10.1007/s00120-009-2197-8. [05.05.2023].
Berridge, Kent/Kringelbach, Morten (2013): Neuroscience of affect: Brain mechanisms of pleasure and displeasure. Current Opinion in Neurobiology 23: 294–303.
Bertrand, Paul/Jenkins, Trisha/Nguyen, Jason/Polglaze, Kate (2016): Einfluss von Tryptophan und Serotonin auf Stimmung und Kognition mit einer möglichen Rolle der Darm-Hirn-Achse. In: DOAJ. 8(1): 56. http://www.mdpi.com/2072-6643/8/1/56 [19.02.2021].
Bertsch, Katja/Herpertz, Sabine/Neumann, Inga/Schmidinger, Ilinca (2013): Reduced plasma oxytocinlevels in female patiens with borderline personality disorder. In: Hormones and Behavior 63(3): 424–429.
Binder, Elisabeth/Bradley, Rebekha/Epstein, Michael/Liu, Wei/Nair, Hemu/Stowe, Zachary/Tang, Ylang/et al. (2008): Influence of child abuse on adult depression: moderation by the corticotropin-releasing hormone receptor gene. In: Archives of general psychiatry 65(2): 190–200.
Binder, Elisabeth/Bradley, Rebekha/Cubells, Joseph/Deveau, Todd/Epstein, Michael/Gillespie, Charles/Heim, Christine/Liu, Wei/Mercer, Kristina/Nemeroff, Charles/Ressler, Kerry/Schwartz, Ann/Tang, Ylang (2008): Association of FKBP5 polymorphisms and childhood abuse with risk of posttraumatic stress disorder symptoms in adults. In: JAMA 299(11): 1291–1305.
Binder, Elisabeth/Provencal, Nadine (2015): The effects of early life stress on the epigenome: From the womb to adulthood and even before. In: Exper. Neurol. 268: 10–20
Birbaumer, Niels/Schmidt, Robert F. (2018): Biologische Psychologie. Sonderausgabe. 7. überarb. und ergänzte Aufl. Heidelberg: Springer Medizin Verlag.
Blackshaw, Seth/Lee, Daniel (2012): Functional implications of hypothalamic neurogenesis in the adult mammalian brain. In: International Journal of Developmental Neuroscience. 30: 615–621.
Blackwell, Aaron/Loftis, Jennifer/Turner, Erick (2006): Serotonin a la carte: Ergänzung mit der Serotonin-Vorstufe 5-Hydroxytryptophan. In: Pharmakologie und Therapeutik. 109(3): 325–338. Amsterdam: Elsevier Inc. https://linkinghub.elsevier.com/retrieve/pii/S016372580500135X [26.5.2020].
Blair, James (2013): The neurobiology of psychopathic traits in youths. In: Nature Reviews. Neuroscience 14(11): 786–799. https://pubmed.ncbi.nlm.nih.gov/24105343/ [21.10.2022].
Bodenmann, Guy/Milek, Anne (2018): Stressbewältigung. In: Margraf, Jürgen/Schneider, Silvia (Hrsg.): Lehrbuch der Verhaltenstherapie, Band 2. Psychologische Therapie bei Indikationen im Erwachsenenalter. 4. überarb. und aktual. Aufl. Berlin/Heidelberg: Springer-Verlag GmbH.
Bohus, Martin/Lieb, Klaus/Linehan, Marsha/Schmahl, Christian/Zanarini, Mary (2004): Borderline personality disorder. In: The Lancat 364(9432): 453–461.
Bohus, Martin (2019): Borderline-Störung. 2. überarb. Aufl. Göttingen: Hogrefe Verlag.
Böker, Heinz/Bösiger,Peter/Ernst, Jutta/Grimm, Simone/Hell, Daniel/Northoff, Georg (2009): Increasedself-focus in major depressive disorder is related to neural abnormalities in subcortical-cortical midline structures. In: Humain Brain Mapping 30: 2617–2627.
Brisch, Karl Heinz (2009): Bindungsstörungen. Von der Bindungstheorie zur Therapie. 9. Aufl. Stuttgart: Klett-Cotta.
Braun, Katharina/Lange, E./Metzger, Martin/Poeggel, Gerd (2000): Maternal separation followed by early social deprivation affects the development of monoaminergic fiber systems in the medial prefrontal cortex of Octodon degus. In: Neuroscience 95(1): 309–318.

Bravo, Juan/Carrupt, Pierre-Alain/Hostettmann, Kurt/Marston, Andreas/Reist, Marianne/van Diermen, Daphne (2009): Monoamine oxidase inhibition by Rhodiola rosea L. roots. In: Journal of Ethnopharmacology. 122(2): 397–401. https://linkinghub.elsevier.com/retrieve/pii/S037887410900021X [26.05.2020].

Buchheim, Anna/Cierpka, Manfred/Roth, Gerhard/et al. (2012): Neuronale Veränderungen bei chronisch-depressiven Patienten während psychoanalytischer Psychotherapie. In: Psychotherapeut 57(3): 219–226.

Buckholtz, Joshua/Meyer-Lindenberg, Andreas (2008): MAOA and the neurogenetic architecture of human aggression. Trend in Neurosciences 31(3): 120–129. https://pubmed.ncbi.nlm.nih.gov/18258310/ [22.10.2022].

Buckholtz, Joshua/Woodward, Neil/Zald, David/et al. (2010): Mesolimbic dopamine reward system hypersensitivity in individuals with psychopathic traits. In: Nature Neuroscience 13: 419–421. https://www.nature.com/articles/nn.2510 [21.10.2022].

Burkhardt, Sausan/Demster, Emma/Meyer, Andreas H./Stähli, Simon/Theil, Nathan/Unternaehrer, Eva et al. (2015): Childhood maternal care is associated with DNA methylation oft he genes for brain-derived neurotrophic factor (BDNF) and oxytocin receptor (OXTR) in peripheral blood cells in adult men and women. In: Stress 18(4): 451–461.

Busse, Anja/Plaumann, Martina/Walter, Ulla (2006): Grundlagen zu Stress. In: KKH Kaufmännische Krankenkasse (Hrsg.): Weißbuch Prävention. Stress? Ursachen, Erklärungsmodelle und präventive Ansätze. Berlin/Heidelberg: Springer Verlag. 3–12.

Buxbaum, Josef/Flory, Janine/Holsboer, Folrian/Ising, Markus/Pratchett, Laura/Yehuda, Rahel (2010): Putative biological mechanisms for the association between early life adversity and the subsequent development of PTSD. In: Psychopharmacology. 212: 405–417.

Canli, Turhan/Lesch, Klaus-Peter (2007): Long story short: The serotonin transporter in emotion regulation and social cognition. In: Nature Neuroscience 10(9): 1103–1109.

Cappi, Carolina/Diniz, Juliana/Lisboa, Garcia/et al. (2016): Epigenetic evidence for involvement of the oxytocin receptor gene in obsessive-compulsive disorder. In: BMC neuroscience 17(1): 79. https://bmcneurosci.biomedcentral.com/articles/10.1186/s12868-016-0313-4 [19.10.2022].

Carson, Dekan S./Garner, Joseph P./Hyde, Shellie A./Keller, Jennifer/Kenna, Heather A./Lembke, Anna/Parker, Karen J./Schatzberg, Alan F./Tennakoon, Lakshika/Yuen, Kaeli W. (2014): Plasma oxytocin concentrations are lower in depressed vs. healthy control woman and are independent of cortisol. In: Journal of Psychiatric Research. 51: 30–36.

Carver, Charles/Johnson, Sheri/Kim, Youngmee (2016): Mu opioid receptor polymorphism, early social adversity, and social traits. Social neuroscience 11(5): 515–524.

Caspi, Avshalom/Craig, Ian/Harrington, HonaLee/Martin, Judy/McClay, Joseph/Mill, Jonathan/Moffitt, Terrie/Poulton, Richie (2002): Role of genotype in the cycle of violence in maltreated children. In: Science 297(5582): 851–854.

Caspi, Avshalom/Craig, Ian/Harrington, HonaLee/Moffitt, Terrie/Poulton, Richie/Taylor, Alan et al. (2003): Influence of life stress on depression: Moderation by a polymorphism in the 5-HTT gene. In: Science 301(5631): 386–389.

Caspi, Avshalom/Craig, Ian/Kim-Cohen, Julia/Moffitt, Terrie et al. (2006): MAOA, maltreatment, and gene-environment interaction predicting children's mental health: new evidence and a meta-analysis. In: Mol Psychiatry 11(10): 903–913.

Chamary, Jean V. (2016): Homöostase. In: 50 Schlüsselideen Biologie. Berlin/Heidelberg: Springer Verlag. https://doi.org/10.1007/978-3-662-48381-7_34 [05.05.2023].

Chen, Frances/Heinrich, Markus/Hummel, Elisabeth/Kumsta, Robert (2013): Epigenetic regulation oft he oxytocin receptor gene: Implications for behavioral neuroscience. In: Frontiers in Neuroscience 7: 83. https://www.frontiersin.org/articles/10.3389/fnins.2013.00083/full [21.10.2022].

Cheung, Natalie/Gibbon, Simon/Khalifa, Najat/McCarthy, Lucy/Völlm, Birgit (2020): Psychologische Interventionen bei antisozialer Persönlichkeitsstörung. In: Cochrane Database Syst Rev. 9(9). https://pubmed.ncbi.nlm.nih.gov/32880104/ [21.10.2022].

Choleris, Elena/Kavaliers, Martin/Matta, Richard (2020): Amygdala In: Zeigler-Hill, Virgil/ Shakelford, Todd K. (Hrsg.): Encyclopedia of Personality and Individual Differences. Cham: Springer Verlag. https://doi.org/10.1007/978-3-319-24612-3_726 [05.05.2023].

Cicchetti, Dante/DeYoung, Colin/Eastman, Maria/Gray, Jeremy/Grigorenko, Elena/Rogosch, Fred (2011a): Sources of cognitive exploration: Genetic variation in the prefrontal dopamine system predicts Openness/Intellect. In: Journal of Research in Personality 45(4): 364–371.

Cicchetti, Dante/Rogosch, Fred/Sturge-Apple, Melissa/Toth, Sheree (2011b): Normalizing the development of cortisol regulation in maltreated infants through preventive interventions. In: Development and Psychopathology 23(3): 789–800.

Cochran, Nick R./Denison, Lydia/Filkowski, Megan M./Haas, Brian W./Isak, Alexanrda/Nishitani, Shota/Smith, Alicia K. (2016): Epigenetic modification of OXT and human sociability. In: Proceedings oft the National Academy of Sciences 113(27): E3816–E3823.

Cole, Steven W./Creswell, David J./Irwin, Michael R./Meyers, Hector F. (2009): Mindfulness meditation training effects on CD4+ T lymphocytes in HIV-1 infected adults: a small randomized controlled trial. Brain Behav Immun. 23(2): 184–188.

Colzato, Lorenza/Hommel, Bernhard/Jongkees, Bryant/Kühn, Simon (2015): Wirkung einer Tyrosin-Supplementierung auf klinische und gesunde Populationen unter Stress oder kognitiven Anforderungen – eine Übersicht. In: J Psychiatr. Res. 70: 50–57. https://linkinghub.elsevier.com/retrieve/pii/S0022395615002472 [20.02.2021].

Dadds, Mark/Ebstein, Richard/Hawes, David/et al. (2014): Methylation of the oxytocin receptor gene and oxytocin blood levels in the development of psychopathy. In: Development and Psychopathology. 26(1): 33–40. https://pubmed.ncbi.nlm.nih.gov/24059811/ [21.10.2022].

Daw, Nathaniel/Dayan, Peter/Kakade, Sham (2002): Opponent interactions between serotonin and dopamine. In: Neural Networks 15(4–6): 603–616.

Dayan, Peter/Montague, Read/Schultz, Wolfram (1997): Ein neuronales Substrat der Vorhersage und Belohnung. In: Wissenscaft 275(5306): 1593–1599. https://doi.org/10.1126/science.275.5306.1593 [03.05.2023].

DeBold, Joseph/Miczek, Klaus/Tornatzky, Walter/van Erp, Annemoon (2002): Alcohol, $GABA_A$-Benzodiazepine Receptor Complex, and Aggression. In: Galanter, Marc (Hrsg.): Recent Developments in Alcoholism. vol 13. Boston: Springer Verlag. 139–171.

De Geus, Eco/Wüst, Stefan (2011): Bedeutung der Genetik für die Psychoneuroendokrinologie und Psychoimmunologie. In: Ehlert, Ulrike/Von Känel, Roland (Hrsg.): Psychoendokrinologie und Psychoimmunologie. Berlin/Heidelberg: Springer-Verlag GmbH. 164–185.

Dia, Si Yuan/Kahouli, Imen/Lomis, Nikita/Prakash, Satya/Singh, Surya/Westfall, Susanne (2017): Mikrobiom, Probiotika und neurodegenerative Erkrankungen: Entschlüsselung der Darm-Hirn-Achse. In: Cellular and Molecular Life Sciences. 74(20): 3769–3787. http://link.springer.com/10.1007/s00018-017-2550-9 [23.02.2021].

Dietrich, Georg/Walter, Hellmuth (1972): Grundbegriffe der psychologischen Fachsprache. München: Ehrenwirth Verlag.

Dimitrova, Nevena/Glatz, Nathalie/Halfon, Olivier/Heinrichs, Markus/Pierrehumbert, Blaise/Torrisi, Raffaela (2009): The influence of attachment on perceived stress and cortisol response to acute stress in women sexually abused in childhood or adolescence, In: Psychoneuroendocrinology 34(6): 924–938.

Dittmar, Volker (2013): Spektrum akuter und chronischer posttraumatischer Störungsbilder. In: Beckrath-Wilking, Ulrike/Biberacher, Marlene/Dittmar, Volker/Wolf-Schmidt, Regina: Traumafachberatung, Traumatherapie und Traumapädagogik. Ein Handbuch für Psychotraumatologie im beratenden, therapeutischen und pädagogischen Kontext. Paderborn: Junfermann Verlag.

Domes, Gregor/Heinrichs, Markus/Kirsch, Peter/Meyer-Lindenberg, Andreas (2011): Oxytocin and vasopressin in the human brain: social neuropeptides for translational medicine. Nature Reviews. Neuroscience 12(9): 524–538.

Domschke, Katharina (2014): Prädiktive Faktoren bei Angststörungen. In: Nervenarzt. 85(10): 1263–1268.

Domschke, Katharina/Schiele, Miriam (2017): Epigenetik an der Schnittstelle zwischen Genen, Umwelt und Resilienz bei Angststörungen. In: Gene, Gehirn und Verhalten. 17(3). https://www.researchgate.net/publication/319499585_Epigenetics_at_the_crossroads_between_genes_environment_and_resilience_in_anxiety_disorders [18.10.2022].

Domschke, Katharina/Schiele, Miriam/Ziegler, Christiane (2017): (Epi)Genetik der Angst. In: Österreichische Gesellschaft für Neuropsychopharmakologie und Biologische Psychiatrie. https://oegpb.at/2017/12/14/epigenetik-der-angst/ [18.10.2022].

Duman, Ronald/Fogaça, Manoela (2019): Kortikale GABAerge Dysfunktion bei Stress und Depression: Neue Erkenntnisse für therapeutische Interventionen. In: Front Cell Neuroscience 13: 87.

Edward, Kate M./Mills, Paul J. (2011): Interaktionen zwischen dem endokrinen, dem zentralnervösen und dem Immunsystem. In: Ehlert, Ulrike/von Känel, Roland (Hrsg.): Psychoendokrinologie und Psychoimmunologie. Berlin/Heidelberg: Springer-Verlag GmbH. 111–127.

Ehlert, Ulrike (2006): Psychoendokrinologie der Angst. In: Psychologische Rundschau. 57(3): 165–175. https://www.fachportal-paedagogik.de/literatur/vollanzeige.html%3FFId%3D761717 [18.10.2022].

Ehlert, Ulrike (2011): Das endokrine System. In: Ehlert, Ulrike/von Känel, Roland (Hrsg.): Psychoendokrinologie und Psychoimmunologie. Berlin/Heidelberg: Springer-Verlag GmbH. 3–36.

Ehlert, Ulrike/von Känel, Roland (Hrsg.) (2011): Psychoendokrinologie und Psychoimmunologie. Berlin/Heidelberg: Springer-Verlag GmbH.

Eidelman-Rothman, Moranne/Feldman, Ruth/Vengrober, Adva/Zagoory-Sharon, Orna (2013): Stress reactivity in war-exposed young children with and without posttraumatic stress disorder: relations to maternal stress hormones, parenting, and child emotionality and regulation. In: Development and psychopathology 25(4pt1): 943–955.

Entringer, Sonja/Hellhammer, Dirk/Koper, Jan/Kumsta, Robert/van Rossum, Elisabeth/Wüst, Stefan (2008): Glucocorticoid receptor gene polymorphisms and glucocorticoid sensitivity of sudermal blood vessels and leukocytes. In: Biological Psychology 79(2). 179–184.

Faller, Hermann (2003): Verhaltensgenetik. In: Psychotherapeut 48: 80-92. https://doi.org/10.1007/s00278-003-0294-5 [03.05.2023].

Falkai, Peter (2022a): Vegetatives Nervensystem. In: Pschyrembel online. Berlin: Walter de Gruyter GmbH. https://www.pschyrembel.de/vegetatives%20Nervensystem/K0F3H/doc/ [01.05.2023].

Falkai, Peter (2022b): Eltern-Kind-Beziehung. In: Pschyrembel online. Berlin: Walter de Gruyter GmbH. https://www.pschyrembel.de/Bindung/P058D/doc/ [03.05.2023].

Favreau, Matthias/Pfeuffer, Simone/Voderholzer, Ulrich (2021): Behandlung von Zwangsstörungen. In: DNP- Der Neurologe & Psychiater 22(2021):27–31. https://link.springer.com/article/10.1007/s15202-021-4672-z [19.10.2022]. Feldman, Ruth (2017): The neurobiology of human attachments. In: Trends in cognitive sciences 21(2): 80–99.

Feldman, Ruth (2017): The neurobiology of human attachments. In: Trends in Cognitive Sciences 21(2): 80–99.

Feldman, Ruth/Gordon, Ilanit/Zagoory-Sharon, Orna (2010): The cross-generation transmission of oxytocin in humans. In: Hormones and Behavior. 58(4): 669–676.

Fernàndez, Guillen/Henckens, Marloes/Hermans, Erno/Joëls, Marian (2014): Dynamic adaptation of large-scale brain networks in response to acute stressors. In: Trends in Neurosciences 37(6): 304–314.

Fernàndez, Guillen/Hömberg, Judith/Kozicz, Tamas (2017): Large-scale network balances in the transition from adaptive to maladaptive stress responses. In: Current Opinion in Behavioral Sciences 14: 27–32.

Fiorillo, Christopher/Schultz, Wolfram/Tobler, Philippe (2003): Discrete coding of reward probability and uncertainty by dopamine neurons. In: Science 299: 1898–1902.

Fox, Nathan/McLaughlin, Katie/Nelson, Charles/Sheridan, Margaret/Tibu, Florin/Zeanah, Charles (2015): Causal effects oft he early caregiving environment on development of stress response systems in children. In: Proceedings oft he National Academy of Sciences 112(18): 5637–5642.

Fredrickson, Barbara/Loftus, Geoffrey/Nolen-Hoeksema, Susan/Smith, Edward (2007): Atkinsons und Hitgards Einführung in die Psychologie. Berlin/Heidelberg: Springer Verlag GmbH.

Gatzke-Kopp, Lisa (2011): The canary in the coalmine: The sensitivity of mesolimbic dopamine to environmental adversity during development. In: Neuroscience and Biobehavioral Reviews 35(3): 794–803.

Glenn, Andrea (2011): The other allele: Exploring the long allele of the serotonin transporter gene as a potential risk factor for psychopathy: A review of the parallels in findings. In: Neuroscience and Biobehavioral Reviews. 35: 612–620.

Graybiel, Ann/Rauch, Scott (2000): Toward a neurobiology of obsessive-compulsive disorder. In: Neuron 28(2): 343–347.

Gunderson, John/Herpertz, Sabine/Skodol, Andrew/et al. (2018): Borderline Persönlichkeitsstörung. In: Nat Rev Dis Primers 4: 18029. https://pubmed.ncbi.nlm.nih.gov/29795363/ [20.10.2022].

Habermeyer, Elmar/Saß, Henning (2018): Psychopathia und antisoziale Persönlichkeitsstörungen im Spannungsfeld zwischen Pathologie und Dissozialität. In: Forens Psychiatr Psychol Kriminol. 12: 183–185. https://doi.org/10.1007/s11757-018-0492-1 [21.10.2022].

Hackermeier, Ursula (2020): Chronobiologie. In: Pschyrembel online. Berlin: Walter de Gruyter GmbH. https://www.pschyrembel.de/Chronobiologie/N00L1/doc/ [02.05.2023].

Hahn, Andreas/Höflich, Anna/Losak, Jan/Mitterhauser, Markus/Wadsack, Wolfgang/Windischberger, Christian et al. (2012): Differential modulation of the default mode network via serotonin-1A receptors. In: Proceedings of the National Academy of Sciences 109(7): 2619–2624.

Hall, Baila/Liston, Conor/Moda, Rachel (2015): Glucocorticoid mechanisms of functional connectivity changes in stress-related neuropsychiatric disorders. In: Neurobiology of stress 1: 174–183.

Hasler, Gregor (2010): Pathophysiology of depression: Do weh ave any solid evidence of interest to clinicians? In: World Psychiatry 9(3): 155–161.

Hausmann, Markus/Jordan, Kirsten (2010): Sexualhormone und Verhalten. In: Müller, Jürgen (Hrsg.): Neurobiologie forensisch-relevanter Störungen. Grundlagen, Störungsbilder, Perspektiven. Stuttgart: Verlag W. Kohlhammer GmbH. 118–127.

Havenaar, Rob (2011): Darmgesundheitsfunktionen von mikrobiellen Metaboliten im Dickdarm: eine Übersicht. In: Benef Microbes. 2(2): 103–114. doi: https://doi.org/10.3920/BM2011.0003. [07.05.2023].

Heim, Christine/Miller, Andrew/Mletzko, Tanja/Nemeroff, Charles/Newport, D Jeffery/Young, Larry (2009): Lower CSF oxytocin concentrations in women with a history of childhood abuse. In: Molecular Psychiatry 14(10): 954–958.

Heinrichs, Markus/Kuppeln, Gregor/von Dawans, Bernadette (2009): Oxytocin, Vasopressin und menschliches Sozialverhalten. In: Neuroendokrinology 30(4): 548-557. https://doi.org/10.1016/j.yfrne.2009.05.005 [04.05.2023].

Henderson, Markus (2010): Verhaltensgenetik. In: 50 Schlüsselideen Genetik. Heidelberg: Spektrum Akademischer Verlag. 88–91. https://doi.org/10.1007/978-3-8274-2381-8_23 [02.05.2023].

Hennig, Jürgen/Netter, Petra (2000): Psychoneuroendokrinologie. In: Spektrum der Wissenschaft. Lexikon der Psychologie. Heidelberg: Spektrum der Wissenschaft Verlagsgesellschaft mbH., Springer Nature. https://www.spektrum.de/lexikon/psychologie/psychoneuroendokrinologie/12129 [19.04.2023].

Hernaus, Dennis/Myin-Germeys, Inez/Vaessen, Thomas/van Amelsvoort, Therese (2015): Die dopaminerge Reaktion auf akuten Stress in Gesundheit und Psychopathologie: Eine systematische Überprüfung. Neuroscience and Biobehavioral Reviews. 56: 241–251. https://doi.org/10.1016/j.neubiorev.2015.07.008 [20.02. 2021]

Holmes, Andrew (2008): Genetic variation in cortico-amygdala serotonin function and risk for stress-related disease. Neuroscience and Biobehavioral Reviews 32(7): 1293–1314.

Hsu, Daphne/Love, Tiffany/Meyers, Kortni/…/Zubieta, Jon-Kar (2013): Response of the m-opioid system to social rejection and acceptance. Molecular Psychiatry 18: 1211–1217

Insel, Thomas/Lyons, Casie/Noble, Pamela/Sterk, Sheila/Winslow, James (2003): Rearing effects on cerebrospinal fluid oxytocin concentration and social buffering in rhesus monkeys. In: Neuropsychopharmacology 28(5): 910–918.

Imeri, Luca/Opp, Marc R. (2009): How (and why) the immune system makes us sleep. Nature Reviews Neuroscience 10: 199–210.

Irwin, Michael R. (2008): Human psychoneuroimmunology: 20 years of discovery. In: Brain Behav Immun 22(2): 129–139.

Irwin, Michael R./Motivala, Sarosh J./Olmstead,Richard (2008): Verbesserung der Schlafqualität bei älteren Erwachsenen mit mäßigen Schlafbeschwerden: Eine randomisierte kontrollierte Studie zu Tai Chi Chih. In: Sleep 31: 1001–1008.

Jans, Thomas/Melfsen, Siebke/Walitza, Susanne/Warnke, Andreas/Wewetzer, Christoph/Zellmann, Henrike (2011): Zwangsstörungen im Kindes- und Jugendalter. In: Deutsches Ärzteblatt. 108(11): 173–179. https://www.aerzteblatt.de/archiv/81312/Zwangsstoerung-im-Kindes-und-Jugendalter [19.10.2022].

Kathmann, Norbert/Staniloiu, Angelica/Vorderholzer, Ulrich/Wahl-Kordon, Andreas/Zurowski, Bartosz/et al. (2022): Leitlinie Zwangsstörungen – Langversion. In: file:///C:/Users/mark/Downloads/038_017l_S3_Zwangsst%C3%B6rungen_2022–07.pdf [19.10.2022].

Keck, Martin (2017): Depression. Wie entsteht sie? Wie wird sie behandelt? Was ist der Zusammenhang mit Stress? In: https://www.psych.mpg.de/2354388/depression_patienten_broschuere_keck.pdf [07.10.2022].

Kennedy, David (2016): B-Vitamine und das Gehirn: Mechanismen, Dosis und Wirksamkeit – eine Übersicht. In: Nutrients 8(2): 68. https://www.6.ncbi.nlm.nih.gov/pmc/articles/PMC4772032/ [03.07.2022].

Kikuchi, Asako/Tanabe, Aya/Iwahori, Yoshihirov (2020): Eine systematische Überprüfung der Wirkung einer L-Tryptophan-Supplementierung auf Stimmung und emotionale Funktion. In: Zeitschrift für Nahrungsergänzungsmittel. 18(3): 316–333. https://www.tandfonline.com/doi/full/10.1080/19390211.2020.1746725 [19.02.2021].

Krähenmann, Rainer/Seiferitz, Erich (2019): Krank durch chronischen Stress. In: DNP 20. Springer Medizin Verlag GmbH. 38–48. https://doi.org/10.1007/s15202-019-2113-z [15.02.2022].

Krueger, James/Obal, Ferenc Jr. (2004): GHRH and sleep. In: Sleep Med Rev. 8(5): 367–377.

Landgraf, Rainer/Neumann, Ida (2012): Balance of brain oxytocin and vasopressin: Implications for anxiety, depression, and social behaviors. In: Trends in Neurosciences 35: 649–659.

Laszig, Parfen/Rieg, Kathy (2004): Recherche zu Zwangsstörungen: Wissenschaftliche Projekte im Internet selten. In: Deutsches Ärzteblatt. 3(2004): 418. https://www.aerzteblatt.de/archiv/43370/Recherche-zu-Zwangsstoerungen-Wissenschaftliche-Projekte-im-Internet-selten [19.10.2022].

Lieb, Roselind (2018): Zwillingsforschung. In: Pschyrembel online. Berlin: Walter de Gruyter GmbH. https://www.pschyrembel.de/Sympathikus/K0M17/doc/ [03.05.2023].

Luerweg, Frank (2019): Wie Geruchssinn und psychische Störungen zusammenhängen. In: Spektrum der Wissenschaft. Medizin. Psychische Krankheiten. Heidelberg: Spektrum der Wissenschaft Verlagsgesellschaft mbH., Springer Nature. https://www.spektrum.de/news/zusammenhang-von-psychische-erkrankungen-und-geruchssinn/1655756 [01.05.2023].

Lück, Monika/Roth, Gerhard/Stüber, Daniel (2008): Sex, aggression and impulse control: An integrative account. In: Neurocase 14(1): 93–121.

Mahlmann, Regina (2020): Gehirnforschung und Psychotherapie – Teil 3: Die sechs psychoneuronalen Grundsysteme. In: Freie Psychotherapie 6/2020. Verband Freier Psychotherapeuten, Heilpraktiker für Psychotherapie und Psychologischer Berater e. V. München: Fulton Akademie GmbH. https://www.vfp.de/magazine/freie-psychotherapie/alle-ausgaben/heft-06-2020/gehirnforschung-und-psychotherapie-teil-3-die-sechs-psychoneuralen-grundsysteme [07.05.2023].

Maier, Wolfgang/Zobel, Astrid (2004): Endophänotypen-ein neues Konzept zur biologischen Charakterisierung psychischer Störungen. In: Der Nervenarzt 75(3): 205–214. Berlin/Heidelberg: Springer Medizin Verlag GmbH. https://www.springermedizin.de/endophaenotypen-ein-neues-konzept-zur-biologischen-charakterisie/8060708 [15.02.2022].

Main, Mary/Solomon, Judith (1986): Discovery of an insecure-disorganized/disoriented pattern. In: Brazelton, T. Berry/Yogman, Michael (Hrsg.): Affective Development in Infancy. Norwood, New Jersey: Ablex Publishing.

Mason, John Wayne (1968): A review of psychoendocrine research on the sympathetic-adrenal medullary system. Psychosomatics Med. 30(5): 631–653.

Mattheisen, Manuel (2018): Genome-wide association analyses identify 44 risk variants and refine the genetic architecture of major depression. In: Nature Genetics. doi: https://doi.org/10.1038/s41588-018-0090-3 und https://www.ukw.de/fileadmin/uk/portal/04_Aktuelles/_Bilder/2018/05_Mai_2018/2018-05-22_-_PI_Uniklinikum_Wuerzburg_44_genetische_Variationen_im_Zusammenhang_mit_Depressionen_identifiziert.pdf [12.10.2022].

Mattioli, Laura/Perfumi, Marina (2007): Adaptogenic and central nervous system effects of single doses of 3% rosavin and 1% salidroside Rhodiola rosea L. – extract in mice. In: Phytotherapy Research. 21(1): 37–43. http://doi.wiley.com/10.1002/ptr.2013 [26.05.2020].

Meerlo, Peter/Sgoifo, Andrea/Suchecki, Deborah (2008): Restricted and disrupted sleep: effects on autonomic function, neuroendocrine stress systems and stress responsivity. Sleep Medicine Reviews 12(3): 197–210.

Meiss, Ortwin (2009): Psychosomatische Störungen. In: Revenstorf, Dirk/Peter, Burkhard (Hrsg.): Hypnose in Psychotherapie, Psychosomatik und Medizin. Manual für die Praxis. Berlin/Heidelberg: Springer-Verlag GmbH. 547–557.

Mocker, Daniela (2022): Eine neue Klassifikation der Krankheiten. In: Spektrum der Wissenschaft. Diagnostik. Heidelberg: Spektrum der Wissenschaft Verlagsgesellschaft mbH., Springer Nature. https://www.spektrum.de/news/icd-11-eine-neue-klassifikation-der-krankheiten/1971949 [06.05.2023].

Morschitzky, Hans (2000): Angststörungen. In: Stumm, Gerhard, Pritz, Alfred (Hrsg.): Wörterbuch der Psychotherapie. Wien: Springer Verlag. 34–35.

Müller, Christian A./Renner, Bertold (2022): Riechstörungen evidenzbasiert diagnostizieren und behandeln. Der unterschätzte Sinn – neue Erkenntnisse belegen die Bedeutung und Leistungsfähigkeit des menschlichen Geruchssinns. In: Wiener Medizinische Wochenschrift. 172: 8–13. https://doi.org/10.1007/s10354-021-00895-x [01.05.2023].

Nelson, Eric E./Panksepp Jaak (1998): Gehirnsubstrate der Bindung zwischen Kind und Mutter: Beiträge von Opioiden, Oxytocin und Norepinephrin. In: Neuroscience and Biobehavioral Reviews, 22(3): 437–452. https://doi.org/10.1016/S0149-7634(97)00052-3 [05.05.2023].

Neumann, Inga D./Peters, Sebastian/Reber, Stefan O./Slattery, David A./Uschold-Schmidt, Nicole (2014): Dosisabhängige Wirkungen einer chronischen zentralen Infusion von Oxytocin auf Angst, Oxytocin-Rezeptorbindung und stressbezogene Parameter bei Mäusen, In: Psychoneuroendokrinologie 42: 225–236. https://doi.org/10.1016/j.psyneuen.2014.01.021 [06.05.2023].

Nienstedt, Monika/Westermann, Arnim (2007): Pflegekinder und ihre Entwicklungschancen nach frühen traumatischen Erfahrungen. Stuttgart: Klett-Cotta Verlag.

Nigg, Joel (2017): Annual Research Review: On the relations among self-regulation, self-control, executive functioning, effortful control, cognitive control, impulsivity, risk-taking, and inhibition for developmental psychopathology. In: Journal of child psychology and psychiatry 58(4): 361–383.

Noll, Jennie G./Putnam, Frank W./Shenk, Chad E./Susman Elizabeth J./Trickett, Penelope (2010): Attenuation of cortisol across development for victims of sexual abuse. In: Development and Psychopathology. 22(1): 165–175.

Olivier, Berend (2010): Serotonin and Aggression. In: Annals of the New York Academy of Sciences 1036(1): 382–392. https://doi.org/10.1196/annals.1330.022.

Pollak, Seth/Seltzer, Leslie/Ziegler, Toni (2010): Social vocalizations can release oxytocin in humans. Proceedings oft the Royal Society B: Biological Sciences 277(1694): 2661–2666.

Pschyrembel Redaktion (2016a): Sympathikus. In: Pschyrembel online. Berlin: Walter de Gruyter GmbH. https://www.pschyrembel.de/Sympathikus/K0M17/doc/ [01.05.2023].

Pschyrembel Redaktion (2022a): Geruchssinn. In: Pschyrembel online. Berlin: Walter de Gruyter GmbH. https://www.pschyrembel.de/Geruchssinn/T01SM/doc/ [01.05.2023].

Pschyrembel Redaktion (2022b): Geschmackssinn. In: Pschyrembel online. Berlin: Walter de Gruyter GmbH. https://www.pschyrembel.de/Geschmackssinn/T01SX/doc/ [01.05.2023].

Purves, Dale/Williams, Stephen (2001) (Hrsg.): Neuroscience. 2. Aufl. Sunderland, Mass: Sinauer Associates. 681.

Rautiainen, MR./Sulkava, S./Tiihonen, J. et al. (2016): Genome-wide association study of antisocial personality disorder. In: Translational Psychiatry. 6(9): e883. https://doi.org/10.1038/tp.2016.155 [07.05.2023].

Ravnkilde, Barbara/Videbech, Paul (2004): Hippocampal volume and depression: a meta-analysis of MRI studies. In: American Journal of Psychiatry 161(11): 1957–1966.

Richter, Kneginja (2021): Chronobiologie. In: Somnologie 25: 87–88. https://doi.org/10.1007/s11818-021-00312-w [02.05.2023].

Riecher-Rössler, Anita (2011): Psychoprotektive Effekte von Östrogenen. In: Journal für Neurologie, Neurochirurgie und Psychiatrie. Zeitschrift für Erkrankungen des Nervensystems. 12(2). Gablitz: Krause und Pachernegg GmbH. 152–156.

Roth, Gerhard (2016): Transgenerationelle Weitergabe von Traumata aus neurobiologischer Sicht. In: Jahrbuch der Kinder- und Jugendlichen-Psychoanalyse. Frankfurt am Main: Brandes und Apsel. 18–32.

Roth, Gerhard/Ryba, Alica (2019): Coaching, Beratung und Gehirn. Neurobiologische Grundlagen wirksamer Veränderungskonzepte. 4. Aufl. Stuttgart: Klett-Cotta Verlag.

Roth, Gerhard/Strüber, Daniel/Strüber, Nicole (2014): Impact of early adversity on glucocorticoid regulation and later mental disorders. In: Neuroscience and Biobehavioral Reviews. 38:17–37.
Roth, Gerhard/Strüber, Nicole (2021): Wie das Gehirn die Seele macht. 4. Aufl. Stuttgart: Klett-Cotta Verlag.
Rotter, David (2021): Serotonin, Dopamin, GABA. Mikronährstoffe für Stimmung und Psyche. Berlin: Dr. Schweikart Verlag.
Schäffler, Arne (2022): Phobie. In: Pschyrembel online. Berlin: Walter de Gruyter GmbH. https://www.pschyrembel.de/Phobische%20St%C3%B6rung/K0GV6/doc/ [06.05.2023].
Schöller, Dorit (2021a): Phänotyp. In: Pschyrembel online. Berlin: Walter de Gruyter GmbH. https://www.pschyrembel.de/Ph%C3%A4notyp/K0GSB/doc/ [03.05.2023].
Schöller, Dorit (2021b): Genotyp. In: Pschyrembel online. Berlin: Walter de Gruyter GmbH. https://www.pschyrembel.de/Genotyp/K08M8/doc/ [03.05.2023].
Selg, Herbert (2000): Aggression. In: Spektrum der Wissenschaft. Lexikon der Psychologie. Heidelberg: Spektrum der Wissenschaft Verlagsgesellschaft mbH., Springer Nature. https://www.spektrum.de/lexikon/psychologie/aggression/337 [05.05.2023].
Spektrum Lexikon der Neurowissenschaft (2000a): Sympathicus. In: Spektrum der Wissenschaft. Lexikon der Neurowissenschaft. Heidelberg: Spektrum der Wissenschaft Verlagsgesellschaft mbH., Springer Nature. https://www.spektrum.de/lexikon/neurowissenschaft/sympathicus/12584 [01.05.2023].
Spektrum Lexikon der Neurowissenschaft (2000b): Parasympathicus. In: Spektrum der Wissenschaft. Lexikon der Neurowissenschaft. Heidelberg: Spektrum der Wissenschaft Verlagsgesellschaft mbH., Springer Nature. https://www.spektrum.de/lexikon/neurowissenschaft/parasympathicus/9522 [01.05.2023].
Spektrum Lexikon der Neurowissenschaft (2000c): Präfrontaler Cortex. In: Spektrum der Wissenschaft. Lexikon der Neurowissenschaft. Heidelberg: Spektrum der Wissenschaft Verlagsgesellschaft mbH., Springer Nature. https://www.spektrum.de/lexikon/neurowissenschaft/praefrontaler-cortex/10178 [05.05.2023].
Spektrum Lexikon der Neurowissenschaft (2000d): Androgene. In: Spektrum der Wissenschaft. Lexikon der Neurowissenschaft. Heidelberg: Spektrum der Wissenschaft Verlagsgesellschaft mbH., Springer Nature. https://www.spektrum.de/lexikon/neurowissenschaft/androgene/608 [05.05.2023].
Spektrum Lexikon der Neurowissenschaft (2000e): GABA. In: Spektrum der Wissenschaft. Lexikon der Neurowissenschaft. Heidelberg: Spektrum der Wissenschaft Verlagsgesellschaft mbH., Springer Nature. https://www.spektrum.de/lexikon/neurowissenschaft/gaba/4441 [05.05.2023].
Spektrum Lexikon der Neurowissenschaft (2000f): Agoraphobie. In: Spektrum der Wissenschaft. Lexikon der Neurowissenschaft. Heidelberg: Spektrum der Wissenschaft Verlagsgesellschaft mbH., Springer Nature. https://www.spektrum.de/lexikon/neurowissenschaft/agoraphobie/235 [05.05.2023].
Spektrum Lexikon der Psychologie (2000a): Bindung. In: Spektrum. Lexikon der Psychologie. Spektrum der Wissenschaft Verlagsgesellschaft mbH., Springer Nature. https://www.spektrum.de/lexikon/psychologie/bindung/2401 [18.02.2022].
Spektrum – Psychische Störungen (2000a): Agoraphobie. In: Spektrum. Psychische Störungen. Heidelberg: Spektrum der Wissenschaft Verlagsgesellschaft mbH., Springer Nature. https://www.spektrum.de/ratgeber/agoraphobie/1146623 [06.05.2023].
Spektrum – Psychische Störungen (2000b): Panikstörung. In: Spektrum. Psychische Störungen. Heidelberg: Spektrum der Wissenschaft Verlagsgesellschaft mbH., Springer Nature. https://www.spektrum.de/ratgeber/panikstoerung/1146615 [06.05.2023].

Spektrum – Psychische Störungen (2014): Antisoziale Persönlichkeitsstörung. In: Spektrum. Psychische Störungen. Heidelberg: Spektrum der Wissenschaft Verlagsgesellschaft mbH., Springer Nature. https://www.spektrum.de/ratgeber/antisoziale-persoenlichkeitsstoerung/1018465 [21.10.2022].

Strüber, Nicole (2016): Die erste Bindung. Stuttgart: Klett-Cotta Verlag.

Tooley, Katie (2020): Auswirkungen der menschlichen Darmmikrobiota auf die kognitive Leistung, die Gehirnstruktur und -funktion: Ein narrativer Überblick. In: Nutrients. 12(10): 3009.

Von Kanäl, Roland (2011): Normaler und gestörter Schlaf. In: Ehlert, Ulrike/von Känel, Roland (Hrsg.) (2011): Psychoendokrinologie und Psychoimmunologie. Berlin/Heidelberg: Springer-Verlag GmbH. 247–266.

Wahl, Klaus (2010): Geerbte Aggression: Gene und Gewalt. In: Aggression und Gewalt. Heidelberg: Spektrum Akademischer Verlag. 91–98.

Yoshimura, Shinpei et al. (2017): Cognitive behavioral therapy changes functional connectivity between medical prefrontal and anterior cingulate cortices. In: Journal of Affective Disorders. 208: 610–614.

Zisapel, Nava (2007): Sleep and sleep disturbances: biological basis and clinical implications. Cell Mol Life Sci. 64(10): 1174–1186.

The Psychological and Psychosocial Counseling Process

3

As a foundation for the eclectic-integrative and biopsychosocial coaching approach "PNES-Coaching" (Chap. 4), the following will delve deeper into the psychological and psychosocial counseling process. Temporary challenges and perspectives will be highlighted, and an overview of selected methods that are relevant to the concept will be provided. The psychological and psychosocial counseling process will be presented, from relevant diagnostics through various counseling approaches and therapy schools, methods as well as training, and the explanation of a professional counseling conclusion, up to the topic of professional relationship building. In the context of defining and explaining psychosocial diagnostics, the biopsychosocial model, which is of particular relevance in this concept, will be described. Furthermore, a brief overview of various counseling approaches and school-specific therapeutic orientations will be presented, followed by a discussion on the topic of methodological pluralism. Additionally, insights into critical considerations of school-specific orientations, based on neuroscientific research findings, will be provided and discussed. Since the implementation of interdisciplinary insights into psychological and psychosocial practice is the focus of this book, interdisciplinary insights are of particular interest. Furthermore, an overview of various intervention models that are of particular relevance to PNES-Coaching will be given. In addition to explaining the counseling conclusion, the importance of evaluation for quality assurance will also be outlined.

J. Wiederhofer, *Psychoneuroendocrinology in Psychosocial and Psychotherapeutic Practice*, https://doi.org/10.1007/978-3-658-46275-8_3

3.1 Counseling Process: Relationship Building, Diagnostics, Interventions, and Counseling Conclusion

After the endocrinological and psychoneuroendocrinological foundation for PNES-Coaching has been laid, the following will establish the psychological and psychosocial basis for the eclectic-integrative counseling concept.

The counseling process will be examined, starting with the enormous importance of the professional relationship and relationship building, which forms the basis for a successful counseling process. Furthermore, psychosocial diagnostics, relevant interventions, as well as the importance of the counseling conclusion and evaluation, will be described. In the section on psychosocial diagnostics, not only will psychosocial diagnostics be explained and defined, but a model that is particularly significant for this concept will be introduced: the biopsychosocial diagnostic model. Additionally, an overview of various counseling approaches and therapeutic schools will be provided, as well as some interventions and methods that are relevant. The effectiveness of the approaches and schools will be critically examined from a neuroscientific perspective. In addition to approaches and interventions, the end of a successful counseling process will also be presented. Here, the importance of evaluation and a successful counseling conclusion will be described.

3.1.1 The Importance of the Relationship

The following will address the relevance of the relationship for successful counseling and psychotherapy. Additionally, techniques for relationship building and relationship design will be described. It will be outlined how a trusting relationship is of enormous importance for success and goal achievement.

> "The relationship between counselors and clients is the most important dimension of any counseling constellation" (Nestmann 2014a, 791).

With this statement, Nestmann briefly and clearly explains what many authors elaborate on, namely the enormous importance of the relationship within psychological counseling (cf. Nestmann 2014a, 791).

> Despite the diverse and varied counseling methods and settings examined, only the counseling relationship has shown a consistent effect in research on successful counseling processes. Any success of psychological or psychosocial counseling is based on the counselor/therapist-client relationship, which is built and shaped within the counseling process. Without a relationship characterized by trust and positive collaboration, the most skillful use of methods will not be successful, according to Nestmann (cf. Nestmann 2014a, 791).

Nestmann (2014a) notes that despite the diverse and varied counseling methods and settings examined, only the counseling relationship has shown a consistent effect in successful counseling processes in research (cf. Nestmann 2014a, 791). A positive relationship is of enormous importance insofar as it enables clients to approach problem-solving without fear, trustfully, and openly (cf. Schmidt-Traub 2006, 111). Borg-Laufs and Wälte (2018b) also point out that psychotherapy research has demonstrated with relevant results the significant impact the relationship has on therapy and counseling effects (cf. Borg-Laufs and Wälte 2018b, 59). The question arises as to how a professional relationship between counselors/therapists and clients can be defined. Sachse (2016) defines a therapeutic professional relationship as a purpose-driven relationship between therapists and clients, which is actively co-created by both parties. This relationship ends when the purpose of the relationship is achieved or it becomes apparent that this purpose cannot be fulfilled (cf. Sachse 2016, 9). A clear position in this relationship can be helpful, especially if counselors are aware that professional counseling is a service (cf. Sanders 2014, 797). Furthermore, Sachse (2016) notes that this relationship is not directly observable but can be inferred from the behavior of the actors. In such a professional relationship, it is relevant that the therapist continuously reconstructs the state of the relationship, as the relationship is subject to recurring changes. The professional relationship between therapists and clients is thus to be seen as a construct that is not objectively definable but only certain reconstructions of the relationship, which in turn are always dependent on the individual perspective and perception of the observers (cf. Sachse 2016, 9 ff.). The core elements of a professional counseling relationship, according to Borg-Laufs and Wälte (2018), are

> "a congruent pattern of verbal and non-verbal communication forms, reflection of the relationship level in communication, mutual punctuation of the conversation flow (…)" as well as the "symmetry between analog and digital communication" (Borg-Laufs and Wälte 2018b, 59).

Communication is a central component of professional relationship building, which depends on how competent counselors are in sending and anticipating clear messages, whether clients have diverse preferences in this regard, and whether possible misunderstandings can be clarified (cf. ibid., 66). Here, the basic skills of conversation management are important, for which Carl Rogers (1942) laid the foundations in "Counseling and Psychotherapy." According to Rogers, the "self-actualization" of clients can be promoted based on the following 3 basic variables. This means that their integrity, autonomy, and appreciation can be optimized (cf. Rogers 1942, cited in Borg-Laufs and Wälte 2018b, 68).

> The 3 basic variables, which are today considered the "classic characteristics" of a supportive counseling relationship, are empathy, warmth or acceptance, and genuineness or authenticity, which were examined and published by Rogers in the context of the development of his client-centered counseling and psychotherapy (1973) (cf. Nestmann 2014a, 792).

- **Empathy:** Empathy is of Greek origin ("empatheia"—understanding with feeling) and "means the ability to put oneself into the thoughts, feelings, and worldview of other people and also to empathize with them" (Borg-Laufs and Wälte 2018b, 68). According to Nestmann, an empathetic attitude means, in particular, the effort to understand another person in their own world, to comprehend their cognitions, their emotions, as well as their actions. Furthermore, it means developing a profound understanding of their subjective and objective possibilities, limitations, and roles. This empathy is a fundamentally sensitive attitude that should characterize the counseling relationship (cf. Nestmann 2014a, 792).
- **Warmth or Acceptance:** This means showing clients positive regard. It is the attempt to express respect and esteem towards the client and to convey to them that they are taken seriously (cf. Borg-Laufs and Wälte 2018b, 69). It is an appreciation that is not conditional. Clients should experience that they are respected as individuals in this counseling relationship just as they are. This is independent of past cognitions, emotions, or actions that may have led them to seek counseling. This counseling relationship, characterized by acceptance and respect, provides clients with security. It can prevent the emergence of fears and enable openness. But above all, it can create the space to restructure cognitions, emotions, and actions.
- **Genuineness or Authenticity:** This attitude enables unadulterated communication (cf. ibid.). Counselors convey genuineness (congruence and self-honesty), which means that their actions also match their emotions. Thus, counselors also serve as a role model for clients (cf. Borg-Laufs and Wälte 2018b, 69). The relationship should be characterized by an open, direct approach, and no masking by the counselors is necessary. Based on this, clients can present their real emotions and cognitions without fear (cf. Nestmann 2014a, 792).

An implementation of these basic variables according to Carl Rogers (1977) can be seen as a guideline in professional relationship building (cf. Borg-Laufs and Wälte 2018b, 59). "Active listening" as well as the "verbalization of emotional experiences" represent the optimization of a professional counseling relationship. However, not all clients are able to speak openly about their emotions, as they may be overwhelmed with emotional processing. Here, there are helpful and proven conversation techniques that counselors and therapists can resort to (cf. ibid., 71). According to Borg-Laufs and Wälte (2018), the following conversation techniques have proven effective:

- **Conversation opening:** In the conversation opening, counselors/therapists provide general information about the counseling/therapy. Based on friendliness and a favorable seating arrangement, the counselor/therapist conveys the course of the counseling as well as the "rules of the game." Anonymity is assured to the clients, and the duration and frequency of the sessions are communicated. At the beginning, all verbal and non-verbal communication offers can be seen as conversation openings. The conversation opening allows for mutual acquaintance and the exchange of relevant information (cf. Borg-Laufs and Wälte 2018b, 72).

- **Asking open questions:** This refers to questions where no specific answer is expected. This way, clients have the opportunity to present their problems and cognitions more broadly. This gives the counselor/therapist a comprehensive overview of the client's situation.
- **Summarizing:** Here, it is important that counselors/therapists summarize the clients' statements as precisely as possible. This way, clients learn whether the counselor/therapist has really understood everything, and the course of the conversation can be well-structured and emphasized (cf. ibid., 72 f.).
- **Paraphrasing:** This refers to a meaningful reproduction (paraphrase) of what was said. This means that the counselor/therapist repeats the client's statements in their own words without interpreting the content. This can be particularly helpful when clients tend to report very extensively. The conversation can be structured immediately, and the client sees whether the counselor/therapist has understood everything (cf. Borg-Laufs and Wälte 2018b, 73).
- **Clarifying by asking follow-up questions:** Here, the counselor/therapist asks targeted questions to obtain a more detailed problem presentation. Targeted questions can eliminate ambiguities. By clarifying the problem, individually suitable solutions can be pursued. Additionally, precise follow-up questions can contribute to de-catastrophizing.
- **Reinforcing:** Here, clients' statements are reinforced using various techniques. This can be achieved, for example, through an attentive body posture, eye contact, and congruent facial expressions and gestures. This is based on the concept of operant conditioning, whereby desired client behavior is shown more frequently. Likewise, highly insecure clients can be encouraged and supported (cf. ibid.).
- **Exploring:** Here, the counselor/therapist addresses the problem aspects very differentiatedly using specific survey techniques, such as the SORKC analysis. The counselor collects information to make a psychosocial diagnosis. Based on this, the counselor/therapist can create an explanatory model for the client. Furthermore, the client can see how intensively the counselor/therapist is dealing with their problems (cf. Borg-Laufs and Wälte 2018b, 73 f.).
- **I-message:** In an I-message, the counselor/therapist expresses their own goals, wishes, assumptions, or emotions. Here, the counselor/therapist realizes congruence (in the sense of Rogers). Clients also receive feedback on how their behavior affects the counselor/therapist. Furthermore, the counselor/therapist serves as a role model, showing that emotions and wishes may be addressed (cf. Borg-Laufs and Wälte 2018b, 74).

Regarding the following techniques, as Borg-Laufs and Wälte (2018) state, it is of enormous importance to mention that the professional counseling relationship must already be established to avoid triggering additional problems (cf. ibid.).

- **Metacommunication:** This means communication about communication. The counselors/therapists establish a common communication level with the clients. Furthermore, feedback is given by the counselors/therapists on how the content was received by them. The clients can learn that their statements—unconsciously—convey different messages to the recipients than intended (cf. Borg-Laufs and Wälte 2018b, 74).
- **Confronting:** The counselor/therapist confronts the clients with cognitions, emotions, behaviors, or various problems that have not yet been addressed by the clients. Based on this, appropriate explanations and suitable coping strategies are sought. The clients are also encouraged to solve problems.
- **Setting Boundaries:** The counselor/therapist verbally distances themselves from the behaviors or statements of the clients. The counselor/therapist clearly distinguishes between their own perceptions and behaviors and those of the clients. However, based on acceptance of the clients' views and behaviors, this is not necessarily required.
- **Negative Feedback:** The counselor/therapist provides a solution-oriented, constructive, mindful, and situation-appropriate response to the client, based on a respectful attitude towards the client. Existing weaknesses are addressed, and a change in behavior is promoted (cf. ibid., 75).

The techniques and attitudes presented here are to be applied both in individual settings and in couple settings as well as in family systems (cf. Borg-Laufs and Wälte 2018b, 75). These basic techniques and methods of conversation are a foundation for shaping a professional counseling relationship, which the counselor/therapist can draw upon throughout the entire counseling process (cf. ibid., 77). These fundamental communication skills make it easier for clients to openly present their problems. It is of enormous importance that the counselor/therapist ensures that the clients do not experience destabilization through their statements. To avoid destabilization based on the necessary exploration of problems, a resource-oriented attitude, which highlights strengths as well as attempts at solutions, is helpful (cf. Borg-Laufs and Wälte 2018b, 78 f.). In summary, as Nestmann (2014) states, the relationship between counselors/therapists and clients is significantly shaped by the implementation of specific methods in the counseling process. A professional therapeutic and counseling relationship also implies individual methodological strategies and procedures (cf. Nestmann 2014a, 795).

> "Relationship and methods are therefore inseparable aspects of the conceptual development of counseling in all fields of action" (ibid.).

Based on a trustful relationship, it is possible to make an adequate psychosocial diagnosis, which is of enormous relevance for the success of counseling and for the concept of PNES coaching. The following section will examine psychosocial diagnostics in more detail, and certain diagnostic foundations and diagnostic procedures will be explained.

3.1.2 Psychosocial Diagnostics: Definition, Foundations, and Methods

The following will examine psychosocial diagnostics, as this is of enormous relevance for PNES coaching. Psychosocial diagnostics will be defined, and the importance of diagnosis in the psychosocial context will be explained. Additionally, some relevant methods and diagnostic tools, which are considered empirically tested diagnostic procedures, will be presented.

The foundation and prerequisite for a successful counseling process are diagnoses (cf. Wälte 2018a, 97). These can be defined as "(…) (empirically) verifiable statements about the problems, burdens, and disorders of the addressee" (ibid.). Diagnostics are relevant for understanding the case and thus for determining the disorder. A balance between disorder and resource diagnostics supports the development of motivation for change as well as the evaluation of the entire counseling process. Therefore, diagnostics are indispensable within the counseling process. They primarily focus at the beginning of the counseling but are also helpful throughout the entire process to optimize the course of treatment (cf. Wälte 2018a, 97).

3.1.2.1 Psychosocial Diagnostics: Definition and Fundamentals

> "Psychosocial diagnostics aim to analyze, classify, and understand life situations, lifestyles, and life crises and their changes, as well as the health situation of individuals, couples, families, and groups under the given contextual conditions" (Gahleitner and Pauls 2020, n.p.).

Gahleitner and Pauls (2020) state that psychosocial diagnostics examine the individual case at the beginning, during, and at the end of psychological, social work, and social psychiatric measures (cf. Gahleitner and Pauls 2020, n.p.). Psychosocial diagnostics must capture individual, social, psychological, medical, economic, and political aspects and processes, as well as their interactions, particularly with regard to the psycho-, socio-, bio-, economic-political focus (cf. Gahleitner et al. 2012, 9). The diagnostics justify the interventions and provide the opportunity to measure and describe goal achievements as well as goal changes (cf. ibid., 10). To professionally argue and substantiate the form of psychosocial intervention, the goal of diagnostics is to understand biopsychosocial life situations, lifestyles, and any life crises and their changes in relation to the given context and conditions. The diagnostic process, which captures the burdens, resources, events, and situations of the clients, can be seen as multidimensional. It is relevant to point out the significance of social-pathological risk factors and the complex biopsychosocial intertwining of the "person in environment," as situations and events, experiences and behaviors, as well as relationships and their systemic context, are analyzed in psychosocial diagnostics as parts of person-environment transactions. It can be helpful in various multiple problem situations to subdivide and structure these into sub-problems, in order to then, if necessary, plan interdisciplinary interventions and substantiate and address them professionally. Furthermore, this is advantageous for evaluating goal achievement. Psychosocial diagnostics can be seen as a communicative process between counselors/therapists and clients and at the same time as an indispensable tool in psychosocial interventions. The term psychosocial diagnostics is to be seen as very comprehensive; it is used both for the designation of the process and for the data collection (this means both anamnesis and exploration as well as tests, observation and questionnaire procedures for data collection, as well as psychosocial findings and psychosocial diagnosis and the goal setting and planning of the individual intervention based on it; cf. Gahleitner and Pauls 2020, n.p.). Wälte (2018) notes in this regard that the diverse psychosocial activities in particular require that counselors/therapists are able to correctly capture and classify various disorders and problems and, based on this, initiate the individual intervention. Therefore, diagnostic knowledge is essential in both the therapeutic and psychosocial fields. Knowledge of classificatory diagnostic systems such as ICD-10, DSM-IV-TR, or DSM-5 is helpful but does not need to be in-depth for the PNES coaching presented here. These classification systems focus particularly on the individual or the single person, which is generally not the case in medicine. However, since psychosocial interventions do not only work individual-centered but include much more in the intervention strategies, psychosocial diagnostics must also go beyond the individual and, for example, illuminate interpersonal interactions (cf. Wälte 2018a, 98). Additionally, real everyday living conditions such as housing, work, and income, as well as neighborhood, are in focus, according to Gahleitner and Pauls (2020). Thus, a psychosocial diagnosis involves the explanations "(…) of behavior and experience in their interaction with the real-life situation" (ibid.). Individual interests and abilities are examined, problem-solving and conflict-resolution skills are analyzed, as well as individual perspectives, values, and beliefs, emotional basic moods, and individual life plans are included in psychosocial diagnostics (cf. Gahleitner and Pauls 2020, n.p.). In summary, it can be stated that psychosocial diagnostics are to be seen as an essential quality criterion for biopsychosocial casework. It is about the multidimensional capture of problem- or disorder-relevant characteristics and the resources of the clients (cf. Gahleitner and Pauls 2017, 680).

In the following, the various forms of psychosocial diagnostics according to Gahleitner and Pauls (2020) are presented.

3.1.2.2 Forms of Psychosocial Diagnostics

Gahleitner and Pauls (2020) divide psychosocial diagnostics into various forms, which diverge in the following aspects:

- **Intuitive diagnostics versus method-based and rationally founded diagnostics:** In psychosocial fields of action, intuitive forms of diagnostics are often observed. Likewise, more or less intuitive conclusions are drawn. Given the complexity of various tasks, experience- and knowledge-based intuition is indeed of enormous importance, but scientific and rationally founded method-based diagnostics are indispensable. The intuition must be methodically verifiable or subject to scrutiny (cf. Gahleitner and Pauls 2020, n.p.).

- **Status diagnostics versus process diagnostics:** The goal of status diagnostics is to clarify temporarily relevant dimensions such as relationship conditions and psychological environmental conditions as well as events and environmental conditions. Process diagnostics, on the other hand, capture change processes and attempt to evaluate them. They refer to processes that arise or should arise, for example, during the intervention (cf. Gahleitner and Pauls 2020, n.p.).
- **Initial diagnostics versus intervention-oriented diagnostics:** Initial diagnostics capture relevant characteristics at the beginning of an intervention. In psychosocial fields of action, diagnoses in interdisciplinary cooperation are often necessary. The goal of clarification before the start of the intervention is, among other things, to find out whether the clients can be treated adequately. In initial diagnostics, the fundamental question is: "What is the case?". Intervention-oriented diagnostics, on the other hand, aim to capture information relevant to goal setting and strategy. Furthermore, it aims to find out which intervention methods and techniques are suitable for the clients. The fundamental question here is: What is this case about?
- **Norm-oriented diagnostics versus criterion-oriented diagnostics:** In norm-oriented diagnostics, the information collected about a person is assigned to a comparison population concerning statistical norms. This classificatory diagnostics, according to the DSM-5 or ICD-10 or ICD-11 system, offers the possibility to assign the symptoms of the clients to a specific diagnosis. This can be particularly helpful for disorder-specific decisions and appropriate procedures. In criterion-oriented diagnostics, the information of the subjects is compared to certain set criteria that are to be achieved (cf. ibid.).
- **Individual-oriented diagnostics versus system-oriented diagnostics:** Individual-oriented diagnostics focus on the client themselves, whereas system-oriented diagnostics deal with the relationships between the person and their environment. These diagnostic procedures have a mutually complementary function. Individual-oriented diagnostics are based on theoretical assumptions and findings about a specific psychological or social problem (e.g., dissocial and borderline problems). System-oriented diagnostics work with network and social support instruments (cf. Gahleitner and Pauls 2020, n.p.).

Based on the forms and various aspects of diagnostics presented here, some diagnostic models and specific diagnostic instruments that are used in biopsychosocial concepts will be explained in the following.

3.1.2.3 Methods of Psychosocial Diagnostics

As already mentioned, psychosocial diagnostics particularly involve the challenge of capturing the multidimensionality of the problems. This means developing a working model that

> "(…) does justice to the multidimensionality of biopsychosocial problems and the interface character between psychological, social, everyday situational, and health dimensions" (Gahleitner and Pauls 2020, n.p.).

To assess these dimensions, for example, the biopsychosocial framework concept can be applied, which can further be complemented by the concept of salutogenesis. To assess the psychosocial baseline situation of the clients, network maps, biography-oriented methods, and test procedures can be used, for example. To identify resources that clients are often unaware of at the beginning of the counseling, it is useful to apply resource diagnostics. This serves both as a diagnostic procedure and as a form of intervention. To find out what function a specific problem behavior has for the clients, the SORKC analysis can be used (cf. Borg-Laufs and Wälte 2018a, 97 f.). In addition to the biopsychosocial model, there are many other diagnostic instruments that have proven helpful in psychosocial interventions. According to Borg-Laufs (2016) and Wälte (2018a, b, c), six levels of analysis have proven significant in psychosocial practice (Borg-Laufs 2016; Wälte 2018, 99 f.):

- functional analysis (e.g., according to the SORKC model),
- relationship analysis (e.g., relationship between counselor and client),
- motivation analysis (e.g., suffering pressure, secondary gain, belief in success),
- system analysis (e.g., interaction, communication),
- resource analysis (e.g., psychological, physical, social, economic/ecological),
- disorder analysis (e.g., according to ICD-10).

The forms of diagnosis, analyses, and instruments are diverse. Some that are relevant for PNES coaching are examined in more detail below.

- **Resource Diagnostics**

> To achieve resource activation in the counseling process, a well-founded and differentiated resource diagnosis is primarily required (cf. Schubert 2018, 114). "Only a resource-diagnostic assessment ensures a methodologically sound case conception" (ibid.).

The foundation of resource diagnostics is the assumption that resources are of central importance for coping with everyday life as well as for managing challenging demands and life tasks. Ultimately, mental and physical health and well-being depend on the available and deployable resources (cf. Willutzki 2008, 129). Schubert sees a thorough resource diagnosis as a prerequisite for professional counseling. It is relevant that it is carried out together with the clients, also involving the social environment, not only at the beginning of the counseling but consistently throughout the entire counseling process (cf. Schubert 2018, 117). According to Schubert (2018), resource diagnostics aim to find concrete indications in the clients and their living environment of:

- available resources and possibilities,
- existing, hidden, or unused resource potentials, and
- necessary, newly to be developed resources.

Often, clients are not aware of their resources at the beginning of the counseling, but they often become aware of them during the course of resource diagnostics. Thus, resource diagnostics can simultaneously be seen as a form of intervention, especially when the diagnostic results and areas of successful life management are discussed with the clients (cf. ibid.). Resources are classified into personal and environmental resources. More specifically, personal or internal, external such as social, material, or sociocultural, and interpersonal, i.e., interpersonal resources, are distinguished (cf. Schubert 2018, 114).

According to Knecht and Schubert (2012), resources are classified as follows:

Classification of Resources

1. **Personal Resources** (individual, intrapersonal resources):
   a. Physical resources: such as fitness, health, physical attractiveness, etc.
   b. Psychological resources:
      - Skills and cognitive resources:
        - intellectual abilities as well as problem-solving skills, aptitudes, and talents
        - availability of coping strategies and life experience
        - education and vocational training, knowledge for managing daily life as well as for meeting professional requirements, reflection, and understanding of self, environment, and contexts
        - positive beliefs and attitudes such as self-efficacy, commitment, confidence, self-esteem, sense of coherence (life meaning), and ambiguity tolerance (the ability to tolerate differences and contradictions)
      - Emotionality and personality traits:
        - emotional stability and emotional intelligence, optimism and reliability, differentiated self- or identity development
        - emotion regulation and well-being, positive handling of emotions and enjoyment

- holding identity-promoting roles and positions in social systems

c. Interactional resources (also called interpersonal resources): are expressed in interaction with significant others (e.g., partners, family, friends) and in extended social systems (e.g., with colleagues or in sociocultural groups)
   - relationship skills, empathy, and social sensitivity, maintaining adequate reciprocity in interaction; the ability to differentiate the expression of emotions and motives
   - conflict resolution skills and ability to handle criticism (the ability to express appropriate criticism and to accept justified criticism)
   - respect, tolerance, reliability, and agreeableness towards interaction partners
   - the ability to express the need for help and to seek social support
   - reciprocity (the willingness and ability to balance received support and to adequately make amends for injuries)

d. Economic (personal) resources:
   - financial and material possessions as universal transformable resources, property, and income from work, stable employment income

2. **Environmental resources (external resources):** include psychosocial, social, cultural, social welfare and legal, physical-technical as well as natural aids and resources in the environment of individuals
   a. Social resources (also called psychosocial or interpersonal resources):
      - Social-emotional relationship resources: emotionally positive, trusting interactions with social-emotional belonging and recognition, emotional participation, and supportive care
      - Contacts, relationships, social integration into (extended) networks with acceptance, opportunities for participation and involvement, and support in coping with everyday life as well as specific demands

   b. Socio-ecological resources:
      - Quality of housing and the living environment, socio-ecological infrastructure
      - Workplace quality: work climate and job content, both prospectively and health-wise

   c. Social welfare and socio-cultural resources:
      - Access to educational, health, and social institutions, cultural offerings, and psychosocial support facilities
      - Opportunities for participation in social and socio-cultural life
      - Experience of helpful cultural and societal evaluation patterns
      - Monetary transfer benefits, social insurance, and services
      - Rule of law, transparency, and influenceability of societal structures and developments (cf. Schubert 2018, 114 ff.)

   According to Hobfoll (1989), the following resources are significant:

Personal Resources Personal resources are understood as the individual characteristics/competencies of clients to achieve their goals and cope with challenging demands. These include, for example, cognitive and professional skills, emotional stability, commitment, social skills, social reputation, and a confident attitude towards life.

Living Conditions Living conditions that are considered resources are particularly those conditions that provide support, such as marriage/partnership, family, interpersonal relationships (friends), health, as well as socially highly valued living conditions such as being appreciated/popular, having a job, recognized social role, and a good professional position.

Energy Resources Energy resources are significant because they enable access to further resources, such as access to money, knowledge, reputation, and having time.

Object Resources Object resources are understood as basic resources such as food, clothing, and housing. Additionally, helpful technical devices like a car or other commercial (object) values play a role (cf. Hobfoll 1989, cited in Schubert 2018, 121).

Willutzki (2008) summarizes:

> "For the content level of resource diagnostics, the differentiation between external, interpersonal, and personal resources can be summarized, whereby the interplay of the various types of resources is complex" (Willutzki 2008, 132).

What can a consideration of resources, as classified here, contribute to psychosocial diagnostics? Buttner and Knecht (2009) note that, on the one hand, capturing these core resources is helpful in describing various deficits of clients, so that situations of scarcity are more clearly presented and thus individual solution strategies become more apparent—especially when it comes to long-term contexts, such as the question of education and training as well as social networks. On the other hand, looking at the available resources can reveal development opportunities (cf. Buttner and Knecht 2009, 102). Furthermore

> "(…) the idea of transformations and their relation to a socio-epidemiologically based bio-psycho-social model can represent a background theory for social diagnosis (…)" (ibid.).

The resources of the various areas are intertwined and reinforce each other both positively and negatively. In particular, with problems that have cross-cutting effects, a better analysis is possible. Additionally, a differentiation between resources that are available on the one hand and their use on the other hand can enable a view of individual problem situations as well as the control of coping behavior. The structure of the problem becomes clearer, and it becomes more understandable whether the problem is more due to a lack of certain resources or rather to a dysfunctional use of individual resources (cf. Buttner and Knecht 2009, 102).

There are numerous methods and instruments for capturing resources. Some diagnostic instruments and methods are presented here in an overview (cf. Schubert 2018, 117).

Resource-oriented diagnostic instruments or diagnostic methods

- Resource interviews (e.g., unsystematic resource questions or systematic resource interviews)
- Questionnaires for resource assessment (e.g., the Bern Resource Inventory)
- Creative self-report methods for resource assessment (e.g., resource treasure chest)
- Biography- and life-world-oriented resource diagnostics (e.g., resource cards)
- Graphical diagnostic methods (e.g., social atom, network drawing, network map, resource genogram, resource ecogram) (cf. Schubert 2018, 118–129).

In summary, Buttner and Knecht (2009) note:

> "The resource-theoretical approach in general and the empirical investigation of transformations in particular require interdisciplinary collaboration in research—with health sciences, sociology, and psychology" (Buttner and Knecht 2009, 108).

The more knowledge about the interrelationships of the clients' resource equipment, the supportive and burdensome environmental factors, and the resulting consequences is known, the more a resource-theoretical diagnosis could lead to a better prognosis of future problems as well as to better planning of individually tailored interventions (cf. Buttner and Knecht 2009, 108 f.). A resource diagnosis can thus be carried out with various diagnostic methods and instruments.

To facilitate the comprehensibility of the clients' social networks for the counselors/therapists, it is also sensible to analyze social networks. Therefore, the diagnostic instrument "network map" is described below.

- **Network map**

Particularly in a biopsychosocial coaching approach, it is of enormous importance to implement their social networks and the various meanings for the clients into the work. Borg-Laufs and Tinkens (2018) note that there is an increasing loss of function of traditional families, which leads to individuals often appearing disoriented and helpless. Additionally, it is relevant here, especially for younger clients, to also consider online networks. For, in general, it can be noted that clients' problems become particularly understandable when one knows their (online) network. Since it is therefore of great relevance for successful counseling to know the life-world references, i.e., the social embedding, as well as the biographical references of the clients, a so-called network map is suitable (cf. Borg-Laufs and Tinkens 2018, 105 ff.). The term network research originates from German. The international term is "social network analysis" (cf. Stegbauer 2008, 11).

The network map is a diagnostic instrument that is based on a solid theoretical background, exhibits all the advantages of graphical methods, opens up interpretative possibilities, and is suitable for cooperative diagnostics (cf. Pantucek 2010, 189).

The unique aspect of network research is that relationship contexts and relationship structures are included in the analysis. The focus of this instrument is primarily on recognizing relationship patterns. To recognize the various relationship patterns and structures, different approaches and perspectives interlock (cf. Stegbauer 2008, 11 f.). Pantucek also emphasizes that with network maps, the clients' relationships with their fellow human beings and their environment are the focus. The social references are thus focused and recorded (cf. Pantucek 2011, 146).

According to Pantucek (2010), the following networks are significant for sector division:

- Friends and acquaintances
- Family
- School and/or work
- Professional/occupational relationships (cf. Pantucek 2010, 190).

The network map, according to Pantucek (2010), is best created together with the clients. The client is usually at the center of this network map. First, the area is divided into 4 sectors. Then, the individually significant people in the social environment are entered, noting that the greater the relevance of this person, the closer the symbol is placed to the anchor point of the client. Contacts between the drawn persons are connected or made visible with lines, creating a network that can be differently pronounced in the various sectors (cf. Pantucek 2010, 189 f.). This tool is versatile, for example in case discussions and supervisions, for reconstructing the social landscape, and for reviewing the intervention strategies of the clients. Likewise, "lifeworld advisors," with whom there may be loose contact or no strong relationship, can be depicted. The interpretation of the network map can be done both together with the clients and within the framework of case discussions. It is also useful to create a so-called "desired network map" together with the clients (cf. ibid., 201 f.). Borg-Laufs and Tinkens (2018) note that a "desired network map" can crystallize which changes in relationship intensities the clients would prefer. It can also be used to further interpret the "actual network map" (cf. Borg-Laufs and Tinkens 2018, 108).

Finally, it should be mentioned that the diagnostic tool of the network map does not have to be executed solely analogously, because a new software—"EasyNWK"—was developed and tested within the framework of the SODIA research project. It was developed at the Ilse Arlt Institute for Social Inclusion Research at the FH St. Pölten under the scientific direction of Peter Pantucek and Sabine Sommer by Nikolaus Kelis. The software allows for the easy creation of an egocentric network map—"EGO-centered networks"—as well as the automatic calculation of key figures. The manual, based on practical experiences within the SODIA research project, can be used for interpretation (cf. Pantucek 2012, n.p.). The software is available for free download. The following section will now explain the biopsychosocial aspect of diagnostics, which is of particular importance for the PNES coaching presented in Chap. 4.

- **Biopsychosocial model**

The combination of biopsychosocial aspects into a diagnostic model or intertwining those insights is of enormous importance for the biopsychosocial coaching approach presented in this book. The concept of biopsychosocial diagnostics allows for the precise observation, analysis, and explanation of the clients' problem constellation. Not only are disorders recorded, but also various crises, stresses, and conflicts, as well as the resources and motivation of the clients (cf. Wälte 2018c, 98). These are analyzed

> "(…) in the interaction between body, psyche, and social situation on different system levels of the clientele (person, couple, family, group, in counseling processes also team and organization)" (Wälte 2018c, 98 f.).

Egger (2008) notes that the biopsychosocial model "is a fundamental theory of the body-soul unity (…)" (Egger 2008, 12), and it enables a scientifically based holistic understanding of illness or health. The foundation is the so-called biopsychosocial disease model. This is now declared as one of the most significant theories for the relationship between body and mind. The biopsychosocial model is superior to the biomedical concept because illness and health are not merely defined as a state but as a "dynamic process" (cf. ibid., 12).

> "It promotes a perspective that allows the problems of clients to be placed in their complex individual biopsychosocial contexts and emphasizes the active status of clients (motivation, resources) in coping with stresses, crises, problems, and disorders" (Wälte 2018c, 99).

Wälte (2018c) further maintains that, based on the biopsychosocial model, psychosocial problems arise because clients can no longer maintain their self-regulatory competencies in problem-solving. Based on the interaction between biological, psychological, and social factors, the etiology of psychosocial problems can be attributed to multiple factors. Due to the inclusion of both psychological and social factors, unlike the biomedical model, it is not only the client themselves who are involved in the development and course of psychosocial problems, but also the social context (cf. Wälte 2018c, 100). Egger (2020) views this extended biopsychosocial model as the

> "(…) most coherent, compact, and also significant theoretical concept within which humans can be explained and understood in health and illness" (Egger 2020, 13).

According to Egger, the focus of this theory is

> "(…) that nature is hierarchically ordered on a continuum, with the more complex, larger units being built upon the less complex, smaller units" (ibid., 14).

Egger states that clients must be recognized in their individual client world in its psychological, eco-social, and organ-biological dimensions (cf. Egger 2008, 18). This means that the implementation of a biopsychosocial diagnosis requires the integration of a multi-level diagnosis. The data are integrated using disorder-specific models to obtain connections between the relevant system levels. The three levels of experiential and behavioral data (thinking, feeling, and acting), eco-social data (social environment and physicochemical environment), and functional areas and organ-biological data are significant here (cf. Egger 2008, 18). The biopsychosocial therapy is a multimodal therapy. It helps on a psychological level cognitively and emotionally, and action-oriented psychological interventions are used. On the eco-social level, it is important to promote a familial and professional network and socio-cultural resources. The organ biological level requires, among other things, interdisciplinary collaboration with pharmacotherapeutic, physiotherapeutic, or medical professions (cf. Egger 2008, 18). The biopsychosocial model describes nature, which follows a hierarchical order of systems, and states that each system is based on qualities and relationships typical for the respective level of organization. All levels are intertwined, so a change in one level results in a change in the other levels. None of the levels or systems thus exist in isolation. An event, therefore, occurs simultaneously on various dimensions based on the network, although not all effects occur at the same time. The various system levels have different temporal processes, which is why some aspects can be perceived quickly and others rather delayed. Thus, this theory is based on the interactions of the various system levels over the entire timeline of the clients (cf. ibid., 14). The psychoneuroimmunological connections in relation to immunological diseases are becoming increasingly well known, which means that, based on these findings, targeted behavioral intervention programs can be developed that influence the entire biochemical network in the body. Expectation effects as well as conditioning processes must therefore be intertwined as additional or supportive therapy with pharmacological or medical interventions (cf. Egger 2008, 14). In summary, Egger (2008) states that according to the biopsychosocial model

> "(…) every event or process involved in the etiology, pathogenesis, symptomatic manifestation, and treatment of disorders is consequently not either biological or psychological, but both biological and psychological" (ibid., 14 f.).

This, in turn, means that the helper must acquire a basic understanding of psychological and eco-social as well as medical or biological influences. Only when a certain basic knowledge is present, and the respective phenomena of the system levels can be classified by the helpers, will they be able to analyze the various interactions. It is therefore of enormous importance to intertwine material-physical and psychological-mental aspects, which is why it would not be a contraindication to refer to psychological therapy as a biological treatment, according to Egger (cf. Egger 2008, 17 f.). Wälte (2018c) also points out how closely neurobiology and mental disorders are interconnected, for example. An example here can be violence within the family. Relationship disorders arise, which cause neurobiological changes in the circuit between the limbic system (emotional center) and the prefrontal brain areas (action regulation centers), which can lead to pronounced aggressiveness on the psychological level. In post-traumatic stress disorder (PTSD), the social level also affects the manifestation of the disorder, which can now also be demonstrated using imaging techniques. Depressive patients, for example, show hyperactivation in the amygdala, the ventral striatum (nucleus caudatus, putamen), and the medial prefrontal cortex in response to negative emotional stimuli. In contrast, the ventral striatum shows underregulation in response to positive emotional stimuli. The evidence of so-called networks is possible in various mental disorders, such as anxiety disorders, using neurobiological findings (cf. Wälte 2018c, 101). It is important to clearly capture the main problem areas of the clients. The neurobiological findings make it clear that both the development and the course of mental disorders can only be understood from the dynamics of the interplay or the intertwined interactions of the system levels of the biopsychosocial situation of the clients (cf. Wälte 2018c, 102).

It should be mentioned, however, that despite the increasing acceptance of biopsychosocial diagnostics, it has not been without criticism. This is particularly to be considered from the pathogenic orientation, where the question is pursued as to what keeps people healthy (cf. Wälte 2018c, 104). In this context, the concept of salutogenesis (health creation) is now briefly presented.

- **Model of Salutogenesis**

The model of salutogenesis was founded by the American-Israeli health scientist Aaron Antonovsky (1923–1994). Salutogenesis was introduced as an alternative to pathogenesis (cf. Faltermeier 2020, n.p.). "(…) it is about the genesis (Greek "genesis") of health (Latin "salus"), not about diseases and their causes" (Dollinger 2006, 173). The model aims to explain the genesis of health and answer the questions of how health arises, how people can stay healthy, and how health can be promoted. Antonovsky argues that advances in understanding human health will only occur if science does not exclusively deal with pathogenesis or merely focus on disease, as maintaining health is the actual task (cf. Faltermeier 2020, n.p.). Dollinger notes that salutogenic perspectives bring with them formulas of hope, as this perspective allows people to free themselves from biomedical and disease-focused one-sidedness. In return, people are given the opportunity to develop health individually. The focus is on the genesis of health, not on disease and its causes (cf. Dollinger 2006, 173).

> "Salutogenesis starts from the positive connotation of health and its conceptualization to distance itself from pathogenic narrowings" (ibid.).

According to Antonovsky, health and disease are to be seen as a processual event in a health-disease continuum (between "health-ease" and "dis-ease") (cf. Wälte 2018c, 104).

> "We are all terminal cases. But as long as we have a breath of life in us, we are all to some extent healthy" (Antonovsky 1989, 53).

The model of salutogenesis, in which health and disease are considered a continuum, aims to explain the movements within this continuum. Stressors and resistance resources are used as determinants of health, for example (cf. Faltermeier 2020, n.p.). Of particular importance is the sense of coherence, which indicates whether clients experience life as comprehensible, manageable, and meaningful. The better this sense of coherence is developed, the more positive it is for health. A lower sense of coherence leads to negative health. The model of salutogenesis thus forms a theoretical foundation for the practice of health promotion, as it reveals what needs to be strengthened to promote health. The model of salutogenesis has inspired research worldwide and contributed to the development of new practical approaches (cf. ibid.). Wälte ultimately notes that the salutogenic concept enriches the biopsychosocial model, especially within psychosocial interventions, by focusing more on healing resources (cf. Wälte 2018c, 104).

- **SORKC Model**

The SORKC model can be traced back to cognitive behavioral diagnostic therapy. It is intended to explain and change problematic behavior. The concept is based on Kanfer and Saslow (1965 and 1974). It is declared as a horizontal behavioral analysis that identifies triggering and maintaining influences (condition analysis) (cf. Heuse 2019, n.p.). It should be noted that behavioral analysis is a frequently used diagnostic procedure, especially in behavioral therapy (cf. Abbruzzese and Kübler 2013, 108). However, Borg-Laufs points out that functional behavioral analysis is also of enormous relevance outside of behavioral therapy and can therefore be extremely helpful for psychosocial counseling, as recognizing problematic behaviors, their conditions, and functions is of great importance (cf. Borg-Laufs 2018c, 130). The behavioral analysis

> "(…) provides a cross-disorder framework for behavior-related and multimodal exploration of the patient's problem and consequently provides an important basis for the development of the case concept" (Abbruzzese and Kübler 2013, 108).

In the SORKC model, it is assumed that the problematic behavior to be treated is triggered and maintained by a previously unknown network of conditions. Based on the diagnostic procedure, these conditions are to be uncovered. The results of this diagnostic process then provide the foundation for the individual treatment strategy. To define the problem-relevant conditions as precisely as possible, it is important to analyze the problematic behavior in various situations (cf. Abbruzzese and Kübler 2013, 109). The focused question that can be answered through the SORKC analysis is what function the problematic behavior has for the clients. The question of "why" a behavior occurs can thus be explained (cf. Borg-Laufs 2018c, 130).

> "To answer this question, it is worked out in which situations (S) the behavior (R) occurs, which other intrapsychic or physical enduring dispositions need to be considered (O), and in what exact way the behavior is reinforced (C, K)" (Borg-Laufs 2018c, 130).

Through this procedure, it can thus be derived which change possibilities are subsidiary (cf. ibid.).

S	**O**	**R**	**K**	**C**
Stimulus	Organism	Reaction (Behavior)	Contingency	Consequences

- Stimulus—S

In behaviorism, S stands for the stimulus (e.g., situation, thoughts), which can be triggered by both external and internal stimuli (cf. Heuse 2019, n.p.). It is the stimulus that immediately precedes the problematic behavior to be treated, i.e., the so-called triggering stimulus (cf. Borg-Laufs 2018c, 130). External stimuli or conditions include physical environmental factors as well as social characteristics. Internal stimuli or conditions include thoughts, emotions, and physical changes. It is of enormous relevance to describe the S variable as precisely as possible and to analyze situational characteristics as well as the quality of the stimulus and to derive the connection between S (stimulus) and R (reaction/behavior) (cf. Abbruzzese and Kübler 2013, 111).

> "The connection between S and R can be classically conditioned, unconditioned (i.e., reflexive, biologically determined), or mediated by stimulus discrimination learning" (ibid.).

Stimuli can determine a behavior, which means that a behavior is exhibited regardless of subsequent consequences. They can be referred to as classical or evaluative conditioning. In evaluative conditioning, the response is less pronounced physiologically and more in terms of emotional evaluation. In operantly conditioned behavior, stimuli stimulate a behavior that is not necessarily executed. One can assume a classically or evaluatively conditioned behavior if it is strongly physiological or emotional. In operant behavior, it involves cues that do not determine a behavior but merely indicate whether a certain behavior is reinforced. The distinction between an unconditioned stimulus and a cue is significant for planning individual interventions (cf. Borg-Laufs 2018c, 130 f.).

- **Organism—O**

The abbreviation O stands for organism variables. This includes individual predispositions such as biological processes, personality traits, experiences, and beliefs (cf. Heuse 2019, n.p.). The organism variables can capture both permanent states (e.g., neurological impairments) and transient states (cf. Röhrle 2008, 97). These psychological or physiological dispositions include:

- **Physical conditions:** Physical impairments due to chronic illnesses or various disabilities can, for example, lead to the avoidance of physical activities being highly reinforcing, as specific fears and concerns regarding one's own performance or social feedback can be avoided.
- **Cognitive schemas/irrational beliefs:** Here, enduring beliefs/cognitive schemas play a significant role. Irrational beliefs such as "I always do everything wrong anyway" lead clients to avoid attempting anything difficult to avoid mistakes.
- **Psychological basic needs:** The non-fulfillment of psychological basic needs, such as attachment, can be particularly behaviorally effective. Those who seek attachment will, for example, endure unpleasantness in the relationship just to feel closeness (cf. Borg-Laufs 2018c, 131 f.).
- **Reaction (Behavior)—R**

The variable R stands for the reaction or behavior, which is described on various levels (motor, affective, physiological, cognitive) (cf. Heuse 2019, n.p.). It can include motor tics as well as complex patterns, for example, in various forms of avoidance. It can also be verbal, overt, or covert (cf. Röhrle 2008, 97 f.). Thus, not only observable behaviors are analyzed. The behavior should be described on the following 4 levels (cf. Borg-Laufs 2018c, 132):

"What does the client do in the situation, what thoughts go through their mind, what physical sensations and what feelings do they experience?" (ibid.).

- **Consequences—C**

The variable C stands for the consequences that feedback on the behavior. The consequences C feedback on the behavior (cf. Heuse 2019, n.p.). The precise description of the consequences is crucial here (cf. Röhrle 2008, 98). Operant behavior is influenced by subsequent consequences. It can lead to a behavior occurring more frequently with reinforcement or less frequently with punishment. Reinforcing or behavior-enhancing consequences are positive reinforcers, where something positive is added, such as praise, gifts, attention, or similar, and in negative reinforcement, a negative state is removed, such as anxiety reduction, tension relief, or the elimination of difficult demands. A punishing or behavior-reducing consequence can be a direct punishment, such as devaluation by others, insults, and unpleasant emotions, or an indirect punishment, such as the removal of a positive state or a pleasant feeling (cf. Borg-Laufs 2018c, 132 f.).

- **Contingency—K**

The variable K represents the contingency between R and C. It indicates how frequently and regularly the consequences follow the behaviors (cf. Heuse 2019, n.p.). The focus here is on the variations in the regularity of reinforcement or punishment, as well as the effects on the probability of behavior. For practical purposes, it is especially significant whether the behavior is continuously rewarded or intermittently, at regular or irregular intervals (cf. Borg-Laufs 2018c, 133). In functional analysis, an explanation of the problem behavior is focused on. Therefore, it is important to describe the behavior (R) in the first step. In the second step, the stimulus conditions (S) are analyzed and in which situations the problem behavior occurs. Subsequently, the consequences of the behavior (C) are recorded and their reinforcing or punishing effect is interpreted. This is done in positive and negative reinforcement as well as in direct and indirect punishment. Furthermore, it is noted how contingent (K) the consequence is, i.e., whether it occurs intermittently or continuously. Organism variables (O), which are relevant to the behavior or favor it, or those that influence the reinforcing effect, are recorded in the last step (cf. ibid., 134).

A joint development of behavior analyses can be of enormous benefit to the clients. It offers them the opportunity to create an individual functional model that explains and makes understandable the connections of inner psychological dynamics and the resulting behavior. A behavior analysis also serves as a hypothetical conditional or working model that needs to be regularly reviewed. It is particularly relevant that the model is understandable and authentic for the clients and that they can identify with the behavior analysis. This can make it easier for the clients to notice and analyze their dysfunctional behavior in everyday life, with the goal of influencing or changing the undesirable problem behavior in the long term (cf. Abbruzzese and Kübler 2013, 113 f.).

With the help of the SORKC model, starting points can be derived that lead to active behavior changes in the clients. Furthermore, the SORKC model, based on the involvement of feedback and feedforward loops (cybernetic feedback loop models) in the emergence and change of behavior, provides the foundation for Kanfer's theory of self-regulation (cf. Heuse 2019, n.p.).

The following section will delve deeper into the analysis of self-regulation.

- **Self-Regulation Model**

Psychotherapeutic practice and psychosocial counseling practice show that clients very often have enormous problems controlling their emotions and affects autonomously (emotion regulation). Clients who, for example, are dependent on psychotropic substances, suffer from obsessive-compulsive disorders, or other psychological behavioral disorders, are severely restricted in their behaviors and emotions, making autonomous everyday coping impossible (cf. Wälte 2018b, 135 f.). However, the goal should be to enable the clients to cope with their problems as autonomously as possible. According to the self-regulation model, clients should receive professional guidance and support to implement everyday coping autonomously. The support provided includes instructions and exercises for restructuring their own thought and behavior patterns. These can be components of the clients' pathological patterns or significant determinants of a disorder (cf. Reinecker 2009, 630). The self-regulation model is based on determinants of the regulation of human behavior, which are visible on various levels (variables):

- **α-Variables:** These include external influences of the physical environment, such as living situation or social situation, but also own and others' behavior, such as instructions.
- **β-Variables:** These refer to the internal cognitive processes of the clients, such as thoughts, expectations, fears, schemas, and various standards. These variables form the core component of self-regulation. They are particularly shaped by one's own biography.
- **γ-Variables:** These variables are biological-somatic, including both temporary and enduring physiological processes. These processes often control our behavior and ensure survival. Examples include the sleep-wake cycle, nutritional and medication influences, and blood pressure regulation (cf. Reinecker 2009, 630).

Normally, the dynamic interaction between the variables occurs unconsciously and automatically. However, when disruptions within the system occur, such as when certain behaviors prevent goals from being achieved or an ongoing activity is interrupted, these processes become conscious to us. Self-regulation can be divided into three phases. In the first phase, the individual captures their own behavior and thus the current state through self-observation (cf. Wälte 2018b, 137). In the second phase, a self-evaluation takes place based on the individual's own standards. Here, a comparison between the current state and a target value occurs. Finally, the third phase of self-reinforcement occurs, in which, depending on the result of the second phase, self-punishment may also occur. The processes of self-regulation can be repeated as often as necessary until a target behavior according to individual standards is achieved. According to Kanfer (2012), there are also two feedback loops and a feedforward loop. The first feedback is received by the individual from themselves, based on the comparison of the action (reaction) and personal standards (current-target comparison). A second feedback loop allows for corrective feedback based on the consequences that followed the behavior. This happens by the individual comparing the consequences with their individual consequence expectation. The consequence expectation refers to the subjective assessment of which specific consequences should follow the exhibited behavior. The feedforward loop describes the individual's situation expectations. Previously experienced situations in similar contexts influence the perception of environmental stimuli here. The situation expectation is thus the subjective assessment that certain situations will occur (cf. Wälte 2018b, 137 f.). This model of self-regulation can also be used for the method of cognitive restructuring (cf. ibid., 139). Kanfer, Reinecker, and Schmelzer (2012) have developed a 7-phase model for the diagnostic-therapeutic process for self-management therapy. In the initial phase, the focus is on creating suitable initial conditions for the diagnostic-therapeutic process. Building a cooperative relationship between the counselor/therapist and the client, as well as promoting work orientation and self-activity, are central themes here. Simultaneously, problem-centered information gathering regarding complaints and expectations takes place. This leads to initial considerations regarding therapeutic approaches (cf. Kanfer et al. 2012, 159 f.). In the second phase, the primary focus is on building adequate motivation for change. Various methods can be used to motivate clients. Among other things, supporting the reduction of demoralization and resignation can help clients gain hope regarding changes and improvements in their temporary state. Various strategies for building motivation can be employed here. These methods aim to create positive stimuli and, furthermore, to ensure that clients have new dreams (cf. ibid., 193 f.). In phase 3, the goal is to conduct an intensive behavior analysis on both the micro and macro levels. The aim here is to achieve a functional conditions model. The situational behavior analysis (micro level) deals with narrowly defined behavior episodes on a microscopic level. The contextual behavior analysis (macro level) examines connections, backgrounds, and the overall context on a broadly gridded level. Social systems are also considered here (cf. Kanfer et al. 2012, 229 f.). In the fourth phase, the focus is on clarifying, analyzing, and agreeing on therapy goals. The clarification of potential goals initially represents a purely mental engagement with the future. In a second step, it is therefore important to critically assess all fantasy perspectives and goal ideas. The criteria for this include concreteness, reality content, and comparison with the clients' existing abilities. In a third step, the agreement on concrete goals follows (cf. ibid., 249). In the fifth phase, the counselor compares the clients' information with the requirements of potential measures. Ideally, such planning results in an individually tailored method (cf. ibid., 271). The sixth phase then deals more deeply with the evaluation of progress. Regarding the type of evaluation, both a narrowly problem-related and a broadly system-related perspective should be pursued. This ensures a flexible capture of relevant variables at various levels of resolution. The focus is primarily on self-management processes (cf. ibid., 293). In the final phase, the seventh phase, the goals addressed so far are optimized, which means active preparation for stabilization and transfer. Additionally, goals that have not yet been addressed are discussed or optimized. Subsequently, the optimization of the meta-goal can take place: learning self-control or self-management as a process. Finally, there is feedback and preparation for follow-up or catamneses (cf. Kanfer et al. 2012, 319).

In summary, the following must be noted:

> "The goal of therapeutic intervention from the perspective of self-management is to optimize the extent of self-regulation and self-control (i.e., β-regulation) within the continuum of other influencing factors. The importance of external (α) and biological (γ) variables is not nullified, but it recedes in favor of an increased significance of variables within the self-regulation system" (Reinecker 2009, 630).

The primary prerequisite for achieving self-regulation or self-control is an adequate level of self-motivation and self-discipline on the part of the clients, as well as the willingness not to be paralyzed by failures. This should be encouraged or promoted through motivational interviewing in psychosocial counseling (cf. Wälte 2018b, 140).

Like self-regulation, psychological basic needs are also of enormous importance. Insights into the psychological basic needs of clients can be of great relevance. Therefore, the following will illuminate the analysis of psychological basic needs.

- **Analysis of psychological basic needs from the perspective of consistency theory**

In 2004, based on his scientific research, Klaus Grawe developed a concept of psychological basic needs. His research demonstrates that psychological basic needs are of enormous relevance for human well-being (cf. Borg-Laufs 2018a, 141). The so-called consistency theory represents a concept of the emergence, maintenance, and change of psychological disorders. The model is based on psychological as well as neuroscientific basic research. The basic assumption is that people strive for the satisfaction and protection of their basic needs. In order to adequately satisfy or protect these needs from harm, people set certain goals and develop ways to achieve these goals, depending on individual life conditions (cf. Grawe and Grosse Holtforth 2004, 1).

Grawe classifies the basic needs as follows:

- Attachment,
- Self-esteem protection or self-esteem enhancement,
- Orientation and control,
- Pleasure gain and pain avoidance.

The term basic needs here means that these are needs whose satisfaction is indispensable for maintaining psychological health and a satisfying life. A lack of satisfaction or violation of these basic needs can lead to an unsatisfactory life and be associated with psychological disorders. This applies not only to adults but also to children and adolescents. An analysis of these basic needs helps in psychosocial as well as psychotherapeutic settings to better understand the behavior of clients (cf. Borg-Laufs 2018a, 141). Additionally, based on this analysis, individual counseling and therapy goals can be developed, which consist of enabling clients to better satisfy their needs in their life situation. Borg-Laufs (2018a, b) points out that often no specific diagnostic tools are necessary here, but rather counselors/therapists should simply put on the “need glasses.” Because when considering the information from clients against the background of these 4 basic needs, it can often quickly become understandable why clients seek advice or how the problem is related to need violations (cf. Borg-Laufs 2018a, 144).

Borg-Laufs (2018a, b) explains these 4 basic needs in the psychosocial context as follows:

1. **Attachment**

This particularly concerns attachment relationships, which represent a deep emotional relationship with significant, not easily replaceable reference persons. The need for attachment was first described by Bowlby (1975). Psychological mechanisms based on this need shape people's relationship behavior throughout their entire biography. Additionally, early childhood attachment disorders can lead to psychological disorders in adolescence and adulthood (cf. Borg-Laufs 2018a, 142).

2. **Self-esteem protection or self-esteem enhancement**

Regardless of age, people prefer individuals who enable them to have self-esteem-enhancing experiences. Likewise, they avoid self-esteem-injuring situations. A negative self-assessment can lead to a variety of problems. For example, in depressive clients, a negative self-assessment is seen as a component of the primary symptomatology (cf. Borg-Laufs 2018a, 143).

3. **Orientation or control**

People want to understand their world, be able to influence it, and to some extent predict what will happen in their lives. Experiencing oneself as a victim confronted with uncontrollable, unchangeable external influences leads to helplessness, passivity, and reduced zest for life. Experiences of loss of control are associated with adjustment disorders and post-traumatic stress disorders as well as anxiety and obsessive-compulsive disorders (cf. ibid., 143 f.).

4. **Pleasure gain or pain avoidance**

People automatically tend to evaluate certain situations or certain experiences as good or bad, which usually leads to approach (in the case of pleasant stimuli) or avoidance (in the case of unpleasant stimuli). Despite biological or cultural influences, it is essential to consider the individual case here. Experiences of pleasure and displeasure always arise through individual emotional-cognitive evaluation processes (cf. Borg-Laufs 2018a, 144).

In summary, it should be noted that it is advisable in psychosocial and psychotherapeutic practice to determine the satisfaction or non-satisfaction or violation of all 4 basic needs. It is important that clients are enabled to have experiences that satisfy their basic needs during counseling and that no fears of violations of psychological basic needs are triggered. Implementing experiences that satisfy basic needs into everyday life without exhibiting habitual problematic behavior must be part of the counseling goals. Because people strive to satisfy their basic needs, and if these are not met, they will continue to seek problematic ways to satisfy their needs and prevent (further) violations (cf. ibid., 148).

3.1.2.4 Summary: Psychosocial Diagnostics

The chapter on psychosocial diagnostics, with the presented analyses, methods, models, and diagnostic instruments, clearly shows the enormous importance of professional diagnostics both in psychotherapeutic practice and in psychosocial counseling. In recent years, concepts and analyses have increasingly developed, and the importance of psychosocial diagnostics has grown. The models range from biography-oriented and life-world-oriented to biopsychosocial and thus interdisciplinary models. Many experts state that a multidimensional and interdisciplinary approach in psychosocial diagnostics, as well as continuous evaluation of the collected information, contributes to the quality assurance of psychological interventions. It is advisable to document the entire process and to discuss the effects with the clients or to explain everything to them in an understandable way. By developing insight and understanding of the connections between their problems or difficult life situations and actively participating in the diagnostic procedures, clients can already view psychosocial diagnostics as a form of intervention. The individual problems and deficits of the clients are the focus, allowing for individually tailored intervention forms to be assembled. It is also important to see which systems are involved. This means it is relevant to know what environment the clients have and to what extent it is involved in the problem. Gahleitner and Pauls (2020) succinctly state that for successful psychosocial diagnostics, it is necessary to

> "(…) represent complexity in a case-understanding manner, but ultimately aim at structuring the complex interweaving of biological, psychological, and social processes and structures in their significance for health and well-being (…) with the goal of an independent and fruitful linkage of the unavoidable ambivalence of complexity acquisition and complexity reduction in diagnostic processes" (Gahleitner and Pauls 2017, quoted in Gahleitner and Pauls 2020, n.p.).

The enormous relevance of psychosocial diagnostics in the psychological and psychosocial counseling process has thus been demonstrated from various perspectives.

The following section will present which counseling approaches or therapy schools and orientations exist, which have also been established from a neuroscientific perspective, and provide an insight into intervention models relevant to PNES coaching.

3.1.3 Forms of Intervention: Counseling and Therapy Approaches, Methods, and Training

> "Methods of counseling are virtually inexhaustible"
> (Nestmann 2014, 783).

This section will address various counseling approaches, therapy schools, as well as methods and training. The goal is to provide readers with an overview of intervention forms that can be applied in PNES coaching. As the variety of methods in psychological and psychosocial counseling, as mentioned in the above quote by Nestmann, is virtually inexhaustible, some counseling approaches, therapy schools, and methods will be briefly described, while others, which are of greater relevance to the presented biopsychosocial concept or the understanding of this concept, will be explained in more detail. Additionally, the various approaches or schools will be critically examined from a neuroscientific perspective to discuss whether certain approaches still correspond to the current state of science and whether approaches whose effectiveness has been questioned neuroscientifically still have their justification. Furthermore, the importance of methodological pluralism will be addressed, and eclecticism, on which biopsychosocial PNES coaching is based, will be explained.

3.1.3.1 Counseling Approaches and School-Specific Therapeutic Orientations

Before I delve into specific methods and training, I will provide an insight into the various counseling approaches and therapy schools. Some orientations will be briefly described, and it will be shown to which therapeutic orientations psychological counseling can be assigned. The methods of psychosocial counseling are based on philosophical dialogue and/or psychological counseling, which can be assigned to one or more of the following orientations:

- "depth-psychological-psychodynamic orientation,
- humanistic-existential orientation,
- systemic-sociodynamic orientation,
- behavior-modifying orientation" (WKO Personenberatung und Personenbetreuung 2013, 1),

- philosophical dialogue.

Since Socrates and Plato, dialogue (Greek "dialogos") has been referred to as the development of an opinion related to the truth, because Socrates, in contrast to the Sophists, was concerned with the formation of a moral attitude in dialogue (cf. Metzler Lexikon Philosophie 2008, n.p.).

> "People should become capable of communicating with others and correcting their own opinions. The principle of dialogue is thus the recognition of the equality and taking seriously of all interlocutors" (ibid., n.p.).

Since the 1990s, the philosophical dialogue as a communication attitude has also been increasingly gaining acceptance in the German-speaking world (cf. Benesch 2020, 7). In this context, the word dialogue is synonymous with conversation. This can be either an oral or written communication between two or more individuals, according to Benesch (2020). The goal of the Socratic dialogue is to support interlocutors in uncovering hidden insights through skillful questioning and thus making coping strategies accessible (cf. ibid., 10). Philosophical dialogue is understood as a communication that serves to determine and convey insights and/or to present and explain problems. The dialogue is based on classical dialectics (thesis and antithesis). The focused goal here is to develop a chosen thought, solve crisis situations, or defend a primarily established position against the views of the opponent. The philosophical dialogue can, as an applied method, be seen as an intersubjective client-counselor/therapist relationship. Based on situation-appropriate questions from the counselor/therapist, fundamental insights are elicited from the client to identify coping strategies (cf. WKO Personenberatung und Personenbetreuung 2013, 1). However, Benesch (2020) points out that there is no uniform framework for the "dialogue." This means there is neither a congruent nor an empirical theory behind it, but many approaches from various orientations (cf. Benesch 2020, 10). However, the fact that there is no empirical "dialogue theory" is an opportunity for everyone to use the dialogue in their own way. This, however, is associated with the necessity that primarily counselors/therapists are aware of what they themselves understand by a philosophical dialogue and how they apply it (cf. ibid., 11).

- **Psychological counseling and school-specific orientations**

Psychological counseling can be assigned to one or more of the following orientations:

a) **Depth-psychological-psychodynamic orientation**

> "The term psychodynamics describes the approach advocated by psychoanalysis to explain psychological phenomena as an interplay of forces attributed to the soul life, most of which are unconscious. Psychodynamic thinking relates to psychological development, healthy experience, and pathological mental processes. It also considers psychosocial phenomena under the aspect of unconscious processes, e.g., processes in social organizations such as groups and institutions" (Ermann and Waldvogel 2022, n.p.).

The depth-psychological-psychodynamic approach is understood as an orientation that pays great attention to unconscious mental processes, which are of enormous importance for human behavior and thinking. The focus of all depth-psychological-psychodynamic counseling approaches is the view that there is a subconscious that is shaped by various processes and has a significant impact on conscious mental life. These approaches focus on interpreting the unconscious. Becoming aware of these unconscious processes is emphasized. Based on the awareness of the unconscious processes, a change in the client's life situation is achieved. Depth-psychological approaches in psychological and psychosocial counseling are particularly based on the teachings of psychoanalysis by Sigmund Freud, individual psychology by Alfred Adler, and analytical psychology by Carl Gustav Jung and are process-oriented in their orientation (cf. WKO Personenberatung und Personenbetreuung 2013, 1 f.).

Psychoanalytic and depth-psychologically based methods can be classified as follows:

I. "Psychoanalytic Methods
   - Analytical Psychology (AP)
   - Group Psychoanalysis (GP)
   - Individual Psychology (IP)
   - Psychoanalysis/Psychoanalytic Psychotherapy (PA)

II. Depth Psychology-Based Methods
   - Autogenic Psychotherapy (AT)
   - Existential Analysis (DA)
   - Dynamic Group Psychotherapy (DG)
   - Hypnosis Psychotherapy (HY)
   - Catathymic Imaginative Psychotherapy (KIP)
   - Concentrative Movement Therapy (KBT)
   - Transactional Analytical Psychotherapy (TA)" (WLP, Wiener Landesverband für Psychotherapie 2021, n.p.)

Characteristic of these methods based on psychoanalysis are generally changes in behavior and experience, which are particularly based on influencing the unconscious psychodynamics of the clients. The manifestation of the unconscious in the client-counselor/therapist relationship is of particular interest here (cf. Ermann and Waldvogel 2022, n.p.).

b) **Humanistic-Existential Orientation**

Humanistic orientations are based on the tendency for self-actualization, which exists in every individual, as well as on the increasing ability for self-responsibility. The foundation of the concepts is primarily built on individual personal fulfillment and the inner consent of the clients to life. Humans are seen as beings capable of arranging their lives meaningfully and overcoming crises based on their own strength (WLP, Wiener Landesverband für Psychotherapie 2021, n.p.). The commonality of humanistic-existential approaches lies in the shared view of humanity rather than in similar counseling/therapy models. However, the foundation of all approaches is the conviction that all people possess an inner potential for development. The focus of these counseling and therapy models is on the individual with the goal of self-actualization. It is important to note that only suggestions are communicated and not advice. The forefront of humanistic-existential approaches is self-experience and self-actualization of the clients. The concentration is on increasing creativity and promoting the ability to make contact, as well as discovering and reclaiming inhibited and/or blocked aspects of personality. Based on this, clients should achieve a self-actualized life (cf. WKO Personenberatung und Personenbetreuung 2013, 2).

Humanistic-Existential Approaches have Developed From

- "Existential Analysis and Logotherapy according to Viktor Frankl
- Gestalt Therapy according to Fritz and Lore Perls
- Integrative Gestalt Therapy and Integrative Therapy according to Petzold,
- Client-Centered Therapy according to Rogers, and
- Psychodrama according to Jakob Levy Moreno" (WKO Personenberatung und Personenbetreuung 2013, 2).

Just like depth-psychological-psychodynamic approaches, humanistic-existential approaches are process-oriented (cf. ibid.).

c) **Systemic-Sociodynamic Orientation**

> "We refer to a system as any group of elements that are connected by relationships and can be delineated from their environments by a boundary. We find such systems almost everywhere—from frogs in a pond to axons and dendrites in a nervous system, communication between parents and children in a family, to the circuits in a computer" (Schweitzer and von Schlippe 2016, 31).

This orientation is similar to the humanistic orientation in terms of its view of humanity; however, in these approaches, the focus is not on individuals but on the social system (family, couple, group, etc.) of the clients. The focus is directed by the counselors/therapists from the system to the client, and the orientation is goal-oriented (cf. WKO Personenberatung und Personenbetreuung 2013, 2).

Known Systemically-Sociodynamically Oriented Approaches, from which Psychosocial Counseling Methods have Developed, are for Example (cf. ibid.):

- "Systemic family therapy according to Virginia Satir as well as
- neurolinguistic programming NLP according to Grinder and Bandler" (ibid.).

d) **Behavior-modifying orientation**

Behavior modification refers to the

> "systematic application of learning psychological and other psychological learning techniques with the aim of behavior change, especially the promotion of desired behaviors and the reduction of problematic behaviors" (Bengel and Warmbrunn 2022, n.p.).

In behavior-modifying counseling and therapy approaches, the behavior of clients is seen as a learned behavior pattern that manifests as a reaction in certain situations. Problematic behavior is therefore not seen as an expression or system of an unconscious or conscious conflict or desire. The aim is to make clients aware of their behavior and change it through learning processes. It is assumed that clients have learned to respond to various situations or problems with a certain behavior over the course of their life history, but this behavior has become a problem. The behavior-modifying approaches are considered goal-oriented (cf. WKO Personenberatung und Personenbetreuung 2013, 3).

Finally, it should be noted that all four psychological basic orientations presented here, depending on the orientation, can be associated with body-, movement-, breathing-, and relaxation-oriented procedures (cf. ibid.).

- **Counseling approaches**

Since the PNES coaching presented in Chap. 4 is a biopsychosocial counseling concept, an overview of various psychosocial counseling approaches is provided below. There is a variety of different counseling approaches such as:

- psychoanalytically oriented counseling,
- cognitive-behavioral counseling,
- client-centered counseling,
- systemic counseling,
- integrative counseling,
- constructivist counseling,
- cooperative counseling,
- lifeworld-oriented social counseling,
- resource-oriented counseling,
- solution-oriented counseling,
- narrative counseling (cf. Engel et al. 2014, 610 ff.),
- biography-oriented counseling.

Depending on the relevance of the approaches for PNES coaching, some are described rather briefly and others are examined in more detail.

- **Psychoanalytically oriented counseling**

Psychoanalytic counseling orientations refer to approaches based on the principles of psychoanalysis. Psychoanalysis is declared an anthropological science that explores behavior and experience as an interaction of unconscious and conscious psychological processes (cf. Ermann and Waldvogel 2022, n.p.). Sigmund Freud (1856–1939) is to be mentioned as the founder of psychoanalysis. Despite scientific changes, Freud's thinking still determines a significant part of psychoanalysis (cf. Roth and Strüber 2021, 347). The core of the psychoanalytic approach is the exploration of the unconscious. This is done through free associations and interpretations of behavior and experience, aiming to resolve unconscious conflicts and compensate for acquired developmental deficits (cf. Ermann and Waldvogel 2022, n.p.). Psychoanalysis is often associated with clients lying on a couch and questioning the meaning of their experiences together with therapists, according to Datler et al. (2014). The basis of this approach is the assumption of a "ubiquitous dynamic unconscious." This assumption is based on the idea that people constantly come into contact with experiential content that they unconsciously perceive as threatening and therefore try to keep away from conscious perception. Various forms of unconscious defense and security mechanisms are activated, which in turn shape thoughts, emotions, behavior, and perception. This means that individual thoughts, emotions, behavior, and perception are based on unconscious defense and security. This theory of the "dynamic unconscious," which is declared "ubiquitous," shows (cf. Datler et al. 2014, 613 f.),

> "(…) that psychoanalysis is not only concerned with psychopathological conditions, their meaning, and the psychotherapeutic treatment of those who suffer from these conditions" (ibid., 614).

The psychoanalytic orientation deals more with the correlation between unconscious processes and various human emotions, cognitions, perceptions, and forms of behavior (cf. ibid.) as well as

> "(…) successful and less successful developmental and relationship processes, including play and work processes, educational and problem-solving processes" (Datler et al. 2014, 614).

The boundaries between various psychoanalytic therapy forms, such as psychoanalytic focal therapies, child, adolescent, and family therapy, as well as various group therapy forms, are often transparent. However, for psychoanalytic counseling, it can be noted that the counselor particularly questions what "unconscious subjective meaning" the problems or circumstances (e.g., income, profession, and family situation) have for the client. Additionally, it is discussed why the client cannot independently find an adequate solution to the problem. The relationship patterns of the clients are also analyzed and reflected upon. Furthermore, for sustainable success in psychoanalytic counseling, the relationship between counselor and client is crucial, as only with an adequate relationship can the client fully open up (cf. ibid., 615).

- **Cognitive-behavioral counseling**

The behavioral counseling approach, like behavior therapy, is based on the findings of learning psychology. The goal of this approach is to achieve a change in behavior. The foundation is solely directly observable behavior; non-observable emotions and cognitions must consistently be disregarded (cf. Borg-Laufs 2014, 629).

Behaviorism is a concept for both human and animal behavior. The crucial approach here is the scientific perspective of behavior. This concept was founded by John B. Watson (early 20th century) and was further developed scientifically in the 1950s by Frederic Skinner. The focus of behaviorism lies in the importance of learning (cf. Bengel et al. 2020, n.p.).

It is important to mention here that, unlike in classical behaviorism, it is no longer disputed that there are genetic predispositions in humans (cf. Roth and Strüber 2021, 371). For behaviorists, two fundamental learning principles are crucial for behavioral change: classical and instrumental conditioning (cf. Borg-Laufs 2014, 629).

- **Classical Conditioning:** Here, "(…) an originally neutral stimulus is presented together with a stimulus that triggers a sensation or behavior (UCS = unconditioned stimulus). As a result, the formerly neutral stimulus also acquires a signaling or triggering function (CS = conditioned stimulus)" (Borg-Laufs 2014, 629). Classical conditioning can arise from a single traumatic experience as well as from chronic stress. Classically conditioned behaviors can often be recognized by their physiological components (arousal) and the stimulus being triggered almost compulsively (cf. ibid.).
- **Instrumental Conditioning:** Here, behavior is not triggered by the preceding stimulus but by subsequent behavioral consequences. Thus, the behavior is under "reinforcer control." This means that a positive consequence increases the likelihood of a specific behavior occurring. The consequence can be either a reward or the removal of a negative state (cf. Borg-Laufs 2014, 629).

- **Client-Centered Counseling**

Since the 1960s, client-centered counseling has been considered an established counseling approach in the German-speaking world. This form of counseling is based on the concept of Carl Rogers (1902–1989), which is both theoretically and methodologically based and has been further developed for various fields of action. Client-centered counseling is also known as person-centered counseling. The focus of this counseling approach is on developments, experiences, and experiential contexts (cf. Straumann 2014, 641). The American Carl Rogers was a psychologist and developed this approach starting in 1942 in the USA. He was influenced by Otto Rank, who came from psychoanalysis and emphasized the relational aspect in his psychotherapeutic work. In the following decades, Rogers intensely explored the question of what conditions lead an individual to talk about their experiences on their own, thereby learning to understand themselves better, which leads to a change in attitude and behavior (cf. Weinberger 2013, 19 f.). The scientific interest in the "interpersonal" or the therapeutic or counseling relationship brought Rogers both outrage and criticism during a time when psychoanalysis dominated and psychotherapy was not openly discussed (cf. ibid., 21).

> "Rogers thus initiated a comprehensive empirical foundation of the client-centered approach, during which the essential variables of the therapeutic or counseling relationship were abstracted and operationalized" (Weinberger 2013, 21).

The client-centered relationship was made more transparent through tape recordings and made learnable and verifiable through scales. Rogers found that change processes can be activated if a relationship is successfully established (cf. ibid.).

> "With this very radical view that the nature of the relationship design is the decisive factor for changes and not the methods applied, Rogers or the client-centered approach stood very much alone until newer psychotherapy research confirmed exactly this over 50 years later" (Orlinsky 2004, cited in Weinberger 2013, 21).

The client-centered counseling approach assumes that individuals respond directly to impulses from their own organism and the environment. The behaviors depend on the individual perception of the impulses. This is declared as a personal "field of experience and perception," which is considered "reality" and "actuality" for those affected. The client-centered counseling approach assumes that individual behavior is triggered by the organism to satisfy its needs (cf. Straumann 2014, 641). The counseling approach always starts "(...) at the interface between person and environment (life or work environment)" (ibid., 642).

> Thus, it can be noted that client-centered counseling is both person-oriented and holistically oriented as well as context-bound. It activates individual resources and social competencies (cf. Straumann 2014, 642).

Client-centered counseling

> "(...) are professional problem, conflict, and crisis counseling to ensure personal and social security (...)" (Straumann 2014, 643).

It is important to note here that this counseling approach clearly distinguishes itself from medical psychotherapeutic assistance. The counseling goal is achieved when the clients can consciously, independently, and responsibly apply the developed decision aids in their daily lives. For this purpose, individually tailored intervention forms from personal and social work, which vary depending on the subject area, are implied in the counseling work (cf. Straumann 2014, 243). Finally, it should be mentioned that in client-centered counseling, since it is both subject-oriented and holistic, it is relevant that the prerequisites for counselors/therapists, in addition to their professional competencies, include individual competencies and social key qualifications (cf. ibid., 652).

- **Systemic Counseling Approach**

The systemic approach is becoming increasingly popular, especially in psychosocial fields of action. The application of this approach is diverse and ranges from individual case assistance to couple and family assistance, supervision, as well as team and organizational counseling (cf. Barthelmess 2014, 11). A paradigm shift is increasingly noticeable, leading from linear to systemic thinking (cf. ibid., 17).

> "Systemic" is derived from the Greek word "to systema"; "system" in its original meaning is the "whole composed and structured from several parts." Thus, it does not only refer to the "systematic" order of things but above all to their (ordered) "networking" (Brunner 2014, 655).

Based on this definition, the systemic counseling approach can be described both as "holistic counseling" and "networking counseling." A fundamental prerequisite in systemic counseling work is "thinking in contexts." In general systems theory, all (social) systems are defined as a totality of relationship units, all of which are intertwined. A social system consists not only of several people but also of the network of relationships that the people form with each other. However, it is not only the existing relationships that are relevant; the perceived relationships are equally crucial. This, in turn, means that in systemic counseling, it is important how people feel connected, perceive relationships, and define them (cf. Brunner 2014, 655 f.). Additionally, in the systemic perspective, there is both the active and passive aspect of being human, which means that on the one hand, one can individually shape and influence the systems, and on the other hand, one is oneself an element of other systems. Being an element oneself means adhering to other rules of play from higher levels (cf. Barthelmess 2014, 21). The modern form of systemic counseling can also be seen as "systemic-constructivist." Radical constructivists believe that an objective observation of the social system—"epistemologically speaking"—is not feasible. However, it is of enormous importance that counselors/therapists adopt a neutral position and behave impartially, i.e., they do not take sides with any person (cf. Brunner 2014, 656 ff.). The methods and techniques are diverse. However, all those techniques are focused on that strengthen the autonomy and self-management of the clients (cf. ibid., 660).

- **Integrative Counseling Approach**

The integrative approach links various counseling approaches together. It does not focus unilaterally but intertwines the diversity of aspects. Based on an integrative perspective, theoretical models simply exist side by side, which is arbitrary and thus "unsatisfactory" for psychological and psychosocial counseling, according to Wagner (cf. Wagner 2014, 663). The integrative approach is therefore to be seen as a combination of various interventions as small elements. A new change model is developed in integrative models (cf. Spektrum 2000, n.p.). Therefore, an overarching perspective on the various theoretical models must be adopted, and then, based on this metatheoretical perspective, the approaches must be compared with each other. What is considered a helpful foundation here, according to Wagner, is the model by Groeben (1986). This model is based on three scientific-theoretical subject units, which he designates as *acting*, *doing*, and *behavior*. The behavior unit can be traced back to the foundation of behaviorism. Here, a very reductive image of humans prevails, and the principles of classical and operant conditioning are considered central concepts (cf. Wagner 2014, 664 f.). The unit of doing represents psychoanalysis. The dissonance theory from social psychology as well as various sub-theories of gestalt therapy can be classified into the unit of doing. Here, the relation of the conscious and the unconscious is a central theme. The standpoint is taken that only a small number of human actions are conscious, the main part of motives and aspirations are subconscious. In the human image of the psychoanalytic model, the drives of human activities are thus in focus (cf. ibid., 666 f.). The unit of acting is based on human images of humanistic psychology, gestalt psychology, or action and decision theories. The reflection, language, and communication abilities of humans play a central role in this approach. In the action level, positive aspects of humans are consciously highlighted. An open reality concept is represented here, which implies an integrative relationship to one's own needs, as well as a connection of cognition and emotion (cf. ibid., 668 ff.). These three anthropological core assumptions form the foundation for integrative counseling, which thus enables counseling work that applies cross-school methods and procedures. Methods that have empirically proven to be successful are focused on (cf. Wagner 2014, 670 f.).

> "From *behavior* through *doing* to *acting* – the reflective aspects of humans are more strongly considered, and thus both counselor and client are modeled in an increasingly balanced, more partnership-oriented position" (ibid., 671).

Integrative counseling is thus to be seen as an "anthropologically non-reductive counseling" that can imply all insights from various theoretical directions (cf. Wagner 2014, 673).

- **Constructivist-oriented counseling approach**

The characteristics of a constructivist perspective can be traced back to a concept by Carl Rogers. The humanistic counseling psychology he developed is based on the concept of a "fully functioning person" (1963). Various processes are significant here, such as the increase in self-acceptance and self-actualization, but also coping strategies that promote reconstruction processes and can be described as relationship-oriented, according to Gerstenmaier (2014). As with most modern counseling approaches, the characteristics of the clients are the focus. These, in turn, focus on their competence for self-active action. Context and situational conditions only play a role insofar as the experiences of the clients are "filtered, interpreted, or reconstructed" and then become the starting point for new experiences (cf. Gerstenmaier 2014, 675 f.). Characteristic of a constructivist perspective are

> "the orientation towards individual experience and its processing, the significance of reality as experienced and constructed reality, and the knowledge acquired in relationships and shared with others" (ibid., 676).

Based on the experiences, reality arises, and the clients carry the competence for constructive change within themselves. However, for empirically working social scientists and psychologists, radical constructivism is rather to be avoided (cf. ibid., 677).

> "In radical constructivism, people and functional areas are mostly understood as informationally closed systems that only process information that is viable and serves structural preservation" (Gerstenmaier 2014, 677).

More significant are social constructivism and the social-cognitive perspective (cf. ibid.). Mary Gergen (2001) and Kenneth Gergen (1999 and 2001) see the starting point of social constructivist approaches in a socially constructed world. Social problems, insights, and what is relevant to us are the results of our reality constructions. Further aspects of social-constructivist approaches include, for example, studies of ethnic minorities and gender studies as well as the significance of the self-concept. The social-cognitive perspective of constructivism is particularly popular in social and developmental psychology (cf. Gerstenmaier 2014, 677).

The social-cognitive approach

> "(…) characterizes cognitive development as a constructive process of knowledge acquisition, which is described with the help of mental models, cognitive schemas, or propositional, semantic networks" (ibid., 678).

In Summary, Constructivist Perspectives have the Following Characteristics

- The basis for the construction of knowledge is the individual's competence for active action and self-regulation.
- Insights are constructed based on experiences, contexts are perceived and applied as diverse.
- Interventions and counseling are used to promote self-active action, to foster self-management, and to deepen shared insights in groups (cf. Gerstenmaier 2014, 678).

Furthermore, a distinction is made between explicitly and implicitly constructivist counseling approaches. Explicitly constructivist counseling approaches are those that also describe themselves as constructivist. Implicitly constructivist counseling approaches also fulfill these characteristics but do not declare themselves as constructivist (cf. ibid.). Gerstenmaier explains that social constructivism and social cognitive theory are extremely valuable for counseling. Based on the self-activity of the clients, constructivism promotes the competence of self-management, "(…) takes into account the effects of cognitive schemas, stereotypes, and action explanations and examines their influence on actions" (Gerstenmaier 2014, 688). Additionally, this approach is suitable as a basis for institutional and organizational counseling, being particularly cognitively oriented and referring to both individual and shared knowledge constructions (cf. ibid.).

- **Cooperative counseling approach**

Cooperations within counseling are steadily increasing. However, cooperation is not only meant as a structural necessity for problem-solving and answering questions but also as an inner attitude. The attitude and mindset between counselors and clients are also relevant. The cooperative counseling approach is to be seen as a kind of meta- or nested theory. The outer shell consists of assumptions about the human image, beneath which lies the framework of the "object conception, i.e., the action and disturbance theory or behavior and deviation theory" (cf. Mutzeck 2014, 691). The core is the counseling method or the *counseling conception,* here the cooperative counseling. The explication of assumptions about the human image is a basic prerequisite for a counseling method that focuses on the human being (cf. ibid., 691 f.). It particularly encompasses

> "(…) potential abilities such as reflexivity, rationality, intentionality, meaning orientation, cognitive ability, emotionality, verbalization and communication ability, action competence, and autonomy" (Mutzeck 2014, 692).

The underlying framework of the cooperative counseling approach includes the attitude and disturbance conception, which is based on the explicated assumption about the human image.

> "A person's action is to be seen as a context-bound event system, whereby the respective person belongs to several systems simultaneously" (Mutzeck 2014, 693).

The action is seen as an inter- and intra-active reciprocal event, whereby it is not the context that determines the action, but the individual's cognitive perception processes, information processing, and action planning. The influence factors concerning the context are also relevant. These inter- and intra-active processing processes lead to an individually constructed reality, which forms the basis for the person's actions. Thus, the action depends on the human's subjective interpretations of the situation, their ideas and expectations, motives and goals, as well as their weighing processes and decisions. The influence of the environment, culture, and society on behavior is seen from a different perspective, namely from the self- and world-view of the clients (cf. ibid., 693). The counseling conception is based on horizontal counseling, which is non-directive, symmetrical, and cooperative (cf. Mutzeck 2014, 695 f.).

The cooperative counseling approach is a non-instructive approach that forms a cooperative and understanding interaction. This horizontal form of counseling supports and promotes the development of the clients' activity. Clients are trusted to activate their individual resources and possibilities in such a way that they can solve problems themselves (cf. Mutzeck 2014, 695 f.).

The consultants/therapists provide impulses and assistance. No advice is given; instead, solutions to problems are sought together under the methodological guidance of the consultants/therapists, and implementations are worked on. The distribution of roles is to be seen as equal, and the clients always become active participants (cf. Mutzeck 2014, 695 f.). Cooperative counseling is to be seen as a client-centered, resource-oriented, and systematic approach to conversation and problem-solving, which shapes a trusting, accepting, empathetic, and congruent relationship between consultants/therapists and clients. Based on a cooperative, goal-oriented, structured, and transparent approach, problems are understood and explained, resources are uncovered, and solutions are developed. The course of action is planned together, and its implementation is accompanied and jointly reflected upon (cf. ibid., 696).

- **Life-world-oriented counseling**

The life-world-oriented counseling approach is a concept of social counseling and has emerged within social work (cf. Thiersch 2014, 699).

> "Life-world is analyzed against the theoretical background of phenomenology and interaction theory, but above all critical everyday theory, which is associated with structural analyses of social conditions" (ibid., 700).

Life-world orientation means focusing primarily on the addressees and their living conditions or their interpretations of their living conditions, their life difficulties, and also their resources (cf. Füssenhäuser 2006, 127).

This life-world-oriented approach aims at the reconstruction of living conditions, institutions, and action arrangements and is used in educational and social science fields of action as well as in health science and inclusive education areas. The so-called life-worldliness is found in various life fields such as family, schools, and training institutions, as well as in work and public life. Working in a life-world-oriented manner means seeing people in their diversity and considering everyday, small, and inconspicuous constellations in complex, social, communicative, as well as technically instrumental tasks. The life worlds, as well as the life-world coping strategies, are shaped by social conditions. The living conditions and problems are closely examined (cf. Thiersch 2014, 700 f.). The life-world-oriented approach "(…) understands the human being (…) in the dialectic of resources and deficits, of coping competence and inadequacy" (ibid., 701). This approach promotes the stabilization of resources, strengthens one's active life management, and is commissioned and determined by the needs, demands, and possibilities of the clients. Participation and integration can be seen as the highest maxims (cf. ibid., 701 f.). However, life-world orientation also refers to the subject-related as well as social possibilities and conditions. In doing so, the strengthening of living spaces, but also the possibilities for self-help, are focused on to optimize everyday coping. In life-world-oriented action, the complexity, problems, and difficulties of everyday life are addressed (cf. Füssenhäuser 2006, 127). Life-world-oriented work is also characterized "(…) by prevention, low-threshold access, regionalization (social spatiality), and networking between different offers" (Thiersch 2014, 702). Life-world-oriented social counseling also acts in the life world of the clients to find problem-solving strategies for everyday coping (cf. ibid., 707).

> "Working in a life-worldly manner means responding to the problems of people found in the life world and developing and supporting a 'vision' of a more successful life together with them" (Füssenhäuser 2006, 127).

- **Resource-oriented counseling**

Psychological and psychosocial counseling is particularly used when individual competencies and resources are lacking. The counseling must support and promote the clients in making use of individual resources from their environment, from themselves, and from the interplay of social and individual potentials. The connection of counseling to individual personal resources is an approach that contributes to change in both deficit-oriented approaches and humanistic and systemic approaches. The premise of all resource-oriented models is that our way of life, everyday design, well-being, and health are dependent on our resources for our successes and failures, as well as our problem and crisis management (cf. Nestmann 2014b, 726 ff.). Thus, it is not surprising that the term "resources" has almost become a magic word, according to Lenz (2003) (cf. Lenz 2003, 234).

The strengths and potentials of individuals form the focused dimension. In contrast to psychotherapeutic resource approaches, which focus on personal resources, in psychosocial counseling, the interaction of individual strengths and forces of the clients and the context-related resources based on social networks is of importance. The guiding principle here is the empowerment approach (cf. Lenz 2003, 234).

For this, both the availability and the successful use of personal and environmental resources are of relevance. Therefore, it is a necessity to have resources and to maintain them. According to Hobfoll and Lilly (1993), resources can be divided into the following categories:

- **Objects:** Resources from our material environment, such as a house, means of transport, or even clothing.
- **Certain living conditions and circumstances:** These are various self-valued states, such as a partnership, through which desired goals can be achieved.
- **Personal characteristics:** Individual traits such as self-esteem, social skills, coping optimism, or a sense of control.
- **Energy resources:** Resources to achieve desired objects, living conditions, or goals, such as financial means, but also a leap of faith in people as well as certain insights (cf. Hobfoll and Lilly 1993, cited in Nestmann 2014, 728 f.).

In psychosocial counseling, constellations of resource threats or feared resource loss are common. Thus, a key feature of counseling is that resource expansion, targeted resource use, and resource deployment to achieve a resource gain are pursued. Resource-oriented counseling also means promoting resource management and supporting the development and expansion of resources. According to the so-called *conservation of resources theory*, resource loss is more significant than resource gain, as resource loss often means a threat to existence. Therefore, especially in counseling where clients are worked with who live in risky life contexts, preventing resource loss is the primary task and primary goal. To prevent resource loss and achieve resource gain, resources are again necessary. People who have more resources are less susceptible to resource loss than people who have fewer resources. Likewise, those with fewer resources find it more difficult to gain resources. It can thus be seen as a spiral of gain and loss: where there is already something, more often comes, and where there is already a lack, more loss often quickly follows. This can create a vicious circle, as further losses require further resource deployment. This vicious circle then also makes the clients increasingly vulnerable (cf. Nestmann 2014b, 729 f.). Resource-oriented counseling focuses "(…) on 'the full part of a half-filled glass' and consciously forms a counterpoint to the prevailing deficit and risk orientations of clinical-psychotherapeutic client images" (ibid., 730 f.). The positive assets of the clients, their development possibilities of individual and contextual resources of life management, as well as everyday and problem-solving skills, are the focus of this counseling. A resource perspective, in particular, expands and complements deficit and disorder analyses and interventions and changes the view of deficiencies. This does not mean that a resource perspective ignores the demands and problems of the clients, but there is no problem fixation, as it turns the focus to the strengths and potentials of the clients. Resource-oriented counseling, in particular, accepts individual weaknesses, deficiencies, and deficits, but the basic assumption is that even in the most severely damaged individual, promotable resources can be found. This requires counselors to have increased resource sensitivity towards individuals as well as the social, institutional, and natural environment. It requires resource diagnostics, which is equated with problem diagnostics (cf. Nestmann 2014b, 731 f.). Methods of resource diagnostics are, for example: "(…) recording personal strengths, network mapping and support analysis, organizational and institutional diagnoses (…)" (ibid., 732).

Resource-oriented support attempts to

- identify and diagnose both personal and environmental resources,
- activate and mobilize resources that are unused,
- expand or supplement resources in individuals and make them usable in their life contexts, and
- adapt existing personal and environmental resources to the demands, problems, crises, and conflicts, according to Nestmann.

The primary goals are resource security and preservation. Additionally, the focus of resource-oriented psychosocial counseling is on individual human development, self-determined and self-controlled everyday and life management, securing and utilizing development opportunities, preventing stress and crises, and constructively coping with them (cf. Nestmann 2014b, 732 f.). Ultimately, it should be noted, where the proponents of the resource concept largely agree, according to Lenz (2003), that resource activation must be accompanied by a relativization of the expert status. This means a departure from the previously common paternalistic model of the help relationship. Thus, the relationship is not based on "knowing" professionals and "unknowing" clients. The resource-oriented approach has therefore supplemented previous perspectives in both psychosocial and psychotherapeutic work and contributed to methodological and professional developments. The aspects of resource orientation, individual potential, and participation represent central dimensions of a counseling understanding (cf. Lenz 2003, 235).

- **Solution-oriented counseling**

The solution-oriented counseling approach goes back to Steve de Shazer (1989). He developed the *"standard intervention of the first hour,"* which is considered one of the most important tools of solution-oriented counseling. It is about promoting a balanced system, not only focusing on the problem but directing attention to what is not a problem, thus creating a counterbalance to the problem complaint. In addition to the "standard intervention of the first hour," the *"miracle question"* has been established, which is considered one of the most significant and effective intervention techniques of solution-oriented counseling. Both intervention techniques focus on what could solve the problem or what could "work" (cf. Bamberger 2014, 737 f.).

> "And that is exactly what solution-oriented counseling is about: the systematic identification of existing potentials and resources, a grid search for behavioral possibilities that can make a difference and thus solve something" (ibid., 738).

This resource-oriented or solution-oriented principle is to be regarded as the credo of the solution-oriented counseling approach. This provides a clear distinction from those counseling approaches that consider an in-depth problem analysis as the foundation to find a solution. According to Steve Shazer, however, it is of enormous importance to conduct an in-depth *resource analysis* from the very beginning. This can often address the problem without the counselor/therapist even knowing the problem. However, they must be well-informed about the solution competencies or solution potentials. The motto of solution-oriented counseling, also known as the "Milwaukee Axiom," states (cf. Bamberger 2014, 739):

"Construct solutions instead of analyzing problems!" (ibid.).

According to Bamberger (2014), the solution-oriented counseling model follows these principles:

- **Principle of solution orientation:** The goal of counseling is to construct a solution, and this consistently from the very beginning.
- **Principle of utilization:** Clients have a variety of resources, they are cooperative, and they themselves are the experts of their lives. Everything that clients bring and contribute is used to gain a solution perspective.
- **Principle of constructiveness:** What we consider reality is something constructed by ourselves. Problems are also constructed. The expertise of the counselors enables something constructed to be reconstructed.
- **Principle of change:** Solutions always mean change—change of perceptions, cognitions, emotions, behavior patterns, as well as life plans. Even a small step of change is enough to initiate a self-dynamic change process.
- **Principle of minimal intervention:** The solution-oriented counseling approach sees itself as a problem that should be ended as quickly as possible. Therefore, the so-called minimal intervention aims for short-term counseling.

The briefly described principles characterize solution-oriented counseling as a method of the systemic concept (cf. Bamberger 2014, 739 f.).

In summary, it should be noted that the solution-oriented counseling approach does not focus on the problem-relevant context or analyze problem behavior, but rather aims for a change in perspective to move from the problem to the "non-problem." Additionally, solution-oriented counseling methods strengthen solution-oriented cognitions and perceptions as well as solution-oriented actions, thereby promoting the solution (cf. Bamberger 2014, 744 f.).

- **Narrative Counseling Approach**

At the beginning, it is important to mention that the narrative counseling approach is not about a new form of counseling or a new school of therapy, but about a different counseling perspective. It is about a certain attitude that the counselor/therapist adopts, in which he/she emphasizes, among other things, the importance of linguistic and narrative aspects. The emphasis on the relevance of language, narratives, and metaphors has been gaining increasing attention since the early 1990s. The foundation of this counseling approach is that the counseling consists of narratives, which are constructed by the clients through language. It is an individually different language, with individual narrative structures, various culturally anchored contexts, metaphors, and the associated meaningfulness. It is known that speaking is implicit in almost all forms of counseling, but the narrative counseling approach has made language the subject of counseling, emphasizing the relevance of language analysis as well as its relevance for the success of a counseling process (cf. Engel and Sickendiek 2014, 749 f.). The term narration (storytelling) is manifested in the social sciences in empirical research. In qualitative research, there are so-called narrative interviews, in which problematic life situations are often reported by the interviewees. In psychology, the so-called narrative psychology has developed (cf. ibid., 752), "(…) which allocates the central space for understanding human actions to the interpretation of narratives" (ibid.). Counselors need a narrativesensitivity. Narrative sensitivity means showing a sensitive attitude towards language.A conscious handling of language further implies maintaining an open and trustingrelationship with the clients, as the counseling relationship is largely shaped bylanguage. Furthermore, a non-knowing perspective is required in a narrative attitude.The role of the counselors/therapists is to create a conversational free space, topromote a joint conversation, and to maintain the dialogue (cf. ibid., 753).

> The focus is not on a specific change in behavior or perception, but on enabling a space for open conversations, "(…) in which changes result as a dialogical development of new narratives" (cf. Engel and Sickendiek 2014, 754).

It is of enormous relevance that the counselors explicitly listen and follow the presentation logic of the clients' narratives from a non-knowing perspective. This means that the narrative form of presentation takes precedence and any school-specific interpretations are avoided. Space is created for the development of new and different narratives and changes in meaning (cf. Engel and Sickendiek 2014, 754).

> "The position of 'being informed' by the client and the joint creation of new meanings presupposes that the narrative understanding takes place in the client's colloquial language and thus creates an atmosphere of respect and (self-)affirmation for the client" (Engel and Sickendiek 2014, 754).

Metaphors are of particular relevance in the narrative counseling approach.

> "A metaphor is a linguistic tool in which special properties of one domain are applied to another domain to explore situations or clarify meanings, and as a rhetorical form to embellish representations" (ibid., 756).

Examples of this are "I am completely off track" or "to hit the brakes on something." Metaphors are irrational forms of language used to interpret and vividly verbalize temporary emotional states. In dealing with metaphors, one often learns significant things about various perspectives, goals, conflicts, as well as unspoken attitudes (cf. ibid., 757). Metaphors can influence our cognition and actions, and they are "(…) the subject of conscious reflection and starting points for changes in counseling processes" (ibid., 759).

- **Biography-Oriented Psychological and Psychosocial Counseling**

In addition to the previously outlined various known counseling approaches and orientations, biography-oriented counseling is also highlighted here. It has increasingly gained acceptance in psychological and psychosocial counseling in recent years.

> "Through biographical work, people experience healing, life orientation, and encouragement" (Klingenberger 2017, 5).

Biographical work enables the recollection, documentation, preservation, and management of past experiences and events, facts, and life experiences together with a trusted person. This gives people the opportunity to understand their history and perceive their present more consciously. Based on this, it is possible to plan the future in a goal-oriented manner (cf. Lattschar and Wiemann 2013, 13). The biographically oriented counseling form implements biographical work in the psychological and psychosocial counseling process, thus opening up opportunities for reflection as well as the exchange of individual experiences and events, as well as the diverse life courses of the clients. The basic assumption of biographically oriented counseling is that a resource-oriented view of the past can promote problem-solving in the present. With the perspective of developing opportunities from problems, various individual future concepts can be developed for the clients. Biographical counseling is increasingly resonating. The goal is to accompany people constructively and solution-oriented to promote their biographical competencies (cf. Klingenberger 2017, 5–11). Through reflection situations, for which there is space in biographical counseling, people can experience healing, life orientation, and encouragement, resulting in a positive attitude towards life. Biographically oriented counseling accompanies people before, during, and after life crises and difficult life transitions. However, biographically oriented counseling is not just a collection of various methods; rather, biographical orientation is to be understood primarily as an attitude (cf. ibid., 27 f.).

"With the thematization of biography, the aspect of education and life management in psychosocial counseling becomes more prominent in dealing with transitions" (Weinhardt 2014, 44).

In biographically oriented counseling, questioned self-world relationships are reflected upon and their transformation is accompanied. Thus, according to Weinhardt (2014), this form of counseling is to be seen as both a biographical educational and coping process (cf. Weinhardt 2014, 45).

- **Eclecticism**

In the following, eclecticism will be explained in more detail. Since PNES coaching is to be classified as an eclectic-integrative approach, eclecticism plays a significant role. As has already become clear in the previous points, there are overlaps with other techniques or approaches in many counseling approaches and methods. Just as a biographical perspective can be implemented in many approaches or intertwined with various methods, one can see that there is a clear trend towards eclectic-integrative action orientations.

Eclecticism can be defined as the combination and mixture of different ideas, styles, or style elements (cf. Duden 2021, n.p.).

Leitner notes that the term eclecticism is often used pejoratively because "eclectic" is equated with "not independent" and thus is not recognized as a therapeutic procedure (cf. Leitner 2010, 113). Nevertheless, the eclectic-integrative orientation, particularly spurred by humanistic therapy approaches in the 1970s, is gaining increasing importance. This orientation is described as comprehensively effective and requires a willingness to open up various method repertoires and implement different concepts and approaches (cf. Nestmann 2014a, 787 f.). Thompson (1996) attributes the increase in eclecticism or pluralism and the frequent use of interdisciplinary methods to the growing diversity of clients and their expectations and needs. Applying only one theory or an intervention method chosen from a single approach, despite the diverse problems and the variety within the entire biography of the clients, the enormous range of interpersonal demands, and the various problem-solving strategies, would not be considered the most effective (cf. Thompson 1996, cited in Nestmann 2014a, 788 f.). Leitner goes further and argues that diverse theory formations could never be "noneclectic" because the various schools have always developed in an already existing field. This is particularly emphasized in the integrative approach. As an example, Leitner cites Freud's psychoanalysis. Freud's thinking was also eclectic, as he combined neuroanatomical-physiological, chemical, physical, and technological insights with philosophical ones in this procedure (cf. Leitner 2010, 113 f.). Nestmann notes that today psychological and psychosocial counseling in most fields of action is multimethodically designed and is to be classified as an eclectic-integrative orientation (cf. Nestmann 2014a, 789).

In an eclectic approach, various methods and procedures from different concepts are used for help and change. However, it is important to mention that this is not a random, haphazard compilation of various methods or elements of various methods, but rather a controlled and planned integration of various procedures adapted to the clients (cf. Nestmann 2014a, 789).

The so-called common factor research has significantly contributed to the discussion about eclecticism and its effects. In common factor research, general dimensions, factors of impact, and effectiveness from various counseling and psychotherapy forms were examined and considered in general, rather than distinguishing the forms individually (cf. ibid.). As early as 1961, Frank stated in his basic thesis that the effectiveness of counseling and therapy is not primarily based on techniques but on functions. These functions offer new learning opportunities, increase a kind of hope for improvement, enable experiences of success, eliminate demoralizing alienation based on the counseling relationship, and have an emotionally stimulating effect (cf. Frank 1961, cited in Nestmann 2014a, 790).

Leitner distinguishes between the following forms of eclecticism:

- "(…) unreflected eclecticism, called syncretism,
- systematic eclecticism, which pays attention to critical and systematic selection,
- technical eclecticism, which is oriented towards the principle of utility and tries to gather the most effective methods from various therapy schools without examining their compatibility with the original theories, and
- theoretical eclecticism, which aims at the integration of various theories and is often used synonymously with the term integration" (Leitner 2010, 114).

In conclusion, Nestmann states that the basis for an effective eclectic-integrative counseling orientation, which is composed in a controlled manner from various therapy schools, is a successful relationship between counselors and clients (cf. Nestmann 2014a, 791).

3.1.3.2 Critical Considerations of School-Specific Orientations

As already shown in this book, there is an enormous variety of counseling approaches as well as various psychotherapeutic orientations. In certain points, the effectiveness of the orientations as well as the pluralism of methods has already been discussed. The effectiveness of psychotherapies or the various orientations has already been empirically researched in neuroscience. However, the effectiveness could not be empirically confirmed for all orientations. Therefore, critical interdisciplinary considerations are presented and discussed below.

The number of school-specific orientations is large. Whether in the psychoanalytic, gestalt therapeutic, or behavior-oriented approach, the possibilities are diverse. As early as 2004, Grawe and his research team had been researching the effects of psychotherapeutic approaches on a neuroscientific basis for years and explained the mechanisms of therapeutic methods on a neuronal level. This led him to a cross-school and neuroscientifically founded approach. Henningsen (2017) critically notes that by the turn of the millennium at the latest, neuroscience was "trending" and was discussed and applied by far more people than those who could actually call neurobiological science their expertise (cf. Henningsen 2017, 7). Skop criticizes that the major breakthroughs of neuroscience within psychotherapy, however, have failed to materialize (cf. Skop 2019, 22). She points out,

> "(…) that a neuroscientific foundation of psychotherapy is problematic because the implicit reductionism of the subjective in client treatment brings no significant progress" (ibid., 20).

She believes that the implication of neuroscience in therapeutic schools has lost its urgency in the last 10 years. She particularly points out that neuroscientific findings in psychotherapy science always play only a subordinate role. Furthermore, she explains that until 2019, there was no attempt to establish a neuropsychotherapeutic school, and such a school has not even remotely established itself in therapeutic practice (cf. Skop 2019, 20). However, in 2021, Roth and Strüber published a revised and expanded edition, in which it is definitively stated that the criticism from neuroscience towards the common approaches and schools has not disappeared. Based on the book or research work by Roth and Strüber (2021), I would now like to present more current critical considerations of school-specific orientations. Roth and Strüber (2021) note that the effectiveness of some models shows significant deficits of various kinds from today's scientific perspective. For example, assumptions are made that are not compatible with the current state of knowledge in neuroscience (cf. Roth and Strüber 2021, 435 f.). This applies, among other things, to the belief in behavior therapy that human behavior is determined entirely or mostly by learning processes. Many experts agree here that genetic-epigenetic influences, as well as prenatal or early postnatal environmental influences, have a highly relevant share in psychological development and personality. Thus, conditions arise that form a framework in which behavioral therapeutic interventions can unfold their effect at all. Equally unscientifically proven is the belief that unwanted behaviors can simply be erased. According to Roth and Strüber, they can at best be dampened or encapsulated by newly learned behaviors. Cognitive behavioral therapy (CBT) assumes that cognitions control our emotions and that, based on this, restructuring of mental schemas can change emotions similarly to behavior. However, a multitude of neuroscientific studies, in which representatives of CBT also participated, showed the opposite (cf. Roth and Strüber 2021, 436). It was shown,

> "(…) that the sole change of cognitive schemas does not bring about emotional and behavioral changes, but that the latter are necessary for the change of the former" (ibid.).

In the psychoanalytic approach, besides Freud's drive theory, one should admit that the relevant part of a positive therapy does not consist of the "power of the word," nor of the clarification of unconscious drives or motives (cf. Roth and Strüber 2021, 436). Füllgrabe (2022) also criticizes the psychoanalysis developed by Sigmund Freud. For him, it is not understandable that psychoanalysis still holds a certain reputation today, although it is not based on a scientifically confirmed foundation. It is also not as successful as a therapeutic method as is often assumed or claimed (cf. Füllgrabe 2022, 1). Füllgrabe notes that psychoanalysis does not clarify the abysses of the human soul but much more often applies superficial terms and does not consider scientifically based psychological processes. He also points out that not only does a healing effect fail to materialize, but instead, a damaging effect can occur (cf. ibid., 14). The humanistic approaches, as well as the gestalt therapeutic approaches, also hold the mistaken belief, according to Roth and Strüber (2021), that merely linguistic-communicative interactions with patients and empathetic talking would be a way to successful therapy (cf. Roth and Strüber 2021, 436). Another area criticized from a neuroscientific perspective is that the interventions of the various counseling and therapy directions are one-sided. They are either on the level of well-being and memories or on the level of behavior. Sometimes the body level is also addressed. However, Roth and Strüber emphasize that moderate to severe mental disorders always affect all three levels. Based on this insight, psychotherapies with mentally ill people should always be directed at all three levels, as otherwise, no profound and long-term improvement occurs. This should not mean that everything about the various schools is bad, as there are extremely valuable components of the different orientations. For example, the further developed CBT and various humanistic orientations should be mentioned (cf. ibid., 437). These "(…) offer effective approaches to mental and affective-emotional restructuring" (Roth and Strüber 2021, 437). Modern psychoanalysis, along with psychodynamic, attachment-based, and developmental psychological approaches, is probably one of the most significant orientations. It is assumed that current mental illnesses are based on negative developmental dynamics of the psyche and personality. Through this approach, the importance of the therapeutic relationship (alliance) for therapeutic success was also recognized. According to Roth and Strüber, the current state of knowledge for general therapy schools and counseling approaches results in,

> "(…) that therapeutic success results from the combination of non-specific factors, especially the therapeutic alliance, and specific factors, which, however, unfold their effect in a highly individualized manner" (Roth and Strüber 2021, 437).

After a counseling or therapeutic relationship or alliance has been established and the counselor/therapist has conducted sufficient analyses, is sufficiently informed about the client's disorders, crises, and current life situations, the counselor/therapist selects appropriate interventions from their toolbox. These cannot be applied without an adequate alliance, whereas the alliance alone does not produce long-lasting, profound effects. Therefore, a fusion with neuroscientific findings is necessary, according to Roth and Strüber (cf. Roth and Strüber 2021, 437 f.). However, just as there are proponents of merging psychotherapeutic approaches with neuroscience, there are also opponents. It sometimes seems as if it is a well-known battle between the humanities and the natural sciences, according to Skop (cf. Skop 2019, 26). For example, Hubert (2006) states that brain research fosters a reductionist view of humanity, in which mind and psyche are not to be separated from material nature but rather reduced to it. He criticizes that neuroscience turns mind and psyche into a matter of nerves (cf. Hubert 2006, 20). Modern psychosomatics, on the other hand, has already implemented an interdisciplinary perspective into everyday psychosomatic practice. The biological-natural scientific level is a significant part of thinking and acting and thus cannot be excluded, according to Rüegg (cf. Rüegg 2011, 2 f.). Eßing states that it would be most sensible to choose and apply those elements that have empirically proven to be effective and successful and are supported by neuroscientific findings (cf. Eßing 2015, 12). In summary, Skop concludes that some consider it sensible to implement neurobiological knowledge into their therapeutic approaches, but only to enhance their own therapeutic school. The fact that no neuropsychotherapeutic school has prevailed to this day speaks, according to Skop, for the persistence of methodological pluralism (cf. Skop 2019, 30 f.).

Summary

This section highlighted the diversity of counseling approaches and school-specific orientations. It also became clear that some approaches overlap or implement some methods from other orientations in their approaches. Furthermore, it was shown that, based on empirically proven effectiveness, more and more counselors/therapists prefer the eclectic-integrative approach, as this allows methods to be individually tailored to clients and their issues. The last part of the section demonstrated how the current state of neuroscientific research disproves the effectiveness of some orientations. However, clear neuroscientific recommendations were also made, for example, for various humanistic orientations, advanced CBT, and modern psychoanalysis, which convinces with attachment-related, developmental psychological, and psychodynamic approaches. Based on empirical neuroscientific research results, interdisciplinary findings should definitely be implemented in both psychosocial counseling and psychotherapeutic interventions. However, these critical considerations also have opponents, giving the impression that it is a recurring "battle" between the humanities and the natural sciences. It seems that the only consensus is that the therapeutic relationship or alliance between counselors/therapists and clients is the foundation for any intervention success. Regardless of these critical considerations and interdisciplinary findings, various methods, tools, and training will be presented in the following to form a certain toolbox for methodological pluralism in practice. Since the diversity, as already mentioned, is enormous, only an overview will be provided here. Some methods and training will be briefly described, and some methods relevant to PNES coaching will be explained in more detail.

3.1.3.3 Methods for Problem Solving in Psychological and Psychosocial Counseling

After providing an overview of therapeutic orientations and various counseling approaches in the previous section and briefly outlining the philosophical dialogue, I will now discuss some methods I have chosen that are relevant to this coaching concept. Additionally, the setting of the various counseling methods will be described, as psychological and psychosocial counseling can be offered in various settings, as mentioned at the beginning of this chapter. Counseling can take place in individual settings as well as with couples, families, and groups (cf. Borg-Laufs and Wälte 2018, 205).

Psychological and psychosocial counseling is characterized by a variety of diverse professional intervention forms, which are influenced by both external and internal factors. The various interventions help clients cope with problems and crises, as well as make decisions. Additionally, clients are supported in generating and optimizing their individual and social life worlds. The following section will outline this versatility as well as adaptability. The enormous spectrum of methods and the associated relationship formations between counselors/therapists and clients, as well as the various counseling settings, contribute to the versatility and multiplexity of psychological and psychosocial counseling. It will be shown that counseling is an open and flexible form of help that addresses individual problem situations and life crises and can be classified as "modern" and timely (cf. Engel et al. 2014, 599).

> "A method is a consciously planned, already tested course of action with which a specific goal is to be achieved"
> (Nestmann 2014a, 784).

According to Nestmann (2014), ultimately, any forms of interpersonal communication and interaction that are not harmful can be potential counseling methods; even the relationship between counselors and clients can be a purposeful "support and change method" (cf. ibid., 783). In addition to many unspecific forms of supportive communication and interaction, there are also many specific methodological procedures derived from theoretical-conceptual concepts or various counseling schools and directions. Equally influential are various disciplines and professional affiliations, institutional and organizational frameworks, as well as diverse fields of action and settings (cf. Nestmann 2014a, 783).

1. **Methods of Individual Counseling**

Nestmann (2014) states that the methods in individual counseling can be classified as follows:

- **Cognitive Restructuring:** The premise of cognitive restructuring is that the psychological distress of clients is shaped by negative thoughts. The goal here is to uncover and change those thoughts to enable clients to have different attitudes about themselves, their life world, and the future.
- **Methods of Affect and Emotion Regulation:** These methods draw on relaxation and mindfulness-based methods as well as methods of activity building.
- **Operant Methods:** These methods are guided by the assumption that human behavior is controlled by its consequences. Various methods have been developed here that serve both the development or stabilization of behaviors and the reduction of negative behaviors (cf. Nestmann 2014a, 783).

1.1 **Methods of Cognitive Restructuring**

In cognitive therapy and counseling

> "(...) it is assumed that psychological distress is often caused by distorted cognitive processes, especially dysfunctional automatic thoughts, cognitive styles, and irrational core beliefs. These often unconscious cognitive processes can be uncovered and changed (restructured), which is why cognitive methods (...) represent a very effective approach" (Beck and Borg-Laufs 2018, 207).

Stavemann (2010) notes that the methods of cognitive restructuring are based on various forms of cognitive behavioral therapy (CBT), which emerged in the second half of the 20th century. The roots of CBT are variously anchored in "orthodox" behavior therapy, psychoanalysis and depth psychology, social psychology, philosophy, linguistics, and neuropsychology (cf. Stavemann 2010, 1). The basic idea is that individuals with psychological impairments or severe psychological stress often have distorted (irrational and/or catastrophic) thoughts, which is why even positive or neutral situations or statements are negated or misinterpreted. In the cognitive model, these automated, negative emotions as well as behaviors become the focus of counseling, with the goal of changing these thought patterns (cf. Beck and Borg-Laufs 2018, 208). The solution to psychological problems, which according to Stavemann (2010) is permanent, is achieved through a targeted change in psychopathological behavior. Special exercise and learning programs are used to build up missing insights, skills, or experiences through relearning or new learning. Furthermore, inappropriate learning experiences are modified or erased. Based on this, psychotic symptoms are reduced and mental health is restored (cf. Stavemann 2010, 2). At the beginning of cognitive counseling, it is essential to identify, understand, and especially determine the origin or emergence of these dysfunctional or irrational beliefs. Common thought patterns are "I can't do anything," "I am stupid," "I never do anything right, and that will never change." Such irrational thought beliefs create a distortion of perception and thus affect all performance-relevant areas of life and life situations of the clients (cf. Beck and Borg-Laufs 2018, 208). After the individual cognitions of the clients have been identified, a work plan is created individually for these clients and their individual problems, with which the clients train new behavioral alternatives and thus develop a new behavioral repertoire. The associated new experiences lead to a sense of achievement and the associated increased self-efficacy and growing self-confidence, which in turn is supposed to resolve existing problems (cf. Stavemann 2010, 2 f.). Beck and Borg-Laufs (2018) note that these problems of the clients are based on cognitions. Human cognitions affect emotions as well as behaviors and can thus cause psychological distress. This often arises not from the situation itself, but due to the dysfunctional and irrational thoughts that had developed over the course of the biography (cf. Beck and Borg-Laufs 2018, 209). The following describes the process of cognitive counseling.

- **Process of Cognitive Counseling**

Beck and Borg-Laufs (2018) note that at the beginning of the counseling process, building a good relationship with the client is of relevance. Based on this, offers are slowly made to reconsider their thought patterns and to independently reassess them. This process of restructuring dysfunctional or irrational thoughts is based on 5 partially overlapping phases according to Beck and Borg-Laufs (cf. Beck and Borg-Laufs 2018, 210):

1. "Conveying the cognitive model (thoughts influence feelings and behavior)
2. Identification of dysfunctional/irrational thoughts
3. Questioning (disputation) of unfavorable thoughts
4. Development of alternative thoughts
5. Practice and further development of alternative thoughts" (ibid., 210).

- **The 4 Disputation Techniques**

After the dysfunctional and irrational thoughts have been identified or worked out, the thoughts are subsequently questioned (disputation) (cf. Beck and Borg-Laufs 2018, 210 f.). According to Stavemann (2006), there are 4 disputation techniques:

- Empirical Disputation: The counselors encourage the clients to research facts and statistics.
- Logical Disputation: This technique is also called reattribution. The clients devalue themselves significantly and should learn to view situations with more objectivity. For

example, one can visualize certain perspectives, i.e., create graphics or scales from 1–100.

- Normative Disputation: This technique is used with clients who suffer from particularly rigid cognitions. It attempts to make the clients recognize the subjectivity of individual norms. "Who determines that it has to be this way?" Working out these differences can lead to significant relief for the clients.
- Functional or Hedonistic Disputation: Reasons for this type of disputation include, for example, unmet goals of the clients, based on the premise of preferring short-term satisfaction over long-term contentment. Long-term satisfaction is contrasted with short-term relief, and the consequences are explained in comparison. Jointly working out goals can also be a meaningful strategy (cf. Stavemann 2006, cited in Beck and Borg-Laufs 2018, 214 ff.).
- Summary and Divergence between Persuasion and Cognitive Counseling

At the end of the method presented here, it should be noted that the various methods of cognitive counseling can change cognitive schemas that cause suffering. However, these are not attempts at persuasion. The counselors/therapists first try to understand the dysfunctional cognitions and schemas, particularly based on their biographical experiences, and then enable the clients to develop alternative perspectives using the described conversation techniques. These alternative perspectives aim, in particular, to cause less psychological suffering for the clients (cf. Beck and Borg-Laufs 2018, 219 f.).

1.2 **Schema Therapeutic Interventions in Counseling**

After briefly addressing schemas, schema therapeutic interventions are now explained, and the term schema is defined at the beginning. In the psychological context, schemas refer to patterns that have developed over the course of life based on individual experiences and events. They influence how the individual perceives themselves and the environment. Such patterns are important for the individual to organize, structure, and understand life (cf. Lübeck and Wälte 2018a, 178 f.).

> Schema therapy originated from cognitive behavioral therapy. It includes elements of gestalt therapy as well as object relations theory. Techniques such as keeping schema diaries, body-oriented procedures, imaginative techniques, life-activating role plays, and general cognitive therapy procedures are used (cf. Margraf and Pschyrembel Redaktion 2016, n.p.).

Schema therapy is primarily used for difficult-to-treat personality disorders, chronic depression, childhood trauma, eating disorders, substance abuse, and other indications. To date, there are 4 significant controlled studies on the effectiveness of schema therapy (cf. Margraf and Pschyrembel Editorial 2016, n.p.). For clients with a (subclinical) personality disorder, psychological and psychosocial counseling is rather a cross-sectional method. This means that counseling here is an intervention among others. In difficult counseling situations, however, the Wälte method of schema therapy can promote the action security of counselors/therapists. As a consequence, the counselor/therapist can better support the clients in solving their problems. Schema therapy was developed by Jeffrey E. Young in the 1990s and is thus still a relatively young approach. The approach is based on a schema model with early maladaptive schemas (cf. Lübeck and Wälte 2018a, 178). Jeffrey Young defines early maladaptive schemas as very comprehensive themes and patterns that are considered significantly dysfunctional and affect the individual as well as relationships with other people. These schemas encompass physical sensations as well as cognitions, memories, and emotions. They originate in childhood or adolescence and continue to develop throughout life (cf. Young et al. 2008, 99). It is not uncommon for an individual to have multiple schemas, which can also be active at the same time. This is especially the case with more complex mental disorders such as borderline disorder. Furthermore, it is the case that based on a disorder, certain schemas do not necessarily have to be present, nor does the presence of certain schemas necessarily lead to a personality disorder. Nevertheless, it should be mentioned that there are many similarities between individual personality disorders and individual schemas (cf. Lübeck and Wälte 2018a, 180). It is important to note that schemas serve to make the world predictable and controllable from an individual perspective and to create a sense of security and stability (cf. ibid., 181). In schema therapy, there are 3 different coping styles that are considered (survival-)necessary in difficult situations during childhood and are adequate to endure neglect of needs. If these coping styles are maintained throughout life despite changing life circumstances, they become dysfunctional (cf. Young et al. 2008, 67).

Coping Styles

> "The coping style as a fundamental tendency of schema coping manifests itself in individual coping reactions, which include, among other things, the specific behaviors of a person" (Lübeck and Wälte 2018a, 182).

The coping style can not only diverge individually but also vary in different situations or different schemas or over the course of life in various ways. This results in a multitude of complex possibilities of how an activated schema can appear. For example, an individual with the schema of inadequacy/shame may completely avoid contact with others (schema avoidance = flight) or seek devaluing partners or overly critical friends (schema surrender) or reject others, excessively criticize them, and present themselves as infallible and grandiose (schema overcompensation = fight). If the individual gives in to the schema, thinks, feels, and acts accordingly, and accepts it, they confirm the schema (schema confirmation = freeze) (cf. ibid.).

Of importance in all techniques of schema therapy is a professional relationship design, which is characterized here by empathic confrontation and “limited reparenting” (limited parental care) (cf. Lübeck and Wälte 2018a, 184).

The techniques include, for example:

- Steps of empathic confrontation,
- Schema or mode memos (schema or mode reminder cards),
- Schema diaries,
- Imaginations (cf. Lübeck and Wälte 2018a, 185–189).

1.3 **Methods of Affect and Emotion Regulation**

As already shown in this book, cognitively oriented methods indirectly influence the emotions of the clients. Other methods address the emotions more directly, which can lead to an ability to control impulses. The following are various methods that particularly promote relaxation, mindfulness, and activity building.

- **Relaxation Methods**

Relaxation methods such as meditation, autogenic training (AT), or progressive muscle relaxation (PMR) can be used to support various methods of problem-solving (cf. Beck and Borg-Laufs 2018, 220).

They promote, for example, concentration and attention as well as stress management, but can also be used for psychosomatic disorders, anxiety, sleep problems, and in conjunction with coping strategies regarding aggression or aggressive behavioral abnormalities. However, it is of enormous importance to mention that relaxation methods can also be contraindicated. This can be the case, among other things, with post-traumatic stress disorder (PTSD), acute psychotic states, specific asthmatic conditions (small-airway asthma), acute fever, chronic gastrointestinal diseases, as well as acute cardiovascular diseases. The goal of relaxation methods is a state that is perceived as calm and pleasant; this is accompanied by neurobiological changes and physiological switching reactions of the autonomic nervous system. Clients should learn to induce this state in themselves. Additionally, the measures serve for acute affect regulation or the initiation of imaginations. Besides more complex relaxation methods such as AT and PMR, there are also simple breathing exercises that can be performed (cf. Beck and Borg-Laufs 2018, 220). For children and adolescents, a “lightning relaxation” can be helpful for affect regulation. In this exercise, all muscles in the body are tensed simultaneously and then relaxed. This exercise serves to regulate affect during increasing arousal (cf. ibid., 221).

- **Mindfulness-based methods**

Mindfulness-based methods are increasingly used in counseling as well as in therapy. Based on a spiritual and cultural concept, Kabat-Zinn (2013) introduced these into the therapeutic and medical field in the 1970s with the method of "mindfulness based stress reduction (MBSR)" (cf. Beck and Borg-Laufs 2018, 221). In mindfulness-based methods, the three aspects "intentional," "non-judgmental," and "focused on the present moment" play a significant role. These methods are based on the theory that the body goes about daily activities on "autopilot," meaning that the mind is occupied with something else during this time. For example, while showering, the water on the skin is no longer perceived, but rather thoughts are already on upcoming tasks. The so-called "autopilot mode" (a term coined by Kabat-Zinn) supports an inefficient preoccupation with the past or future and impairs situationally appropriate and conscious responses. To counteract this autopilot mode, intentional action is required. According to Zarbock et al. (2012), this intentional action requires practice and constant repetition, otherwise mindfulness is lost. These perceived sensations are not classified as positive or negative. Naming the perceptions can then be helpful in minimizing escape tendencies such as avoidance, suppression, or the urge to change. Meibert (2013) notes that mindful perception helps to accept the moment as it is and to accept the state. From this acceptance, it is then possible to discover new ways and deal with the situation (cf. Beck and Borg-Laufs 2018, 222 f.).

> A mindful attitude promotes conscious engagement with the contents of the present. This attitude can help to recognize falling into negative cognitions earlier and to feel pleasant situations more consciously. This, in turn, can have a positive effect on self-image, and the attitude towards negative cognitions can change, making it easier to accept these cognitions (cf. Beck and Borg-Laufs 2018, 222 f.).

An accepting attitude towards difficult experiences can, in the long run, according to Meibert (2013), have both stabilizing and healing effects. Through breathing exercises and techniques like body scan, mindfulness-based methods not only work cognitively but are also body-oriented, thereby promoting a mindful approach to one's own body (cf. ibid., 223 f.). In breathing exercises, it is important to guide the clients. The spine should be upright, with lying down or standing being particularly suitable. The breathing should be accompanied by words from the counselors/therapists, making the clients aware that if thoughts arise, they should pass by like clouds in the sky. Thoughts should neither be judged nor held onto. After a few minutes, the end of the exercise should also be consciously initiated and announced, indicating that the exercise is over and the client should return to the here and now (cf. ibid., 224). The body scan exercise can also be performed lying down or standing, and it is important that the client remains awake throughout the entire exercise. If this is difficult due to various circumstances, the person should better keep their eyes open. During the exercise, the focus is on directing attention to specific body parts, such as the toes, feet, legs, or the rising of the abdominal wall while breathing, the contact with the ground, etc. It is observed what can be perceived. If thoughts arise, it is beneficial to redirect attention to the breath and then return to the body region. Here too, at the end of the exercise, it is important to consciously guide back to the here and now. It is of enormous importance to note that before starting such mindfulness-based methods, it should be clarified whether the client is in acute psychotic or suicidal crises, as this method would be contraindicated in such cases. Additionally, Heidenreich and Michalak (2009) note that in cases of trauma, it must first be clarified to what extent body-oriented exercises might overwhelm the clients. Mindfulness-based work places high demands on the counselors, which is why it is important that the counselors performing the exercises also have a willingness to engage in mindfulness-based exercises and practice them regularly, such as yoga, breathing meditation, etc. (cf. Beck and Borg-Laufs 2018, 224).

- **Activity Building**

Many clients are in a counterproductive cycle because their mood is bad, and as a result, they are only minimally active. According to Hautzinger (2012), this is typical for depressive disorders. Due to the low level of activity, they have few mood-enhancing experiences, which makes them even less motivated to engage in activities (cf. Beck and Borg-Laufs 2018, 225).

> Activity building plays a significant role in clinical depression and resource-oriented counseling approaches. Activity building promotes the collection of positive and mood-enhancing experiences (cf. Beck and Borg-Laufs 2018, 225).

To support activity building, a weekly log in which all activities and the emotions experienced during them are recorded with a scale from one to ten is helpful. The activity log can serve both in the area of goal setting, for diagnostics, and as an intervention measure. Here, the counselor/therapist should also be persistent and motivate the client to keep the log. Activities that have provided particular pleasure should be discussed in counseling, and activities that previously brought joy should be recalled and carried out again. To minimize the possibility of overwhelming the clients, it is advisable to build up activities slowly, take time for them, and plan them in detail. Possible problems, difficulties, or fears before carrying out the activities should also be discussed. In the following counseling session, the activities, even those that provided only minimal pleasure, are discussed. Reflecting on mood-enhancing activities increases a positive perspective towards further activities (cf. Beck and Borg-Laufs 2018, 225).

1.4 **Operant Methods**

Operant methods are based on Skinner's (1904–1990) paradigm of operant conditioning, according to Linderkamp (2009). However, there are divergences from classical conditioning (cf. Linderkamp 2009, 210).

> Operant conditioning requires an active behavior of an individual, which triggers environmental reactions that, in turn, affect the individual's behavior, in contrast to classical conditioning, which describes reactive behavioral processes (cf. Linderkamp 2009, 210).

To a large extent, human behavior is shaped by the consequences that this behavior entails. In everyday life, operant conditioning, especially in the field of education, occurs unplanned. In counseling, a conditioning process must be consciously implemented over a fixed period of time and based on a plan. Particularly in working with children and adolescents, operant methods are of enormous importance in supporting behavioral changes. These operant procedures are largely transparent, and children and adolescents have a strong influence on the change processes. Crucial for operant conditioning are reinforcers of both negative and positive behavior, whereby the operant methods diverge depending on the goal of the procedure. The operant procedures depend on whether the goal is to build up a certain behavior, reduce it, or stabilize a certain behavior (cf. Beck and Borg-Laufs 2018, 227). These procedures were empirically proven by learning research at the beginning of the last century, according to Linderkamp. This means that operant conditioning is based on empirically proven studies that are adequate for both disruptive behavior and appropriate behavior (cf. Linderkamp 2009, 210). According to Beck and Borg-Laufs (2018), the following points are indispensable for the successful use of operant methods:

- A reinforcement plan should not record too many behavioral changes (a maximum of 3 behaviors).
- It is also of great relevance that the rewards are of great value to those affected and that the sanctions are displeasing.
- To achieve the effect of the reinforcers, they must only be attainable through the desired behavior.
- Both rewards and sanctions must be applied promptly. Rewards that are set over a longer period require, for example, token allocations (e.g., smileys), which must also be awarded promptly.

- Primarily, it must be discussed in detail with all involved which behavior will be reinforced and which will be sanctioned.
- Reinforcement must not be made dependent on other, unrecorded behavior.
- The starting point must be the previous and temporarily shown behavior to achieve the targeted goals. If these are difficult to achieve, motivation quickly decreases.
- The agreed goals should be documented, and a list should be created. Additionally, it is beneficial to continuously record the respective behavioral developments (cf. Beck and Borg-Laufs 2018, 230 f.).

The following provides an overview of various operant methods for both behavior building and behavior reduction.

1.4.1 Strategies for Behavior Reduction

For behavior reduction, according to Beck and Borg-Laufs (2018), the following strategies are used:

- **Extinction:** This involves the removal of reinforcers that previously reinforced negative behavior. Initially, it is of enormous importance to identify these reinforcers. A so-called extinction must be carried out particularly consistently because if the reinforcers are only achieved in exceptional cases, the behavioral problem can be intermittently reinforced and thus become particularly resistant to extinction.
- **Checking:** This form is sometimes referred to as "graduated extinction." Through screaming and crying, children achieve the attention of their parents. However, parents should not let their children scream but should give them attention at regular intervals, even when the child is not screaming or crying. As a result, the attention occurs independently of the child's problem behavior and thus is not reinforced (cf. Beck and Borg-Laufs 2018, 231 f.).
- **Punishment:** "Punishment is defined as the consistent application of an aversive stimulus after the display of problem behavior" (Beck and Borg-Laufs 2018, 232). It is of great importance to mention that punishment should only be administered when self-harming or other-harming behavior cannot be immediately prevented otherwise.
- **Response Cost (Reinforcer Removal):** Initially, a certain number of reinforcers are given, which are withdrawn in case of misbehavior. This must be explicitly communicated beforehand. In case of misbehavior, an immediate and consistent removal of reinforcers must occur. This method is sometimes more successful than a rewarding procedure (cf. Beck and Borg-Laufs 2018, 232).

1.4.2 Strategies for Behavior Development

Suitable strategies for behavior development are declared according to Beck and Borg-Laufs (2018) as follows:

- **Shaping (Behavior Shaping):** Often, a desired behavior is complex and not easy to achieve. In shaping, the desired overall behavior is divided into partial behaviors. This is used, for example, when the goal is to complete homework independently. Whenever the child has achieved a part of the goal, the next independently achieved step is expected after a few days. If the child achieves this, a reinforcer is used. In this way, the child gradually learns the complex overall behavior desired by them.
- **Chaining (Behavior Chaining):** In chaining, the approach is the opposite of shaping. This method is often used with cognitively impaired individuals. It is expected that the person performs the last link of this behavior chain alone, and they are then rewarded for it. In the next step, the last and second-to-last behavior sequences are expected, and if they manage these alone, they are rewarded, and so on.
- **Token System:** Here, so-called generalized reinforcers are used. These can be, for example, smiley stickers or similar items. After reaching a certain number of these reinforcers, they can be exchanged for a reward. This method has significant advantages (cf. Beck and Borg-Laufs 2018, 233):
  - Since the reinforcers can be changed over time, they do not lose their positive incentive through frequent goal achievement.
  - Tokens can always be given immediately after the desired behavior is performed.
  - Very individual reinforcement plans can be agreed upon.
  - It can be agreed that a different number of tokens can be given as different rewards. For example, one token is a candy, and several tokens are a cinema visit.
  - It is motivating if the tokens are visible to the individuals (cf. Beck and Borg-Laufs 2018, 233 f.).

1.4.3 Motivation for Implementing Operant Methods

It has been shown that in the upbringing of children and adolescents, reinforcers are often used unintentionally, which, however, reinforces misbehavior in many cases.

> In the context of counseling with operant methods, a reinforcement plan is consciously created, and the desired target behavior is clearly defined, so that over an agreed period, the target behavior can be systematically built up or misbehavior can be reduced based on these reinforcers.

It should also be mentioned that these methods may only need to take place within an agreed period, as in most cases, self-motivation occurs (cf. Beck and Borg-Laufs 2018, 234 f.).

1.4.4 Confrontational Techniques

Confrontation primarily means a confrontation between two people, but it can also mean that a person is placed in a certain situation so that they have to deal with a topic that is unpleasant for them, for example, due to feelings of fear, or because they would otherwise not expose themselves to this situation (cf. Sieben and Wälte 2018, 167).

In settings where psychological and psychosocial counseling is offered, this type of confrontation as a technique is not uncommon. In behavioral therapy, the term "stimulus confrontation" is used more specifically for this. This means that patients are frequently and sufficiently long exposed to external or internal stimuli according to established rules with the goal of modifying behavior. These confrontational techniques can be used to reduce avoidance behavior, such as in problems based on fears, or to minimize behavioral excesses, such as shopping addiction. Additionally, confrontational techniques are considered essential parts of therapy for mental disorders such as obsessive-compulsive disorder or post-traumatic stress disorder. In psychological and psychosocial counseling, many clients are affected by avoidance behavior or behavioral excesses. Here, confrontational techniques can be adequately utilized (cf. Sieben and Wälte 2018, 167). Bengel and Margraf (2020) also note that the effectiveness of confrontation therapy in anxiety and obsessive-compulsive disorders, as well as in PTSD and other trauma-related disorders, is considered established (cf. Bengel and Margraf 2020, n.p.). However, Hand notes that exercises aimed at eliminating avoidance behavior, where the reduction of negative cognitive-emotional reactions to specific situations is sought, belong to both the potentially most helpful and the most dangerous psychotherapeutic procedures. Confrontation or exposure to feared or avoided stimulus conditions can occur both in the "symptom area" and in deeper areas, for example, through meditation ("self-confrontation") (cf. Hand 1993, 139). A distinction is made between "flooding," which means that the situation chosen for exposure is the one that clients find hardest to cope with, and graduated confrontation, also called habituation training. Here, clients approach the highest stimulus intensity in small steps. Both methods aim for clients to no longer show avoidance behavior in real situations (in vivo). This means they must remain in the situation until the feeling of fear or the fear reaction significantly decreases. Only under these conditions can habituation or expectation change occur (cf. Sieben and Wälte 2018, 170).

The following section outlines and explains some confrontation techniques. Sieben and Wälte recommend starting all techniques with a SORKC analysis, followed by psychoeducation (cf. ibid., 171).

• Systematic Desensitization

Wolpe (1958) already pointed out systematic desensitization in vivo (cf. Sieben and Wälte 2018, 170). Systematic desensitization can be described as a form of counterconditioning, where clients are confronted with increasingly stronger anxiety-provoking stimuli while in a pleasantly perceived, relaxed state. The theoretical basis for systematic desensitization is classical conditioning (cf. Hedlund 2021, n.p.).

> Systematic desensitization is graduated, and the focus is on preventing the occurrence of anxiety feelings or reactions through relaxation (in children through distraction) (reciprocal inhibition). In graduated confrontation, the anxiety is supposed to occur and be endured (cf. Sieben and Wälte 2018, 170).

This procedure is particularly used to decouple isolated stimuli from anxiety reactions. Through multiple graduated confrontations with the anxiety-provoking stimulus, habituation of the anxiety reaction is intended to occur. The confrontation takes place in sensu (cf. Linden 1993, 307). Initially, relaxation training such as progressive muscle relaxation is conducted with clients, and then an anxiety hierarchy from neutral to maximally anxiety-provoking items is created together with the clients. In the following step, an increasing escalation of stimulus confrontation (in sensu) is coupled with relaxation. Unlike in graduated confrontation, it is important to ensure that clients do not experience anxiety based on the feeling of relaxation. As soon as anxiety occurs, the anxiety imagination is terminated, and the relaxation exercise is continued. Only when clients are completely relaxed again and the anxiety feelings have disappeared is the anxiety-provoking stimulus resumed (cf. Sieben and Wälte 2018, 171). Linden notes that positive treatment outcomes were achieved with systematic desensitization for the following anxieties:

> "Anxieties about heights, open spaces, sharp objects, closed spaces, flying, fire, contact with certain people, driving, dental visits, swallowing anxieties, and also post-traumatic stress reactions" (Linden 1993, 307).

For more complex disorders, such as complex agoraphobias or anxieties associated with depression, fewer treatment successes were observed. However, Linden cautions that in unsuccessful desensitization attempts, the phobic reaction to the anxiety-provoking stimulus may be reinforced (cf. ibid.). Finally, it is important to note that the procedure is rarely used today and that cognitive-behavioral exposure is primarily used for phobias (cf. Hedlund 2021, n.p.).

- **Flooding**

> "Overstimulation, a procedure in intensified stimulus confrontation with anxiety-inducing stimuli" (Psychology Textbook 2023, n.p.).

Flooding is a method of exposure therapy in which patients are exposed to real, highly anxiety-inducing stimuli (cf. Margraf and Pschyrembel Editorial Team 2021, n.p.). It is considered an effective treatment method, particularly in the treatment of panic disorders with and without agoraphobia, as well as specific phobias. This anxiety-inducing approach can be used on several consecutive days and for several hours. This requires a massive effort from the patients. It is worth mentioning positively that patients intensely confront their fears and can thus make significant progress very quickly. However, indispensable alongside good preparation is a good therapeutic relationship. Without a good quality of alliance, these procedures often lead to therapy dropouts, based on the frequently strong anxieties that arise. Above all, it is important that patients are given a sense of security. However, there is also criticism of this confrontation method, which is particularly based on ethical aspects. Many patients also prefer graduated procedures because they are concerned that they might not be able to endure the emerging anxieties. Flooding is considered an effective treatment method, particularly in the treatment of panic disorders with and without agoraphobia, as well as specific phobias (cf. Hauer et al. 2014, 159).

- **Cue Exposure**

> "Cue Exposure Therapy (CET) is a behavioral psychological approach to the treatment of substance use disorders (…)" (Juhl et al. 2017, 195).

Cue Exposure (stimulus exposure) is part of exposure therapy, but here the focus is not on anxiety or obsessive-compulsive disorders or the reduction of escape or avoidance behaviors; instead, it deals with disorders of approach and consumption behaviors, as found in addictive behaviors, for example. A cue can be considered a stimulus here. The classical confrontation therapy served as the basis for the development of this method. Clients are confronted with stimuli and situations that trigger craving, i.e., the urge or desire for addiction or greed. A motivational state is thus triggered, which promotes relapses. Through confrontation with the cues, the craving is supposed to be extinguished over time, thereby reducing the risk of future addictive behavior. Cue Exposure represents a meaningful addition to multimodal treatment programs, according to Lörch (cf. Lörch 2015, 93–96).

After behavioral therapy methods have now been examined, an insight into systemic methods will be presented below.

2. **Methods of Systemic Counseling**

Systemic methods are often associated with couple and family counseling/couple and family therapy. However, since the coaching approach presented in this book is intended for individual settings, the topic of couple and family counseling will not be explored in depth. Systemic foundations as well as basic attitudes will be explained, systemic hypothesis formation will be examined, and standard methods of systemic counseling will be presented.

In the systemic approach, techniques have been developed that primarily respect the individual reality constructions of the clients. They are based on neutrality and impartiality, and the hypotheses serve to expand the scope of action. The foundation of the systemic approach is the creation of favorable initial conditions by the counselors/therapists. This is done according to concepts such as "joining," "clarification of the assignment," and "reframing." Systemic questions can be used to uncover relationship patterns in the client system. Techniques such as the genogram, timelines, family board, and family sculpture are used for this purpose. To provide feedback to clients on a meta-level, the "reflecting team" can be used as a method. To resolve problematic communication and interaction patterns in the client system, concluding comments are helpful (cf. Borg-Laufs and Wälte 2018c, 205 f.).

> "Systemic counseling emphasizes the social context of problems, as they are related to social connections and influence each other ("circularity")" (Meyer et al. 2018, 235).

This means that not only the individual clients (index clients or index patients) are part of the counseling, but also people who are relevant to the clients in the social system. This often refers to the clients' families, which is why systemic therapy often takes place in a family setting (cf. Meyer et al. 2018, 235).

> The methods of systemic counseling are based on the disruption (influence) of communication and interaction patterns in the system to activate changes (cf. ibid.).

Systemic Foundations

The systemic way of thinking and acting is inspired by the system-theoretical-constructivist theory. Meyer et al. (2018) describe this, among other things, as follows:

1. "Reality is a subjective construct of our perception and is created and defined through social interaction, as knowledge is constructed based on experience and is context-sensitive. (…)

2. Systems are constructed through observation, whereby observation is the application of a distinction.
3. Each system is a necessary environment for the other systems. Additionally, each system is a subsystem of a larger system and, in turn, integrates several subsystems within itself.
4. Social systems arise and sustain themselves through communication. (…) Perception and communication with the environment do not occur directly but selectively and refer to one's own internal image (construct) of the world. Autopoietic systems repeatedly attempt to handle their way of thinking and living in their own, same manner (functional structural determinacy and operational closure). (…) Thus, an influence or change of psychological and social systems can only be achieved from the outside through structural coupling, e.g., through the process of perturbation" (Meyer et al. 2018, 236).

Systemic Attitudes

Systemic action is guided by various rules.

- **Understanding Circularity:** It is relevant to think in a networked manner and to recognize complex patterns and implement them in the counseling process.
- **Context and Relationship Orientation:** It requires an understanding from the counselors/therapists of various life contexts, life models, and family forms, as well as the often-discrepant influencing factors (cf. Meyer et al. 2018, 237 f.) and an "(…) understanding of the meaning of the problem in the given relationship and life context. This attitude is based on a critical distance from ideological as well as politically and fundamentally religiously motivated societal models" (ibid., 238).
- **Multiperspectivity:** This requires the implementation of various perspectives, beliefs, and realities of all system members (including those of the counselors/therapists). This means understanding, bringing to discussion, and accepting them.
- **Respect for the Autonomy and Self-Organization of the Client System:** This demands, among other things, recognizing the problem from the autopoiesis of the entire system.
- **Client Orientation:** The counselors/therapists orient themselves exclusively to the goals and life concepts of the clients, regardless of their own life concepts or desired counseling outcomes.
- **Expansion of Possibilities and Scope for Action:** This is based on the activation of various resources, solution orientation, and perspective change.
- **Resource Orientation:** This means seeking and activating available resources that contribute to coping strategies and problem-solving.
- **Solution Orientation:** This approach does not focus on the problems in detail but on the solutions and goals of the clients.
- **Neutrality and Impartiality:** Since systemic counseling is directed at multiple persons within the system, a certain neutrality is required. This means that the

counselor/therapist is empathetic and attentive to all system members, does not represent a one-sided concern, and maintains the objective perspective from the outside (cf. Meyer et al. 2018, 238).

- **Hypothesizing:** As a fundamental procedural rule, the so-called hypothesizing applies, which will be explained in more detail in the following section (cf. ibid., 239).

Systemic Hypothesis Formation

The generation of systemic hypotheses is a specific basic attitude and procedure in systemic practice (cf. Meyer et al. 2018, 239).

> "It takes the form of assumptions and explanations about the emergence, mutual effects, and function of problematic structures, relationship patterns, and beliefs that can be observed in the client system as well as in interaction with other involved systems" (ibid.).

This means that not only the individual or the individual clients or the environment are captured separately, but all perceptible circular interactions, patterns, and processes within and between the system levels (individual, subsystem, (family) system, and environmental system). Additionally, it is important to mention that systemic hypothesis formation is not primarily to be seen as a diagnostic survey instrument (cf. Meyer et al. 2018, 239).

Goals of Systemic Counseling

The focus of systemic counseling is to disrupt and deconstruct the disturbance within the system and the intertwined behavior and relationship patterns as well as beliefs (constructs), if possible, together with the system. Within the system, more positive solutions, patterns, and constructs should be discussed (cf. Meyer et al. 2018, 246).

Standard Methods of Systemic Counseling

Structural and strategic methods (joining, clarification of assignments, hypothesis formation, and reframing), symbolic-metaphorical methods (genogram, timeline, family board, and family sculpture), systemic questions (circular questions, solution-oriented questions, differentiation questions, problem-oriented questions, questions about reality and possibility constructions, and hypothetical questions), narrative methods, as well as the reflecting team, are frequently used in systemic counseling (cf. Meyer et al. 2018, 246). The extent to which narrative methods play a role in systemic counseling is explained below.

3. **Narrative Methods**

When people repeatedly tell negative biographical experiences, relationships, or behaviors from a negative perspective, this can become cognitively entrenched and have negative effects on everyday life. In the narrative counseling approach, these narratives are questioned, allowing for new constructions of life narratives (cf. Meyer et al. 2018, 252 f.). According to Epston and White (2013), the following is important for the narrative approach in family therapy: The focus is on the client with their lived experiences.

> "A therapy that relies on the narrative mode of thinking should take a form that (...) promotes the perception of a changing world by linking lived experiences in the dimension of time" (Epston and White 2013, 88 f.).

Furthermore, the following is of relevance:

- Various perspectives are created and implicit meanings generated with the help of the subjunctive.
- The use of polysemiotics, an everyday as well as figurative language, to support the embedding of new stories.
- Challenging a reflective attitude.
- Conveying to the client a sense that they are the author of their own life by rewriting and telling the story.
- Stories are each co-productions, and conditions must be created for the client to become the privileged author.
- Always using the pronouns "I" and "you" when describing events (cf. Epston and White 2013, 89).
- Final Intervention

At the end of the counseling, a final comment can be used to make another intervention. This final intervention usually takes place after the last break. It is relevant that it begins with something positive, such as praise or expressed recognition. This can be both verbal and written. This method summarizes what has been discussed, worked on, the hypotheses, and other impressions. Here, final impulses and motivation for restructuring can be given (cf. Meyer et al. 2018, 254).

In summary, it should be noted that the field of systemic couple and family counseling is a very large area with different and well-developed methods and techniques. Method pluralism is also appreciated in this counseling/therapeutic area, and well-known methods and training are applied. In addition to narrative methods, these include role-playing, for example. Therefore, the following two sections will explain role-playing and then various training methods.

4. **Role-Playing**

> Role-playing is used as a method in many therapeutic schools. In this process, a problem is not merely addressed but is also implemented into the counseling through role-playing (cf. Borg-Laufs 2018b, 162).

Role-playing was referred to as psychodrama by Moreno (1959) and was first used as a therapeutic method. Today, it is employed in a variety of schools or orientations, such as psychodynamic, systemic, gestalt therapy, transactional analysis, and behavioral therapy orientations. Role-playing is also used in various training programs, such as training to promote social skills (cf. Borg-Laufs 2018b, 162). Schaller also notes that role-playing is a significant technique in both behavioral therapy orientations and psychodrama. However, he mentions differences here, as almost exclusively structured role-plays are used in the behavioral-oriented field. These are referred to as "top-down processing," whereas, for example, spontaneous role-plays are more frequently used in psychodrama, which are referred to as "bottom-up role-plays" (cf. Schaller 2014, 211). The goal of using role-playing within psychosocial counseling or various therapies is, on the one hand, to practice and learn new behaviors and, on the other hand, to update existing behaviors that are not being used for various reasons. Role-playing can also be used for diagnostics, for example, to reenact problem situations to make them more understandable. When clients switch roles, that is, take on the role of their interaction partners, role-playing is also a good technique to promote perspective-taking and empathy (cf. Borg-Laufs 2018b, 163). Wagner also notes that both treatment techniques, the role-playing method and role-switching, are significant. The range of indications for both treatment techniques is broad. The goals are, on the one hand, to expand the range of perception and, on the other hand, to acquire new behavior patterns (cf. Wagner 2003, 69). Borg-Laufs explains that the focus of role-playing is on social problems of all kinds. Aggressive behavior disorders or behavioral problems involving social insecurity can be addressed in role-playing. Social problems are of particular importance in various counseling contexts, such as parenting counseling or addiction counseling, and in many other counseling contexts. The goal of the clients is always to be able to show appropriate behaviors in social situations, that is, to behave appropriately (cf. Borg-Laufs 2018b, 163).

> Role-playing promotes the ability of people to empathize with others, which represents a significant resource (cf. Wagner 2003, 69).

The goal, according to Wagner, is for clients to be able to approach themselves and the world more openly and tolerantly (cf. Wagner 2003, 69).

Now that role-playing has been presented as a method used in various orientations and counseling approaches, the following will highlight some training programs that are also used in different counseling approaches and orientations.

5. **Training Programs**

Structured training programs can be used for various conflict and problem areas, which are specifically tailored to the individual topics as well as the target groups. Parent training, communication training, self-confidence training, social skills training, and stress management training are particularly in demand. The training programs are focused on specific topics such as (cf. Borg-Laufs and Wälte 2018c, 206) “stress, relaxation, communication, emotions, concentration, self-confidence, problem-solving, health” (ibid., 255).

Furthermore, the training programs are tailored to various target groups, selected age groups, and also areas of psychological disorders (cf. Borg-Laufs and Wälte 2018c, 255).

In psychological and psychosocial counseling, training programs for problem-solving are primarily used. The techniques applied in the training programs often originate from behavioral therapy (cf. Borg-Laufs and Wälte 2018c, 255).

The maxim of the training programs is that not only insight leads to success, but especially practice is the foundation of problem-solving. Clients learn to better cope with their problems, and new ways open up (cf. Borg-Laufs and Wälte 2018c, 255).

> “Problem updates often go hand in hand with exposure, where clients are encouraged to give up their avoidance behavior. Habituation, extinction, and expectation changes in problems can occur as a result” (Borg-Laufs and Wälte 2018c, 255).

Through role-playing, clients learn to apply the various techniques in everyday life (cf. ibid.). Furthermore, it is important to note that the process of the training programs can be divided into at least three phases: “diagnostics, psychoeducation, and exercises” (Borg-Laufs and Wälte 2018c, 255).

The following will briefly explain some relevant training models.

- **Parent Training Programs**

The availability of various programs for parent training is steadily increasing. The occasion for parent training can involve both acute crises and chronic conflicts within the family. The goal is to strengthen the parents in their parenting skills (cf. Borg-Laufs and Wälte 2018c, 206). In recent years, the availability of programs to strengthen parenting skills has increased enormously. They were targeted at various groups, parents with children or adolescents, with or without specific problems (cf. ibid., 255).

By strengthening the parenting skills of the parents, the psychological condition of the children and adolescents should also improve (cf. Borg-Laufs and Wälte 2018c, 255).

Empirically proven programs include: Triple P., THOP, KES, The Incredible Years, Helping the Noncompliant Child, STEP, Gordon Parent Training, and Strong Parents—Strong Children (cf. Hahlweg und Heinrichs 2009, cited in Borg-Laufs and Wälte 2018c, 255). It is important to mention that programs for parent training are extremely valuable for psychosocial and psychotherapeutic practice. They can be held in various settings and do not always have to be completed in full. Often, an adaptive approach is necessary to adjust to both the individual clients and the given settings (cf. Borg-Laufs and Wälte 2018c, 262).

- **Progressive Muscle Relaxation (PMR)**

The following section will explain the PMR method, a very well-known relaxation method.

> The concept of this training is based on psychophysiological findings (cf. Borg-Laufs and Wälte 2018c, 262) which state that

> "(…) people with problems often suffer from a permanent sympathetic arousal, which is accompanied by a constant muscular tension aimed at maintaining posture and performance" (ibid.).

The goals of PMR are:

- a minimization of physical as well as psychological arousal readiness,
- recognizing tension and learning to relax oneself in a goal-oriented manner,
- an improvement in problem-solving during relaxation.

The procedure is as follows:

- Maximum physical tension for a few seconds followed by relaxation of the limbs and trunk muscles; starting with the arms, then legs, respiratory and abdominal muscles, and facial muscles.
- Subsequently, an active withdrawal is required (cf. Borg-Laufs and Wälte 2018c, 262).
- **Communication Training**

> These are specifically designed to teach special speaking and listening skills in cases of couple and family problems, in order to promote constructive communication between the interactants (cf. Borg-Laufs and Wälte 2018c, 206).

Particularly conflict-laden parent-child relationships are often based on parental problems. In these cases, the focus of counseling should primarily be on the parental conflicts and only secondarily on the disturbed parent-child relationship. These problem constellations are almost always due to communication problems or are accompanied by them. Therefore, communication training is of particular relevance in these cases (cf. Borg-Laufs and Wälte 2018c, 263).

- **Self-assertiveness Training and Social Skills Training**

These are applied by counselors when clients suffer from a lack of social skills as well as low self-esteem and self-confidence (cf. Borg-Laufs and Wälte 2018c, 206).

> Psychosocial problem constellations often go hand in hand with reduced self-esteem, self-confidence, and self-assurance and are often accompanied by socially incompetent behavior, which is why self-assertiveness training is often used in psychological and psychosocial counseling (cf. Borg-Laufs and Wälte 2018c, 264).

The clients do not always have to suffer from subclinical or mild cases of social insecurity. These trainings can also be conducted with individuals who do not have problems but wish to improve their social competence in various situations. The focus of assertiveness training is on behavior change in complex social situations. Salter (1949) is considered the founder of assertiveness training. His "expressive training" focused on communicating emotions and needs. This lack of communication competence was often learned. It was not until 1958 that Wolpe took up this concept and developed "assertiveness training" based on the concept of assertiveness. For him, the foundation of insecurity was social anxiety (cf. Borg-Laufs and Wälte 2018c, 264). Based on this view, various programs have developed, focusing on anxiety in the training. Programs such as ATP (Assertiveness Training Program) and GSK (Group Training of Social Skills) were originally designed for adults. However, for children and adolescents, there are similar programs based on developmental psychological findings. Most of these programs target group settings, which have advantages but also disadvantages. However, individual parts of these programs can still be used for counseling work in individual settings. In a group setting, participants see that they are not the only ones with such problems, which can protect against self-stigmatization. In an individual setting, however, the program can be more individually adapted to the respective client and is particularly helpful when these clients feel overwhelmed in a group setting (cf. Borg-Laufs and Wälte 2018c, 263–267).

According to Durlak et al. (2010), the success of training to optimize social competence is highest, especially in children and adolescents, when they meet the "SAFE" criteria:

- "Sequenced (building on each other),
- Active (role-playing, active practice, behavior orientation),
- Focused (not everything at once),
- Explicit (transparent goals)" (Durlak et al. 2010, 294; Borg-Laufs and Wälte 2018c, 267).

- **Stress management training**

Since stress is a significant topic in the field of psychoneuroendocrinology and thus of enormous importance for the PNES coaching outlined in Chap. 4, I will take a closer look at Kaluza's stress management training.

In stress management training, individual stress management strategies are learned to stabilize clients in everyday life and also to prevent burnout and other stress-related illnesses (cf. Borg-Laufs and Wälte 2018c, 206).

The concept of stress has become increasingly popular over the last 40 years. There is hardly any area in everyday life that is not associated with stress (cf. Kaluza 2011, 12).

> "The term stress here marks an interdisciplinary field of research that, in the broadest sense, deals with the significance of socio-emotional stress experiences for physical and mental health" (ibid.).

There are various stress management strategies, but a distinction can be made between individual coping strategies, i.e., what the affected person can do themselves, and structural or situational stress management, i.e., what the respective organization or employer can do (cf. ibid., 50). To get an idea of what stress training as an intervention can look like, I would like to briefly introduce the program "Calm and Confident in Stress" by Kaluza (2011). According to Kaluza, this method is an individual-oriented intervention aimed at promoting the physical health and mental well-being of participants. The goal is to reduce the frequency and intensity of everyday stressors, based on optimizing individual coping skills. Existing skills should be strengthened, and new skills developed (cf. Kaluza 2011, 60). "Instrumental, mental, and palliative-regenerative strategies of stress management are to be conveyed" (Kaluza 2011, 60). The content involves

> "(…) reducing cognitions of helplessness and hopelessness, unrealistic assessments of situational demands or threat evaluations, as well as developing self-efficacy beliefs, relativizing or meaningful cognitions" (ibid.).

The elaborate manual "Calm and Confident Under Stress" includes an introductory module, 4 training modules, and 5 supplementary modules, which are briefly explained below:

- **Introductory Module:** The introductory module focuses on psychoeducation about stress: "Stress—what is it actually?" is the primary topic of this module. Additionally, clients are to learn to recognize their resources through a group activity on the topic "My Competencies for Stress Management" (cf. Kaluza 2011, 178).
- **Training Module 1:** Relax and Let Go—Relaxation Training: Every person has the ability to relax, and this ability can be optimized through training. This is relevant because the ability to cognitively switch off as well as physically relax is a significant component of regenerative stress competence. First, participants learn to become aware of tension sensations. They learn to experience the transition from tension to relaxation (see PMR according to Jacobsen) and then the so-called "switching," as it is called in autogenic training, as intensely as possible. The next goal is to consciously enjoy the relaxation and maintain it over a certain period. The ultimate goal of this training module is to use and regulate the trained relaxation ability in everyday life. Clients should be able to implement the positive feeling of relaxation into their daily lives whenever and wherever they want. The result of this relaxation ability is a relief of functional symptoms. This increasingly leads to psychological ease, calmness, and serenity, as well as a feeling of recovery and mental freshness (cf. ibid., 80). Additionally, it can "contribute to a higher degree of self-confidence and a reduction in anxiety and depression" (Kaluza 2011, 80). This competence can also be used in acute stress situations as a kind of self-control technique. The feeling of control gives a sense of reduced vulnerability, which in turn can lead to increased resilience. Thus, regular relaxation training serves not only for recovery and stress compensation (cf. ibid.) but also "as a short-term coping strategy in acute stress situations" (Kaluza 2011, 80).
- **Training Module 2:** Developing Beneficial Ways of Thinking and Attitudes—Mental Training: The goals of this module are the "reflection of stress-intensifying evaluation patterns and attitudes and their transformation into stress-reducing, beneficial mental processes and content" (Kaluza 2011, 104). Here, participants learn to apply methods of mental stress management. It is about stress-reducing ways of thinking through cognitive restructuring. Cognitions should be directed towards positive aspects, opportunities, and positive consequences (cf. ibid.). Additionally, clients should "develop a self-distancing and relativizing mental approach to everyday stress situations" (Kaluza 2011, 104).
- **Training Module 3:** Perceiving, Accepting, and Changing Stressful Situations—Problem-Solving Training: Here, participants are confronted with specific stressors. Coping strategies for the individual stressors of the participants are to be developed and implemented. They should learn the competence to cope with stressors, thus strengthening problem-solving ability and adopting a problem-solving mindset. Emotional distancing from stressors should be achieved, and feelings of helplessness and hopelessness should be revised. Participants should move from the role of victims to the role of actors. The foundation for this is that clients loosen self-imposed

boundaries and entrenched viewpoints as well as blockages and keep the search space open in which coping ideas are developed (cf. Kaluza 2011, 120).

- **Training Module 4:** Recover and Enjoy—Enjoyment Training: This is about "compensating for existing stressors and strengthening regenerative stress competence" (Kaluza 2011, 140). The balance between stress and recovery, i.e., the balance between work and leisure, must be maintained. Often, the awareness for this is lacking. Peak performance is based on systematically planned recovery times. An intact social network is particularly noteworthy here. Social interactions offer both practical and emotional support, especially in coping with stressors (cf. ibid.).
- **Supplementary Modules:** The manuals are accompanied by various supplementary modules:
  - "Supplementary Module 1: Stress Management through Sports and More Physical Activity in Everyday Life
  - Supplementary Module 2: Social Support
  - Supplementary Module 3: Clarifying and Defining Goals
  - Supplementary Module 4: No Time?—Meaningful Time Management in Everyday Life
  - Supplementary Module 5: Quart-A Strategy for Emergencies: Accepting the Situation, Cooling Down, Analyzing, Distraction or Action" (Kaluza 2015, cited in Borg-Laufs and Wälte 2018c, 269).

In summary, it should be noted here that stress management training is intertwined or supplemented with various procedures and methods, for example, through psychophysiological relaxation techniques such as progressive muscle relaxation according to Jacobson. In addition, methods of cognitive restructuring, self-management techniques, as well as training elements for self-confidence and social competence, and methods for emotion regulation are used to adequately cope with stressful situations (cf. Borg-Laufs and Wälte 2018c, 269).

- **Conclusion: Training in psychological and psychosocial counseling**

All the presented training programs are classically applied both in psychosocial counseling and psychotherapy. However, it should be noted that in both fields of action, rarely only one of these training programs is used (cf. Borg-Laufs and Wälte 2018c, 270). To adapt to the individual problems and needs of the clients, it is beneficial if the counselor/therapist applies components from various programs. This is particularly true for problem-solving training or relaxation training (cf. ibid., 206). For example, communication training can be a significant component of parent counseling; however, it cannot be reduced to that, as other methods of family counseling are also applied (cf. Borg-Laufs and Wälte 2018c, 271).

After various methods and training programs have been presented, the conclusion of the counseling process is still a significant phase. Therefore, the following will address a professional conclusion of counseling and the importance of evaluation within the framework of quality assurance.

6 **Conclusion and effectiveness of the methods and training programs**
In the previous explanations, various forms of interventions, methods, and training were described. Even if the effectiveness of some methods or counseling approaches has been scientifically disputed from a neuroscientific perspective, I would still like to emphasize in this conclusion that this does not mean that these approaches and methods do not work at all, because the effectiveness of a professional trust relationship between counselors and clients is scientifically substantiated. Roth and Strüber (2021) state that large-scale meta-studies have clearly shown that the most significant factor in successful counseling or therapy is a positive relationship between clients and counselors or patients and therapists, which means a professional relationship based on trust, a collaboration in which the practitioner has the competence to grasp, communicate, and understand the emotions and mental states as well as the general well-being of the clients, as well as a relationship in which the clients trust the practitioner and their approach. Thus, it can be assumed that the quality of the professional relationship is probably the most effective factor in psychosocial counseling or psychotherapy, although it must be considered that some clients are unable to form such an alliance due to deep-seated disorders (cf. Roth and Strüber 2021, 390 f.). Regarding effectiveness research, I would also like to refer to the latest findings of Roth and Strüber (2021), as these are based on neurobiological insights and are of enormous relevance for the coaching concept that follows in Chap. 4. Thus, I would like to present his findings on the effectiveness of methods, training, or various schools as a conclusion:

1) Effectiveness is definitely present in all treatment methods, albeit less effective than sometimes stated. In psychotherapies, regardless of which treatment method is applied and which disorders are present, about one-third of the interventions show good to very good effects as well as long-term effects. Another third of the clients show minor and short-term effects, and the last third shows no effectiveness. However, the same picture emerges under pharmacotherapy. This is referred to as the "one-third rule." At this point, I would like to point out that no distinction was made here between "healing" or, for example, "coping with everyday life," as in my view, the healing of a mental illness presents a different challenge than psychosocial support for coping with everyday life for mentally healthy clients (cf. Roth and Strüber 2021, 392).
2) Contrary to what is often claimed, there is no orientation or approach that is fundamentally superior to other directions in terms of success rate, as each approach seems to have a different effect individually on certain clients and certain disorders as well as on certain counselors or therapists (cf. ibid.).

3) Regarding psychotherapeutic interventions, effectiveness is determined by 30–70% by factors that cannot be clearly identified, which are therefore nonspecific factors (cf. Roth and Strüber 2021, 392). These consist of
   a) the clients' belief in the art of the counselors/therapists,
   b) the counselors'/therapists' belief in their ability to help the clients, and
   c) the belief of both in a particular form of intervention (cf. ibid.).

Roth summarizes these factors as "(…) factors for therapeutic alliance" (Roth and Strüber 2021, 392).

This does not mean that the effectiveness of certain interventions is generally excluded, but it cannot be proven whether the effectiveness is due to the therapeutic alliance or the effectiveness of certain interventions. It also cannot be ruled out that the effectiveness is solely based on the alliance (cf. ibid.). However, the effectiveness of the alliance or the relationship, as well as the effect of, for example, certain stress training, can be explained psychoneuroendocrinologically.

At the end of this chapter, the conclusion of the counseling and its connection with quality assurance will be addressed.

3.1.3.4 Conclusion of Counseling: Evaluation and Quality Assurance

At the end of the psychological and psychosocial counseling process lies the conclusion of the counseling. The following outlines the tasks associated with the conclusion of counseling, what is meant by evaluation, and how it becomes possible to contribute to the quality assurance of psychological and psychosocial counseling. To begin with, I would like to point out that this discussion will focus solely on evaluation as an optimization of the counseling services, meaning evaluation that is relevant to both counselors and clients in practice, and not specifically on evaluation research, which, for example, in the USA is a distinct discipline with its own chairs, journals, textbooks, developed professional standards, and its own professional association (cf. Heiner 2014, 825). The practice-relevant methods of evaluation presented here serve particularly to ensure the quality of the counseling services (cf. Vogel 2014 and Heiner 2014, 835). This can range from the communicative evaluation of the counseling session through systematically documented follow-up questions, the assessment of clients' developmental progress, the analysis of appropriateness, to the acceptance and effectiveness of the counseling (cf. Heiner 2014, 835). However, since the practice-relevant methods of interest for this biopsychosocial coaching approach are particularly the satisfaction of clients and the prevention of relapses, a more detailed description of evaluation research is omitted, and the conclusion of counseling as a phase of the counseling process is examined more closely, addressing the handling of emotions and possible relapses.

According to Meyer and Wälte (2018), every psychosocial counseling process is individually different and unique and depends on various factors and conditions: factors such as the psychosocial conditions of the clients, the setting in which the counseling takes place (individual/group or other settings), institutional conditions, and the nature of the clients' problems. The conclusion of counseling does not merely refer to the last appointment; rather, it is advantageous if the conclusion of counseling is a phase of the counseling process and clients are informed about it at the first appointment. It is recommended to conduct a feedback session during the concluding phase, at the latest in the final session. This involves the clients' satisfaction, where the entire counseling process should be reflected upon. It is of enormous importance to make clients aware that criticism is explicitly desired and that it has no impact on the relationship between counselor/therapist and clients. Clients with social insecurity, in particular, should be encouraged to provide honest feedback. Additionally, it is discussed which goals were achieved, which steps were necessary for this, what worked well, and what could have worked better. There should also be room to discuss failures, as the goal after counseling is for clients to independently manage life and everyday challenges and problems with the techniques and self-management learned in counseling, for which it is essential to know what helped and what did not. Clients should also receive feedback from the counselor/therapist, focusing particularly on the clients' resources and progress. Another task of the conclusion of counseling, which can also be understood as evaluation, is the writing of a report documenting the entire counseling process (cf. Meyer and Wälte 2018, 281 ff.). This report records information about the initial situation or counseling assignment, the symptoms present, the goals set, and the steps taken in the timeline (cf. ibid., 283).

> It should be noted here that, in general, the term evaluation refers to "(…) the systematic, data-based, and criteria-related assessment of programs, projects, and individual offerings (…)" (Heiner 2014, 825).

In the evaluation of counseling, a distinction can be made between the

- evaluation as proof of performance and utilization and
- evaluation as concept clarification and process reflection (cf. Heiner 2014, 832).

For the practice-relevant evaluation of counseling, not only the satisfaction of the clients is important, but also the evaluation of the results. The evaluation of the counseling process contributes to professional action, and a clarification of the concept serves to specify the assignment and the goals. It forms the foundation for the operationalization of goal-related evaluation criteria (cf. ibid., 832 f.). McLeod (2004) notes that, based on the evaluation surveys, possible recommendations for action can also be given to the clients, such as the initiation of psychotherapy (cf. Meyer and Wälte 2018, 283). It is also important to offer the possibility of contacting the counselor/therapist again in case of recurring problems (if the conditions allow it). Even if there is initially no need for this at the end of the counseling, it is reassuring for the clients to know that they are allowed to come back. Accompaniment over several years, even if the clients need only a few sessions within a year, can certainly occur. Likewise, to ensure that the counseling has a long-term benefit, it is relevant in the final phase to jointly review with the clients whether additional interventions are needed to stabilize success and cope with everyday life, in addition to the techniques and methods used so far. An important point in the phase of concluding counseling is relapse prevention. It is important to note that the conclusion of counseling is not merely about saying goodbye to the clients, but also about ensuring that they leave the counseling with the greatest possible benefit for themselves and their future (cf. ibid., 283 f.). McLeod (2004) mentions how important it is to anticipate and openly discuss future problematic situations to minimize the likelihood of relapse. Preventively, to reduce relapses and failures, the counselor/therapist should explain to the clients that old problems can resurface after the end of counseling, which is why it is important to discuss which acquired strategies can help to get out of a possible low. The clients should be discharged with the knowledge that while problems in the future cannot be prevented, dealing with these problems will be easier through the techniques acquired in counseling (cf. Meyer and Wälte 2018, 284). Additionally, as a relapse prevention measure, it is helpful if theoretical problem situations are not only discussed but also practiced, allowing the clients to try out their learned knowledge. A list of thoughts and actions can also be helpful to have anchor points and a structured approach. Furthermore, it is important to discuss the likelihood of problems occurring. This way, the clients can look to the future with confidence, understanding that difficulties will not constantly arise and that they will be able to manage without a counselor/therapist in the future. Often, strong feelings of separation arise at the end of the counseling process, which can be caused by habit and fears about the future, or because the counseling was a significant constant for the clients. These feelings can be very painful, and it is important that the counselor/therapist takes them seriously and does not downplay them. These feelings of separation can occur not only in clients but also in counselors/therapists. If this is the case, the counselor/therapist should not be ashamed, but it is important to work through these feelings in supervision. It is important to examine what feelings the client triggers and why this is the case. Addressing these emotions is a relevant part of professional reflection. An alarm signal should be particularly noted if a counselor/therapist not only has these feelings but also accepts offers of friendship, which is considered extremely unprofessional (cf. ibid., 286 f.).

In summary, to prevent problems at the conclusion of counseling, it is best if the termination of counseling is initiated gradually. Recommended measures and techniques for this are:

- At the beginning of the counseling, clients receive an overview of the process as well as the number, duration, and frequency of appointments, making the end of the counseling foreseeable for the clients.
- The session frequency is thinned out in the final phase of counseling, for example, from once a week to once a month.

- In the last third of the counseling, there is an open discussion about what the clients associate with the conclusion of the counseling.
- Addressing any emotions that may arise at the end of the counseling can facilitate the actual farewell or enable better handling of the emotions.
- If clients have few social contacts, it is particularly relevant that the counselor/therapist supports the clients in expanding their social resources.
- A regular breakdown of the agreed counseling goals can help to see how far the counseling has already approached the goals or that they have already been achieved.
- As already mentioned, clients can be offered the opportunity to return if the conditions allow it. However, it is important to ensure that the offered follow-up appointments are not misinterpreted as counseling with an open end (cf. Meyer and Wälte 2018, 284 f.).

Finally, it should be mentioned that all the aforementioned methods and techniques, the evaluation, documentation, and, if necessary, the supervision with professional colleagues contribute to the quality assurance of psychological and psychosocial counseling. Quality assurance and internal quality management here mean a systematic reflection of the counseling process, the prerequisites and goals, as well as the changes in individual cases by the counselor/therapist. Based on this, conclusions can be drawn for further counseling planning and implementation. It should also be mentioned that the transparency and goal orientation gained through quality assurance often lead to highly relevant developmental impulses for further counseling processes (cf. Vogel 2014, 845).

3.2 Summary

In this chapter, the psychological and psychosocial counseling process and various related topics were described and discussed. The importance of psychosocial diagnostics was explained, and, particularly relevant for PNES coaching, the biopsychosocial diagnostics were highlighted. The significance of interdisciplinarity was already discussed in psychosocial diagnostics, which is recommended not only for psychological or social fields of action but also in the medical field. In the further explanation of the various counseling approaches and school-specific therapeutic orientations, it becomes clear that there are overlaps and boundaries are sometimes to be considered transparent. The increasing importance of methodological pluralism and the associated eclecticism as well as the openness to interdisciplinarity were explained. Furthermore, in this chapter, not only the positive aspects of the various counseling approaches and therapy schools were presented, but also critical considerations were discussed. Neuroscientific critiques were particularly mentioned, which, however, are also subject to criticism or have opponents. It feels like this is a veritable debate, comparable to the "battle" between natural sciences and humanities. The only consensus that can be mentioned here, which can be found in all counseling approaches, orientations, psychotherapy schools, as well as current neuroscientific findings, is the enormous importance of the relationship or alliance between the counselor/therapist and the client. A professional relationship is considered the foundation for both successful psychological and psychosocial counseling and successful psychotherapy. The question of which methods should be applied and whether only one method or various methods should be applied, however, leads to the next dilemma. Methodological pluralism and eclecticism are the keywords here. Although the term "eclectic" was also used negatively because it did not stand for a unified orientation, more and more counselors/therapists are turning to an eclectic-integrative counseling approach. This means that the methods and orientations are individually tailored or selected for the clients and their problems. Neuroscientific findings also lead to the methods being individually adapted. However, methodological pluralism also results in an additional requirement for counselors/therapists, as this means being specialized in more than one counseling approach/therapy school or more than one method. This brings certain quality requirements. Regarding the quality assurance of psychological and psychosocial counseling, this chapter also described the conclusion of counseling as well as the evaluation of the counseling process, which in my view is a very significant component, regardless of the chosen counseling approaches or methods. For me, I conclude that there are many, also neuroscientifically empirically researched counseling approaches or orientations, which should be individually adapted to the clients. Based on the knowledge presented here, I consider it particularly promising to transfer an eclectic-integrative coaching concept, which is based on interdisciplinary scientific findings, into psychological, psychosocial, and psychotherapeutic practice. Furthermore, in my view, based on the literature presented here, it is to be seen as a quality enhancement if modern psychological and psychosocial counseling and psychotherapy align with current interdisciplinary scientific findings and implement these findings in their activities.

In Chap. 4, the biopsychosocial coaching approach "PNES Coaching" will now be presented, with the main pillars of this concept to be illuminated.

References

Abbruzzese, Elvira/Kübler, Ulrike (2013): Verhaltensanalyse in der Verhaltenstherapie. In: Verhaltenstherapie, 23(2): 108–116. https://www.zora.uzh.ch/id/eprint/85956/1/352030.pdf [11.12.2021].

Antonovsky, Aaron (1979): Health, Stress, and Coping: New Perspectives on Mental and Physical Well-Being. San Francisco: Jossey Bass.

Antonovsky, Aaron (1989): Die salutogenetische Perspektive: Zu einer neuen Sicht von Gesundheit und Krankheit. In: Meducs 2. 51–57.

Bamberger, Günter (2014): Beratung unter lösungsorientierter Perspektive. In: Engel, Frank/Nestmann, Frank/Sickendiek, Ursel (Hrsg.): Das Handbuch der Beratung. Band 2: Ansätze, Methoden und Felder. 3. Aufl. Tübingen: dgvt-Verlag. 737–748.

Barthelmess, Manuel (2014): Systemische Beratung. Eine Einführung in psychosoziale Berufe. 4. Aufl. Basel/Weinheim: Beltz Juventa Verlag.
Beck, Barbara/Borg-Laufs, Michael (2018): Methoden der Einzelberatung. In: Borg-Laufs, Michael/Wälte, Dieter (Hrsg.): Psychosoziale Beratung. Grundlagen, Diagnostik, Intervention. Stuttgart: W. Kohlhammer GmbH. 207–235.
Benesch, Michael (2020): Der Dialog in Beratung und Coaching. Wien: Facultas Verlags- und Buchhandels AG.
Bengel, Jürgen/Margraf, Jürgen (2020): Konfrontationstherapie. In: Pschyrembel online. Berlin: Walter de Gruyter GmbH. https://www.pschyrembel.de/Konfrontationstherapie/K0QF0/doc/ [31.05.2023].
Bengel, Jürgen/Margraf, Jürgen/Pschyrembel Redaktion (2020): Behaviorismus. In: Pschyrembel online. Berlin: Walter de Gruyter GmbH. https://www.pschyrembel.de/Behaviorismus/K03JQ/doc/ [24.05.2023].
Bengel, Jürgen/Margraf, Jürgen/Pschyrembel Redaktion (2020): Konfrontationstherapie. In: Pschyrembel online. Berlin: Walter de Gruyter GmbH. https://www.pschyrembel.de/Konfrontationstherapie/K0QF0/doc/ [31.05.2023].
Bengel, Jürgen/Warmbrunn, Angelika (2022): Verhaltensmodifikation. In: Pschyrembel online. Berlin: Walter de Gruyter GmbH. https://www.pschyrembel.de/Verhaltensmodifikation/T03WC/doc/ [23.05.2023].
Borg-Laufs, Michael (2014): Verhaltensberatung nach dem kognitiv-behavioristischen Modell. In: Engel, Frank/Nestmann, Frank/Sickendiek, Ursel (Hrsg.): Das Handbuch der Beratung. Band 2: Ansätze, Methoden und Felder. 3. Aufl. Tübingen: dgvt-Verlag. 629–639.
Borg-Laufs, Michael (2016): Störungsübergreifendes Diagnostik-System für die Kinder- und Jugendlichenpsychotherapie (SDS-KJ). 3. Aufl. Tübingen: dgvt-Verlag.
Borg-Laufs, Michael (2018a): Analyse psychischer Grundbedürfnisse. In: Borg-Laufs, Michael/Wälte, Dieter (Hrsg.): Psychosoziale Beratung. Grundlagen, Diagnostik, Intervention. Stuttgart: W. Kohlhammer GmbH. 141–148.
Borg-Laufs, Michael (2018b): Rollenspiel. In: Borg-Laufs, Michael/Wälte, Dieter (Hrsg.): Psychosoziale Beratung. Grundlagen, Diagnostik, Intervention. Stuttgart: W. Kohlhammer GmbH. 162–167.
Borg-Laufs, Michael (2018c): Verhaltensanalyse nach dem SORKC-Modell. In: Borg-Laufs, Michael/Wälte, Dieter (Hrsg.): Psychosoziale Beratung. Grundlagen, Diagnostik, Intervention. Stuttgart: W. Kohlhammer GmbH. 130–135.
Borg-Laufs, Michael/Tinkens, Julia (2018): Psychosoziale Ausgangssituation. In: Borg-Laufs, Michael/Wälte, Dieter (Hrsg.): Psychosoziale Beratung. Grundlagen, Diagnostik, Intervention. Stuttgart: W. Kohlhammer GmbH. 105–113.
Borg-Laufs, Michael/Wälte, Dieter (2018a): Analyse und Klärung der Probleme im Kontext von Ressourcen. In: Borg-Laufs, Michael/Wälte, Dieter (Hrsg.): Psychosoziale Beratung. Grundlagen, Diagnostik, Intervention. Stuttgart: W. Kohlhammer GmbH. 97–154.
Borg-Laufs, Michael/Wälte, Dieter (2018b): Gestaltung einer professionellen Beziehung in der Beratung. In: Borg-Laufs, Michael/Wälte, Dieter (Hrsg.): Psychosoziale Beratung. Grundlagen, Diagnostik, Intervention. Stuttgart: W. Kohlhammer GmbH. 59–77.
Borg-Laufs, Michael/Wälte, Dieter (Hrsg.) (2018c): Psychosoziale Beratung. Grundlagen, Diagnostik, Intervention. Stuttgart: Verlag W. Kohlhammer.
Bowlby, John (1975): Bindung. Eine Analyse der Mutter-Kind-Beziehung. München: Kindler.
Brunner, Ewald Johannes (2014): Systemische Beratung. In: Engel, Frank/Nestmann, Frank/Sickendiek, Ursel (Hrsg.): Das Handbuch der Beratung. Band 2: Ansätze, Methoden und Felder. 3. Aufl. Tübingen: dgvt-Verlag. 663–673.

Buttner, Peter/Knecht, Alban (2009): Wege der Ressourcendiagnostik in der sozialen Arbeit – ein ressourcentheoretisch fundierter Überblick. In: Pantucek, Peter/Röh, Dieter (Hrsg.): Perspektiven Sozialer Diagnostik. Über den Stand der Entwicklung von Verfahren und Standards. Münster-Hamburg-London: LIT Verlag. 99–110. Egger, Joseph W. (2008): Grundlagen der „Psychosomatik"- Zur Anwendung des biopsychosozialen Krankheitsmodells in der Praxis. In: Psychologische Medizin. 19 (2). Wien: Facultas-Universitätsverlag. 19–22. https://www.researchgate.net/publication/265652429_Egger_JW_2008_Grundlagen_der_Psychosomatik_-_Zur_Anwendung_des_biopsychosozialen_Krankheitsmodells_in_der_Praxis_Psychologische_Medizin_Wien_Facultas-Universitatsverlag_2008_19_2_12-22 [14.07.2021].

Datler, Wilfried/Gstach, Johannes/Steinhardt, Kornelia (2014): Psychoanalytisch orientierte Beratung. In: Engel, Frank/Nestmann, Frank/Sickendiek, Ursel (Hrsg.): Das Handbuch der Beratung. Band 2: Ansätze, Methoden und Felder. 3. Aufl. Tübingen: dgvt-Verlag. 613–626.

Dollinger, Bernd (2006): Salutogenese. Macht über die eigene Gesundheit? In: Dollinger Bernd/Raithel, Jürgen (2006): Aktivierende Sozialpädagogik. Ein kritisches Glossar. Wiesbaden: VS Verlag für Sozialwissenschaften/GWV Fachverlage GmbH. 173–191.

Duden (2021): Eklektizismus. In: Bibliographisches Institut GmbH. https://www.duden.de/rechtschreibung/Eklektizismus [29.11.2021].

Durlak, Joseph A./Pachan, Molly/Weissberg, Roger P. (2010): A Meta-Analysis of After-School Programs That Seek to Promote Personal and Social Skills in Children and Adolescents. American Journal of Community Psychology, 45 (3–4). 294–309.

Egger, Josef W. (2008): Grundlagen der „Psychosomatik"- Zur Anwendung des biopsychosozialen Krankheitsmodells in der Praxis. In: Psychologische Medizin. 19 (2). Wien: Facultas-Universitätsverlag. 19–22. https://www.researchgate.net/publication/265652429_Egger_JW_2008_Grundlagen_der_Psychosomatik_-_Zur_Anwendung_des_biopsychosozialen_Krankheitsmodells_in_der_Praxis_Psychologische_Medizin_Wien_Facultas-Universitatsverlag_2008_19_2_12-22 [14.07.2021].

Egger, Josef W. (2020): Die Einheit von Körper und Seele. Die bio-psycho-soziale Perspektive auf Krankheit und Gesundheit. Baden-Baden: Deutscher Wissenschafts-Verlag.

Engel, Frank/Nestmann, Frank/Sickendiek, Ursel (2014): Das Handbuch der Beratung. Band 2: Ansätze, Methoden und Felder. 3. Aufl. Tübingen: dgvt-Verlag.

Engel, Frank/Nestmann, Frank/Sickendiek, Ursel (2014): Statt einer „Einführung": Offene Fragen „guter Beratung". In: Engel, Frank/Nestmann, Frank/Sickendiek, Ursel (Hrsg.): Das Handbuch der Beratung. Band 2: Ansätze, Methoden und Felder. 3. Aufl. Tübingen: dgvt-Verlag. 599–607.

Engel, Frank/Sickendiek, Ursel (2014): Narrative Beratung: Sprache, Erzählungen und Metaphern in der Beratung. In: Engel, Frank/Nestmann, Frank/Sickendiek, Ursel (Hrsg.): Das Handbuch der Beratung. Band 2: Ansätze, Methoden und Felder. 3. Aufl. Tübingen: dgvt-Verlag. 749–762.

Epston, David/White, Michael (2013): Die Zähmung der Monster. Der narrative Ansatz in der Familientherapie. 7. Aufl. Heidelberg: Carl-Auer Verlag. In: https://www.researchgate.net/publication/331951308_Die_Zahmung_der_Monster [21.06.2021].

Ermann, Michael/Waldvogel, Bruno (2022): Psychodynamische Psychotherapie – Grundlagen und klinische Anwendungen. In: Psychiatrie, Psychosomatik, Psychotherapie. E.Medpedia: Springer Verlag und Springer Medizin Verlag. https://www.springermedizin.de/emedpedia/psychiatrie-psychosomatik-psychotherapie/psychodynamische-psychotherapie-grundlagen-und-klinische-anwendungen%3Fepedia. https://doi.org/10.1007/978-3-642-45028-0_37 [09.03.2022].

Eßing, Gabriele (2015): Praxis der Neuropsychotherapie: Wie die Psyche das Gehirn formt. Berlin: Deutscher Psychologen Verlag.

Faltermaier, Toni (2017): Gesundheitspsychologie. Grundriss der Psychologie. Band 21: 2. Aufl. Stuttgart: Kohlhammer.

Faltermeier, Toni (2020): Salutogenese. In: BZgA. Bundeszentrale für gesundheitliche Aufklärung. https://leitbegriffe.bzga.de/alphabetisches-verzeichnis/salutogenese [02.12.2021].

Frank, Jerome D. (1961): Persuasion and healing. Baltimore: John Hopkins Publ.

Füllgrabe, Uwe (2022): Eine kritische Betrachtung der Psychoanalyse. In: http://www.xn–uwe-fll-grabe-hlb.de/mediapool/42/428554/data/Artikel/Therapie/Psychoanalyse.pdf [06.03.2022].

Füssenhäuser, Cornelia (2006): Lebensweltorientierung in der Sozialen Arbeit. In: Dollinger, Bernd/Raithel, Jürgen (Hrsg.): Aktivierende Sozialpädagogik. Wiesbaden: VS Verlag für Sozialwissenschaften. 127–144.

Gahleitner, Silke-Brigitta/Glemser, Rolf/Hahn, Gernot (Hrsg.) (2012): Psychosoziale Diagnostik. Klinische Sozialarbeit. Beiträge zur psychosozialen Praxis und Forschung. Band 5. Köln: Psychiatrie Verlag.

Gahleitner, Silke Brigitta/Pauls, Helmut (2017): Psychosoziale Diagnose. In: Deutscher Verein für öffentliche und private Fürsorge, Hrsg.: Fachlexikon der sozialen Arbeit. 8., völlig überarb. u. akt. Auflage. Berlin: Deutscher Verein, S. 682–683. ISBN 978-3-8487-2374-4 [Rezension bei socialnet]

Gahleitner, Silke-Brigitta/Pauls, Helmut (2020): Psychosoziale Diagnostik. In: Socialnet Lexikon. Bonn: Socialnet. Das Netz für die Sozialwirtschaft. https://www.socialnet.de/lexikon/Psychosoziale-Diagnostik [11.07.2021].

Gerstenmaier, Jochen (2014): Konstruktivistisch orientierte Beratung. In: Engel, Frank/Nestmann, Frank/Sickendiek, Ursel (Hrsg.): Das Handbuch der Beratung. Band 2: Ansätze, Methoden und Felder. 3. Aufl. Tübingen: dgvt-Verlag. 675–688.

Grawe, Klaus/Grosse Holtforth, Martin (2004): Konfliktdiagnostik aus der Perspektive der Konsistenztheorie. In: https://www.researchgate.net/profile/Martin-Grosse-Holtforth/publication/215549712_Konfliktdiagnostik_aus_der_Perspektive_der_Konsistenztheorie/links/5dd25bf692851c382f46f5ec/Konfliktdiagnostik-aus-der-Perspektive-der-Konsistenztheorie.pdf [27.12.2021].

Hahlweg, Kurt/Heinrichs, Nina (2009): Elterntrainings zur Steigerung der Erziehungskompetenz. In: Margraf, Jürgen/Schneider, Silvia (Hrsg.): Lehrbuch der Verhaltenstherapie. Bd. 3. Berlin: Springer Verlag. 255–276.

Hand, Iver (1993): Expositionsbehandlung. In: Hautzinger, Martin/Linden, Michael (Hrsg.): Verhaltenstherapie. Techniken und Einzelverfahren. Berlin/Heidelberg: Springer Verlag GmbH. 139–150.

Hauer, Marion/Reisenzein-Hirsch, Elisabeth/Voderholzer, Ulrich (2014): Konfrontationsverfahren in der Behandlung psychischer Störungen. In: PSYCH up2date 8(03): 157–172. https://doi.org/10.1055/s-0034-1370010. https://www.researchgate.net/publication/275194790_Konfrontationsverfahren_in_der_Behandlung_psychischer_Storungen [31.05.2023].

Hautzinger, Martin (2012): Depressive Störungen. In: Margraf, Jürgen/Meinlschmidt, Gunther/Schneider, Silvia (Hrsg.): Lehrbuch der Verhaltenstherapie. Bd. 4. Berlin: Springer Verlag. S. 313–322.

Hedlund, Susanne (2021): Systematische Desensibilisierung. In: Pschyrembel online. Berlin: Walter de Gruyter GmbH. https://www.pschyrembel.de/Systematische%20Desensibilisierung/K05RR [31.05.2023].

Heidenreich, Thomas/Michalak, Johannes (2009): Achtsamkeit. In: Margraf, Jürgen/Schneider, Silvia (Hrsg.). Lehrbuch der Verhaltenstherapie. Bd.1: Grundlagen, Diagnostik, Verfahren, Rahmenbedingungen. Heidelberg: Springer Verlag. 569–578.

Heiner, Maja (2014): Evaluation in der Beratung. In: Engel, Frank/Nestmann, Frank/Sickendiek, Ursel (Hrsg.): Das Handbuch der Beratung. Band 2: Ansätze, Methoden und Felder. 3. Aufl. Tübingen: dgvt-Verlag. 825–836.

Henningsen, Peter (2017). Geleitwort. In: Brunner, Jürgen: Psychotherapie und Neurobiologie: Neurowissenschaftliche Erkenntnisse für die psychotherapeutische Praxis. Stuttgart: Kohlhammer Verlag. 7–8.

Heuse, Silke (2019): SORKC-Modell. In: Wirtz, Markus A. (Hrsg.): Lexikon der Psychologie. Bern: Dorsch Hogrefe AG. https://dorsch.hogrefe.com/stichwort/sorkc-modell [11.12.2021].

Hobfoll, Stevan E. (1989): Conservation of resources: A new attempt at conceptualizing stress. In: American Psychologist, 44. 513–524.

Hobfoll, Steven E./Lilly Roy S. (1993): Resource cservation as a strategy for community psychology. In: Journal of Community Psychology, 21. 128–148.

Hubert, Martin (2006): Ist der Mensch noch frei? Wie die Hirnforschung unser Menschenbild verändert. Düsseldorf: Walter Verlag.

Juhl, Carsten/Mellentin, Angelina/Nielsen, Anette S./Nielsen, Bent/Schippers, Gerard M./Skot, Lotte/Stenager, Elsebeth (2017): Cue-Expositionstherapie zur Behandlung von Alkoholkonsumstörungen: Eine metaanalytische Übersicht. In: Clinical Psychology Review. 57: 195–207. https://doi.org/10.1016/j.cpr.2017.07.006. [01.06.2023].

Kabat-Zinn, Jon (2013): Gesund durch Meditation: Das große Buch der Selbstheilung mit MBSR. München: Knaur MensSana.

Kaluza, Gert (2011): Stressbewältigung. Trainingsmanual zur psychologischen Gesundheitsförderung. 2. Aufl. Berlin, Heidelberg: Springer Verlag.

Kaluza, Gert (2015): Stressbewältigung. Trainingsmanual zur psychologischen Gesundheitsförderung. 3. Aufl. Berlin, Heidelberg: Springer Verlag.

Kanfer, Frederick H./Saslow, George (1965): Behavioral Analysis: An Alternative to Diagnostic Classification. In: Archives of General Psychiatry, 12. S. 529–538.

Kanfer, Frederick H./Saslow, George (1969): Behavioral diagnosis. In: Franks CM: Behavior Therapy: Appraisal and Status. New York: McGraw-Hill.

Kanfer, Frederick H./Saslow, George (1974): Verhaltenstheoretische Diagnostik. In Schulte (Hrsg.): Diagnostik in der Verhaltenstherapie. München: Urban und Schwarzenberg Verlag.

Kanfer, Frederick H./Reinecker, Hans/Schmelzer, Dieter (2012): Selbstmanagement-Therapie. Ein Lehrbuch für die klinische Praxis. 5. Aufl. Heidelberg: Springer Verlag.

Klingenberger, Hubert (2017): Biografiearbeit in Beratung und Coaching. München: Don Bosco Medien GmbH.

Klosko, Janet/Weishaar, Marjorie/Young, Jefferey (2008): Schematherapie. Ein praxisorientiertes Handbuch. 2. Aufl. Paderborn: Junfermann Verlag.

Knecht, Alban/Schubert, Franz-Christian (2012): Ressourcen – eine Einführung in Merkmale, Theorien und Konzeptionen. In: Knecht, Alban/Schubert, Franz-Christian (Hrsg.): Ressourcen im Sozialstaat und in der Sozialen Arbeit. Zuteilung – Förderung – Aktivierung. Stuttgart: Kohlhammer. S. 15–41.

Lattschar, Birgit/Wiemann, Irmela (2013): Mädchen und Jungen entdecken ihre Geschichte. Grundlagen und Praxis der Biografiearbeit. 4. Aufl. Weinheim und Basel: Beltz Juventa.

Lehrbuch Psychologie (2023): Flooding. In: Springer Lehrbuch Psychologie. Berlin, Heidelberg: Springer Verlag GmbH. https://lehrbuch-psychologie.springer.com/glossar/flooding [31.05.2023].

Leitner, Anton (2010): Handbuch der integrativen Therapie. Wien und New York: Springer Verlag.

Lenz, Albert (2003): Ressourcenorientierte Beratung – Konzeptionelle und methodische Überlegungen. In: PsyDok. Praxis der Kinderpsychologie und Kinderpsychiatrie. 52 (4). Vandenhoeck und Ruprecht Verlag. 234–249. https://psydok.psycharchives.de/jspui/bitstream/20.500.11780/2680/1/52.20034_3_44324.pdf_new.pdf

Linden, Michael (1993): Systematische Desensibilisierung. In: Hautzinger, Martin/Linden, Michael (Hrsg.): Verhaltenstherapie. Berlin, Heidelberg: Springer Verlag. 307–310.

Linderkamp, Friedrich (2009): Operante Methoden. In: Margraf, Jürgen/Schneider, Silvia (Hrsg.): Lehrbuch der Verhaltenstherapie. 3. Band: Störungen im Kindes- und Jugendalter. Berlin/Heidelberg: Springer Verlag. 209–220.

Lörch, Bernd (2015): Cue-Belichtung (Reizexposition). Hautzinger, Martin/Linden, Michael (Hrsg.): Verhaltenstherapie. Berlin, Heidelberg: Springer Verlag. 93–96. https://doi.org/10.1007/978-3-642-55210-6_18 [01.06.2023].

Lübeck, Anja/Wälte, Dieter (2018a): Schematherapeutische Interventionen in der Beratung. In: Borg-Laufs, Michael/Wälte, Dieter (Hrsg.): Psychosoziale Beratung. Grundlagen, Diagnostik, Intervention. Stuttgart: W. Kohlhammer GmbH. 178–189.

Lübeck, Anja/Wälte, Dieter (2018): Was ist psychosoziale Beratung? In: Borg-Laufs, Michael/Wälte, Dieter (Hrsg.): Psychosoziale Beratung. Grundlagen, Diagnostik, Intervention. Stuttgart: W. Kohlhammer GmbH. 24–41.

Margraf, Jürgen/Pschyrembel Redaktion (2016): Schematherapie. In: Pschyrembel online. Berlin: Walter de Gruyter GmbH. https://www.pschyrembel.de/Schematherapie/K00KR/doc/ [27.05.2023].

Margraf, Jürgen/Pschyrembel Redaktion (2021): Flooding. In: Pschyrembel online. Berlin: Walter de Gruyter GmbH. https://www.pschyrembel.de/Flooding/K0JMJ/doc/ [31.05.2023].

McLeod, John (2004): Counselling. Eine Einführung in die Beratung. Tübingen: dgvt-Verlag.

Meibert, Petra (2013): Zugang zu achtsamen Gewahrsein inmitten von Leid und Schmerz. In: Anderssen-Reuster, Ulrike/Meibert, Petra/Meck, Sabine (Hrsg.). Psychotherapie und buddhistisches Geistestraining. Methoden einer achtsamen Bewusstseinskultur. Stuttgart: Schattauer. 177–198.

Metzler Lexikon Philosophie (2008): Dialog. In: Spektrum – Lexikon Philosophie. Berlin Heidelberg: Springer Verlag. https://www.spektrum.de/lexikon/philosophie/dialog/450 [09.03.2022].

Meyer, Melanie/Schubert, Franz-Christian/Wälte, Dieter (2018): Methoden der systemischen Paar- und Familienberatung. In: Borg-Laufs, Michael/Wälte, Dieter (Hrsg.): Psychosoziale Beratung. Grundlagen, Diagnostik, Intervention. Stuttgart: Verlag W. Kohlhammer. 235–254.

Meyer, Melanie/Wälte, Dieter (2018): Beratungsabschluss. In: Borg-Laufs, Michael/Wälte, Dieter (Hrsg.): Psychosoziale Beratung. Grundlagen, Diagnostik, Intervention. Stuttgart: Verlag W. Kohlhammer. 281–287.

Mutzeck, Wolfgang (2014): Kooperative Beratung. In: Engel, Frank/Nestmann, Frank/Sickendiek, Ursel (Hrsg.): Das Handbuch der Beratung. Band 2: Ansätze, Methoden und Felder. 3. Aufl. Tübingen: dgvt-Verlag. 691–697.

Nestmann, Frank (2002): Verhältnis von Beratung und Therapie. In: Psychotherapie im Dialog, 3 (4). Stuttgart/New York: Georg Thieme Verlag. 402–409.

Nestmann, Frank (2014a): Beratungsmethoden und Beratungsbeziehung. In: Engel, Frank/Nestmann, Frank/Sickendiek, Ursel (Hrsg.): Das Handbuch der Beratung. Band 2: Ansätze, Methoden und Felder. 3. Aufl. Tübingen: dgvt-Verlag. 783–795.

Nestmann, Frank (2014b): Ressourcenorientierte Beratung. In: Engel, Frank/Nestmann, Frank/Sickendiek, Ursel (Hrsg.): Das Handbuch der Beratung. Band 2: Ansätze, Methoden und Felder. 3. Aufl. Tübingen: dgvt-Verlag. 725–734.

Orlinsky, David E./Ronnestad, Helge/Willutzki, Ulrike (2004): Fifty Years of Psychotherapy Process-Outcome Research: continuity and Change. In: Lambert, Michael J. (Hrsg.): Bergin and Garfield's Handbook of Psychotherapy and behavior Change. 5. Aufl. New York: Wiley. S. 307–389.

Pantucek, Peter (2010): Soziale Diagnose: Netzwerkkarte. 189–202. In: http://www.pantucek.com/diagnose/netzwerkkarte/netzwerkkarte_manual.pdf [04.12.2021].

Pantucek, Peter (2011): Netzwerke erheben, darstellen und diskutieren. Die Software easyNWK ermöglicht die Analyse persönlicher Kontakte im Sozialraum. In: Blätter der Wohlfahrtspflege (BdW), Jg. 158/4. Baden-Baden: Nomos Verlagsgesellschaft GmbH. & Co. KG. 146–149. https://www.nomos-elibrary.de/https://doi.org/10.5771/0340-8574-2011-4-146/netzwerke-erheben-darstellen-und-diskutieren-jahrgang-158-2011-heft-4?page=0 [04.12.2021].

Pantucek, Peter (2012): Netzwerkkarte digital: EasyNWK. In: Pantucek, Peter (2013): Soziale Diagnostik: Verfahren. http://www.pantucek.com/index.php/soziale-diagnostik/verfahren/13-nwk-digital [04.12.2021].

Reinecker, Hans (2009): Selbstmanagement. In: Margraf, Jürgen/Schneider, Silvia (Hrsg.) (2009): Lehrbuch der Verhaltenstherapie. Band 1: Grundlagen, Diagnostik, Verfahren, Rahmenbedingungen. 3. Erweiterte Aufl. Heidelberg: Springer Medizin Verlag. 630–644.

Rogers, Carl (1942): Die nicht direktive Beratung. Counselling and Psychotherapy. Boston, münchen: Kindler Studienausgabe 1972.

Rogers, Carl (1977): Therapeut und Klient. Grundlagen der Gesprächspsychotherapie. Münschen: Kindler.

Roth, Gerhard/Strüber, Nicole (2021): Wie das Gehirn die Seele macht. 4. Aufl. Stuttgart: Klett-Cotta Verlag.

Röhrle, Bernd (2008): Verhaltenstheoretisch orientierte Modelle. In: Caspar, Franz/Röhrle, Bernd/Schlottke, Peter F. (Hrsg.): Lehrbuch der klinisch-psychologischen Diagnostik. Stuttgart: W. Kohlhammer GmbH. 89–113.

Rüegg, Johann Caspar (2011): Gehirn, Psyche und Körper: Neurobiologie von Psychosomatik und Psychotherapie. 5. Aufl. Stuttgart: Schattauer Verlag.

Sachse, Rainer (2016): Therapeutische Beziehungsgestaltung. 2. Aufl. Göttingen: Hogrefe Verlag.

Sanders, Rudolf (2014): Die Beziehung zwischen Ratsuchendem und Berater. In: Engel, Frank/Nestmann, Frank/Sickendiek, Ursel (Hrsg.): Das Handbuch der Beratung. Band 2: Ansätze, Methoden und Felder. 3. Aufl. Tübingen: dgvt-Verlag. 797–807.

Schaller, Roger (2014): Rollenspiel in Verhaltenstherapie und Psychodrama. In: Zeitschrift für Psychodrama und Soziometrie. 13. Schweiz: Springer Nature Schweiz AG. 211–223.

Schmidt-Traub, Sigrun (2006): Therapeutische Beziehung – ein Überblick. In: Psychotherapeutische Praxis, 3 (3), Göttingen: Hogrefe Verlag. 111–129.

Schubert, Franz-Christian (2018): Ressourcendiagnostik. In: Borg-Laufs, Michael/Wälte, Dieter (Hrsg.): Psychosoziale Beratung. Grundlagen, Diagnostik, Intervention. Stuttgart: Verlag W. Kohlhammer, 113–129.

Schweitzer, Jochen/von Schlippe, Arist (2016): Lehrbuch der systemischen Therapie und Beratung I: Das Grundlagenwissen. 3. Aufl. Göttingen:Vandenhoeck & Ruprecht Verlag.

Sieben, Lara/Wälte, Dieter (2018): Konfrontative Techniken (Verhaltensexperimente). In: Borg-Laufs, Michael/Wälte, Dieter (Hrsg.): Psychosoziale Beratung. Grundlagen, Diagnostik, Intervention. Stuttgart: Verlag W. Kohlhammer, 167–178.

Skop, Karin (2019): Psychotherapie und Neurowissenschaften – Quo vadis? In: SFU Forschungsbulletin SFU Research Bulletin 7(2). 20–32.

Spektrum Lexikon der Psychologie (2000): Integrative Therapie. In: Spektrum der Wissenschaft. Heidelberg: Spektrum der Wissenschaft Verlagsgesellschaft mbH., Springer Nature. https://www.spektrum.de/lexikon/psychologie/integrative-therapie/7253 [09.03.2022].

Stavemann, Harlich H. (2006): Differentialindikation für Disputationstechniken und Sokratische Dialoge in der Kognitiven Verhaltenstherapie. Verhaltenstherapie und psychosoziale Praxis, 38. 337–349.

Stavemann, Harlich H. (2010): Einführung in die KVT: Die Therapie emotionaler Turbulenzen. 4. Aufl. Weinheim: Beltz Verlag.

Stegbauer, Christian (2008): Netzwerkanalyse und Netzwerktheorie. Einige Anmerkungen zu einem neuen Paradigma. In: Stegbauer, Christian (Hrsg.): Netzwerkanalyse und Netzwerktheorie. Ein neues Paradigma in den Sozialwissenschaften. 1. Aufl. Wiesbaden: VS Verlag für Sozialwissenschaften/GWV Fachverlage GmbH. 11–21.

Straumann, Ursula E. (2014): Klientenzentrierte Beratung. In: Engel, Frank/Nestmann, Frank/Sickendiek, Ursel (Hrsg.): Das Handbuch der Beratung. Band 2: Ansätze, Methoden und Felder. 3. Aufl. Tübingen: dgvt-Verlag. 641–653.

Thiersch, Hans (2014): Lebensweltorientierte Soziale Beratung. In: Engel, Frank/Nestmann, Frank/Sickendiek, Ursel (Hrsg.): Das Handbuch der Beratung. Band 2: Ansätze, Methoden und Felder. 3. Aufl. Tübingen: dgvt-Verlag. 699–708.

Thompson, Rosemary A. (1996): Counseling techniques. Washington: Accelerated Development.

Vogel, Heiner (2014): Qualitätssicherung von Beratung. In: Engel, Frank/Nestmann, Frank/Sickendiek, Ursel (Hrsg.): Das Handbuch der Beratung. Band 2: Ansätze, Methoden und Felder. 3. Aufl. Tübingen: dgvt-Verlag. 837–856.

Wagner, Rudolph F. (2003): Rollenspiel und Rollentausch in der kognitiven Verhaltenstherapie. In: Zeitschrift für Psychodrama und Soziometrie. Vol. 2. Springer Nature Schweiz AG. 69–77.

Wagner, Rudolph F. (2014): Integrative Beratungsansätze. In: Engel, Frank/Nestmann, Frank/Sickendiek, Ursel (Hrsg.): Das Handbuch der Beratung. Band 2: Ansätze, Methoden und Felder. 3. Aufl. Tübingen: dgvt-Verlag. 663–673.

Wälte, Dieter (2018a): Analyse und Klärung der Probleme im Kontext von Ressourcen. In: Borg-Laufs, Michael/Wälte, Dieter (Hrsg.): Psychosoziale Beratung. Grundlagen, Diagnostik, Intervention. Stuttgart: Verlag W. Kohlhammer. 97–154.

Wälte, Dieter (2018b): Analyse der Selbstregulation. In: Borg-Laufs, Michael/Wälte, Dieter (Hrsg.). Psychosoziale Beratung. Grundlagen, Diagnostik, Intervention. Stuttgart: Verlag W. Kohlhammer. 135–140.

Wälte, Dieter (2018c): Diagnostische Grundlagen zum Fallverständnis nach dem bio-psycho-sozialen Modell. In: Borg-Laufs, Michael/Wälte, Dieter (Hrsg.): Psychosoziale Beratung. Grundlagen, Diagnostik, Intervention. Stuttgart: Verlag W. Kohlhammer. 98–104.

Weinberger, Sabine (2013): Klientenzentrierte Gesprächsführung. Lern- und Praxisanleitung für psychosoziale Berufe. 14. Aufl. Basel/Weinheim: Beltz Juventa Verlag.

Weinhardt, Marc (2014): Biographie, Lebenslauf und Übergänge in der Beratung. In: Resonanzen. E-Journal für biopsychosoziale Dialoge in Psychotherapie, Supervision und Beratung, 2(1), 34–48. https://www.researchgate.net/publication/301688491_Biographie_Lebenslauf_und_Ubergange_in_der_Beratung [07.07.2021].

Willutzki, Ulrike (2008): Ressourcendiagnostik in der Klinischen Psychologie und Psychotherapie. In: Klinische Diagnostik und Evaluation, 1. Jg. Göttingen: Vandenhoeck & Ruprecht, 126–145. https://docplayer.org/110481177-Ressourcendiagnostik-in-der-klinischen-psychologie-und-psychotherapie.html [28.12.2021].

WKO, Personenberatung und Personenbetreuung (2013): Methodenkatalog Lebens- und Sozialberatung. https://www.wko.at/branchen/w/gewerbe-handwerk/personenberatung-betreuung/Methodenkatalog-LSB.pdf [31.05.2021].

WLP, Wiener Landesverband für Psychotherapie (2021): Tiefenpsychologische Orientierung. https://www.psychotherapie-wlp.at/informationen/psychotherapie/methoden/tiefenpsychologische-orientierung [31.05.2021].

Wolpe, Joseph (1958): Psychotherapy by Reciprocal Inhibition. Stanford: Stanford Univeritsy Press.

Young, Jeffrey/Klosko, Janet S./Weishaar, Marjorie E. (2008): Schematherapie. Ein praxisorientiertes Handbuch. 2. Aufl. Paderborn: Junfermann Verlag.

Zarbock, Gerhard/Ammann, Axel/Ringer, Silka (2012): Achtsamkeit für Psychotherapeuten und Berater. Weinheim, Basel: Beltz.

4 Psychoneuroendocrinology (PNE) in Psychosocial and Psychotherapeutic Practice: "PNES Coaching"

Before the biopsychosocial coaching approach "PNES-Coaching" is introduced, the first section of this chapter discusses to what extent psychoneuroendocrinology (PNE) and its findings can be transferred into psychosocial and psychotherapeutic practice.

4.1 Psychoneuroendocrinology in Psychosocial and Psychotherapeutic Practice

This section of the book demonstrates why the integration of psychoneuroendocrinological findings into psychosocial and psychotherapeutic practice is significant. Since there is currently no biopsychosocial coaching approach based on psychoneuroendocrinological findings, the question arises as to what extent these findings are applicable in psychosocial and psychotherapeutic practice and in which areas they can be helpful for clients. Of particular interest is the connection between psychoneuroendocrinology and the psychosocial everyday life, psychosocial health, and mental disorders of clients. It is also important to consider whether the psychoneuroendocrinological findings obtained so far, which are primarily rooted in the genesis of diseases, are suitable for psychosocial or psychological interventions at all.

4.1.1 Relevant Topics for Psychosocial and Psychotherapeutic Practice

The following sections link significant findings of PNE with relevant topics in psychosocial and psychotherapeutic practice. It is explained whether and to what extent the implementation of PNE findings in psychosocial and psychotherapeutic practice is helpful.

J. Wiederhofer, *Psychoneuroendocrinology in Psychosocial and Psychotherapeutic Practice*, https://doi.org/10.1007/978-3-658-46275-8_4

▶ Psychosocial Influences and Hormone Release

To what extent do psychosocial influences in our daily lives affect our hormone release? Relevant examples and the exploration of this topic are the focus here.

The findings of various researches and studies presented in this book clearly show that psychosocial influences have enormous effects on our hormone release. It is important to understand that our entire behavior, experiences, genetics, and environment influence our hormone secretion. These findings are scientifically substantiated and are now well measurable in laboratory research. Hormonal changes are measurable both in stressful situations and in various emotional situations (e.g., aggression). In PNE, there is a strong interest in stress and cortisol release. There are also numerous studies on aggression and findings on testosterone release. Notably, results from competitive situations between men, where testosterone levels change, are well known. However, it is important to mention that aggression does not always increase testosterone levels. The first two chapters of this book have also extensively discussed how stress or individual burdens affect our endocrine system in daily life. Ultimately, it is important to note that all psychosocial influences and interactions, along with the associated individual emotions, impact our hormone release and thus our psyche and behavior. However, the extent to which hormone release affects our psyche depends on individual gene-environment interactions. Epigenetic influences, individual experiences, and perinatal influences should not be overlooked here.

▶ Hormonal Influence on Psyche, Behavior, and Psychosocial Everyday Life

To what extent do hormones influence our psyche and behavior in psychosocial everyday life? The hormone secretions we are exposed to daily continuously influence our behavior, psyche, cognition, and thus our entire psychosocial everyday life. It is important to mention that hormones are not only relevant for people with mental disorders but also influence the psyche, behavior, and psychosocial everyday life of healthy individuals daily. For example, in everyday stressful situations, norepinephrine and adrenaline help us perform certain daily tasks better. However, if stressful situations result in excessively high cortisol concentrations, this affects the intake and consolidation of information into memory. Another well-known example from everyday life, also discussed in Chap. 1, is PMS (premenstrual syndrome). Hormones have both psychological and physiological effects that influence our entire life, daily routine, emotions, and individual behavior. Again, it is important to mention that the effects are individually different and that individuals are individually burdened or affected by the effects of hormone release due to, for example, their resilience, genetic predispositions, and experiences. It should also be noted that positive psychosocial influences, such as social interactions, also have an individual impact on the psyche and behavior of individuals. Ultimately, it is important to note that we are confronted daily with psychosocial influences and interactions, which always affect our hormone release and thus our psyche and behavior in everyday life.

▶ Psychoneuroendocrinology and Mental Disorders

The connection between PNE and mental disorders was extensively discussed in Chap. 2 of this book. Examples were used to illustrate which diseases are psychoendocrine and to what extent psychoneuroendocrinological findings are significant in this context.

Hormones can be referred to as biomarkers in many mental illnesses. However, in the case of 2 mental disorders, causality can clearly be spoken of: depression and PTSD. In particular, PTSD (post-traumatic stress disorder) is a psychoendocrine-mediated disease because, without an initial stressor (the trauma), which is associated with massive hormone release, there would be no disease. The flashbacks characteristic of the disease are related to the massive stress reaction that the affected person had during the experience. There are also unique findings in depression. In the case of depression or depressive symptoms, changes in hormone levels are clearly measurable. If there is an improvement in the symptoms, cortisol regulation also normalizes again. However, it is important to mention here that hormone administration does not lead to an improvement in symptoms. Furthermore, PNE findings are of enormous importance in anxiety states, as these are also associated with extreme hormone releases. In general, it can be observed that the HPA axis is often involved in stress-related diseases. Additionally, this book has explained how important a healthy thyroid is for our mental health or psychological well-being. Based on these findings, professional psychological diagnostics always ask whether there are already thyroid findings.

These findings are particularly important for psychotherapists who work with patients suffering from mental disorders, but they are also of enormous importance in psychosocial work with, for example, complexly traumatized people. Ultimately, every psychosocial and psychotherapeutic work that accompanies people with mental disorders or impairments benefits from psychoneuroendocrinological findings.

▶ Psychoneuroendocrinology and Behavioral Genetics

The following discusses the relationship between PNE and behavioral genetics. To what extent does PNE require behavioral genetic findings? What is heritability? Do genes influence our behavior, and to what extent do we have influence over our genes? A topic that cannot be ignored in connection with a modern biopsychosocial approach. It has long been known that genetics influence our behavior. However, a lot of misinformation is spread here, which needs to be eliminated, such as the spread of the idea that we are all puppets of our genes. No, we are not. Genetics in the field of psychology and psychiatry primarily ask about the extent of genetic influence. And with this knowledge, one can clearly say, no, we are not puppets of our genes; heritability is influenceable. This finding is of enormous importance, especially for psychological interventions, behavior, or mental disorders. Heritability is a quotient, meaning if you change the environmental variance, you change the heritability. Or explained differently, if you change society, in terms of less stress or earlier recognized depressive symptoms, you also change depressiveness.

The genetic influence can be well researched, especially through family and twin studies. The genetic influence is particularly well researched in depression, schizophrenia, and bipolar disorders. Polymorphisms are important here; they are, for example, the reason why people look different. Which genes are responsible for the disease is also being researched in smaller research projects. However, modern molecular genetics identify genes and hope to develop therapeutic concepts based on them. These research projects can only be implemented globally in terms of size, complexity, and cooperation (also concerning subjects). In this research area, there are always surprises, but also frustration because much is still not understood. It is also important to mention that genetics is a method for PNE to gain insights that would not be researchable otherwise. Much is researched with animal experiments because this research is not allowed on humans and will not be allowed in the future. An example of this is the administration of Neuropeptide-S (NPS) to a rat. The rat became extraordinarily fearless from NPS. Since this cannot be tried on humans, it is important to apply these findings to humans, considering human anxiety and stress sensitivity. Thus, it can be stated that behavioral genetics is of great importance for the findings of PNE as well as for psychology and psychiatry.

▶ **Psychoneuroendocrinology and the Maintenance of Psychosocial Health**

Salutogenesis is an important keyword here, and whether the concept of salutogenesis, based on current scientific findings, is not already outdated. Furthermore, it is of interest how PNE findings can be used to maintain our psychosocial health.

From a modern scientific perspective, the concept of salutogenesis is clearly outdated in light of current findings. Important for the maintenance and preservation of psychosocial health, based on well-founded psychoneuroendocrinological findings, are terms such as resilience, protective factors, and vulnerability factors. Hormones clearly function as biomarkers. Additionally, these terms imply the importance of genetic questions. Even though this takes time and, for example, stress resilience cannot be built up in a short time, this book has shown that it is possible to strengthen resilience. A multidimensional psychosocial and psychotherapeutic work, in connection with emotive-cognitive (reflection of feelings, affects), cognitive-emotive, and cognitive-behavioral interventions, which include practical, individually adapted exercises/homework, show positive effects. Furthermore, educating clients—keyword psychoeducation—is important here. By making simple content, such as the importance of sleep (circadian rhythm), the importance of nutrition (precursors and co-factors), and the negative impact of harmful substances (e.g., alcohol) understandable to clients, it is possible to promote homeostasis and thus the maintenance of psychosocial health.

▶ **Positively influencing hormones yourself**

Do we release opioids by consuming chocolate? It is important to note how it is possible to influence hormones, especially "happiness hormones," yourself. What are the possibilities to positively use hormones in everyday life as well as in psychological disorders or pain? There is a widespread rumor: chocolate produces opioids. However, a general no would be the wrong answer. There are many things one can do to influence hormone release. These are things like ensuring that one feels safe and secure, as well as avoiding situations of fear and uncontrollability. Additionally, exercise is beneficial (physical activity, especially endurance sports). However, it is important to ensure that the extent is individually adequately adjusted. Furthermore, a healthy and balanced diet, in which nutrients, vitamins, and especially amino acids play a significant role, has positive effects on biosynthesis and thus on homeostasis. For example, L-tryptophan is the precursor of the sleep hormone melatonin as well as the neurotransmitter serotonin. Another good example is L-tyrosine. This non-essential amino acid can increase the levels of the neurotransmitters dopamine, adrenaline, and noradrenaline. Both substances can be supplied through a balanced diet or supplemented with dietary supplements. Additionally, music, looking at photos, art, good sexual behavior, social interactions, and any hobbies have a positive influence on our endocrine system and thus on our behavior and psyche.

▶ **Psychoneuroendocrinology and psychological interventions**

Ultimately, the question arises whether it is possible to implement PNE findings into psychological, psychosocial, and psychotherapeutic interventions, and what significance interdisciplinarity has in this context.

Psychoneuroendocrinological laboratory research has clearly advanced to the point where findings can be applied to reality or everyday life. This means it is possible to transfer the findings into practice. For this, one needs precise data, information, or a precise biopsychosocial diagnosis from the clients, as well as the answers to some genetic questions. The basis for successful interventions requires knowledge of how clients immediately experience, feel, or think. For a detailed biopsychosocial diagnosis and the implementation of a biopsychosocial coaching approach, interdisciplinarity and transnational approaches are important. A multimodal therapy/counseling combined with PNE findings is thus goal-oriented. The information presented in this book clearly demonstrates how important it is to transfer PNE findings into psychosocial and psychotherapeutic practice. Based on the findings obtained here, the biopsychosocial coaching approach "PNES-Coaching" is presented in Sect. 4.2.

4.1.2 Conclusion: Psychoneuroendocrinology in Psychosocial and Psychotherapeutic Practice

Besides much misinformation that is spread about hormones, it is indeed the case that we all know the effects of hormones. Hormones influence our behavior, our psyche, our health, and our psychosocial everyday life. But our psychosocial everyday life and our behavior, our environment, and our environmental interactions also influence our hormone secretions. Additionally, behavioral genetics play a significant role, although misinformation is also spread here, because we are not puppets of our genetics; rather, we have an influence on our genes. Environmental influences, (early childhood) experiences, and our society have an impact on this. The findings presented in this book clearly show the enormous importance of interdisciplinarity. Hormones influence not only people with mental disorders but also healthy people, which means that knowledge about hormones and the targeted and conscious application of this knowledge is beneficial in both cases. Hormones function as biomarkers, both in people with disorders such as PTSD, depression, anxiety, and much more, as well as in people with, for example, exam anxiety or enormous stress in everyday life, and people who are in temporary crisis situations. The findings of this still young scientific discipline are definitely advanced enough to be implemented in psychological interventions. Additionally, some previously recognized concepts, based on scientifically sound findings, are currently already considered "outdated." It is possible to influence our hormone secretions ourselves and thus promote our well-being and our physical as well as mental health, even if this requires openness to interdisciplinarity. In terms of implied psychoneuroendocrinological findings in psychological interventions, both in the health-promoting and health-maintaining areas, terms such as resilience, protective factors, vulnerability factors, and behavioral genetics play a significant role. The findings of PNE are sufficiently advanced, and the connection with our psychosocial health, our emotion and behavior regulation, as well as various mental illnesses, are clearly proven, so that the findings of PNE can be implemented without hesitation in a modern, scientifically based biopsychosocial coaching concept, which can be applied both in psychosocial counseling and psychotherapy. The implementation of these findings can be helpful in specifically promoting or facilitating the management of psychosocial everyday life through the influence of our hormones, regardless of whether the clients are healthy individuals in crisis situations or people with mental disorders. The targeted use of behavior that leads to the release of endogenous hormones can definitely positively influence the management of psychosocial life. On the other hand, based on the findings of PNE, the individual resilience of clients can be trained, whereby the body gradually learns to cope better with stress situations and thus reduce the negative effects of stress. Psychoneuroendocrinological findings are particularly important in PTSD, depression, and anxiety disorders, but also in people who have difficulties with stress management or loss of control. Activating the body's own calming system can be individually trained. Additionally, understanding our psychoneural basic systems as well as behavioral genetics and knowledge about heritability can be helpful in finding individual coping strategies. Many of the PNE findings presented in this book are findings that we are confronted with daily, that we have all experienced at some point, and that should naturally be part of all our lives. However, reality shows that much of this is not (any longer) self-evident in our society. We have all experienced how good fun with friends feels and how social interactions can enhance our well-being. We have all experienced how positive it is for our mood when we do something we enjoy. Anyone who has already enjoyed a loving touch, whether from partners, parents, or friends, knows what wonderful feelings this can trigger in a person. Perhaps the dissemination of knowledge about the enormous importance of hormones on our psyche can lead to doing things for oneself more often, to benefit from the body's own forces, consciously recover in challenging times, and achieve individual goals. However, the basic prerequisite for the targeted use of this knowledge is an interdisciplinary openness on the part of psychosocial counselors and psychotherapists. It requires openness to accept critical considerations as well as scientific progress and to implement modern scientifically based findings in already empirically proven psychosocial/psychotherapeutic interventions. Neuroscientific findings show that not all counseling approaches or orientations have an empirically verifiable effect. However, a pluralism of methods or an eclectic-integrative approach, where the methods are individually tailored to the clients, has proven effective. Besides critical considerations, areas of tension between various disciplines, and demarcation debates, I do not see modern psychosocial counseling and psychotherapy under the aspect of hostility, "fighting," or demarcation. In my view, modern psychosocial counseling as well as modern psychotherapy, in terms of successful assistance and quality assurance, show openness to cooperation as well as current scientifically based, including interdisciplinary, findings. Ultimately, my conclusion is that modern psychological or psychosocial interventions should implement interdisciplinary scientifically based findings (both psychoneuroendocrinological and others) in their interventions, as these contribute to the quality of the interventions and promote successful psychological and psychosocial assistance. A biopsychosocial coaching approach, based on interdisciplinary findings and a pluralism of methods, seems effective to me in promoting the quality of psychological/psychotherapeutic as well as psychosocial interventions and achieving a quality improvement.

The following describes a biopsychosocial coaching approach that combines empirically proven counseling approaches/therapy forms with psychoneuroendocrinological findings.

4.2 PNES Coaching: The Implementation of Psychoneuroendocrinological Insights into an Eclectic-Integrative Biopsychosocial Coaching Approach

In the last chapter of this book, the biopsychosocial coaching approach "PNES Coaching" is introduced. This coaching implies the relevant interdisciplinary insights presented in this book. The following concept is based on an eclectic-integrative counseling approach, in which neuroscientifically empirically proven forms of intervention and therapeutic orientations are linked with psychoneuroendocrinological insights. The interventions, methods, and applied techniques are individually adapted to the problems and difficulties as well as the personality of the clients.

Eclectic-Integrative Coaching Approach In an eclectic-integrative coaching approach, different repertoires of methods, concepts, and approaches from various therapy schools are controlled and linked together. A combination of different interventions is created.

At this point, I would like to emphasize that although an eclectic-integrative counseling approach draws on diverse methods and procedures from different concepts and approaches to achieve the individually needed assistance and change, these methods are not assembled arbitrarily or randomly. This coaching approach is based on the so-called technical eclecticism.

Technical Eclecticism The most effective methods from different therapy schools are intertwined. The integration of these procedures is planned and controlled and individually adapted to the clients.

PNES Coaching is a controlled and planned concept based on various "pillars" (phases), in which different approaches, methods, or interdisciplinary insights are implemented to ensure individual interventions and coping strategies. Depending on what the goal of the respective pillar is, or what is needed to achieve the goal of the respective pillar, the scientifically empirically proven, most effective methods from various therapy schools and counseling approaches are linked together. Since the various methods and approaches are applied in different pillars (phases) of the coaching, compatibility of the different orientations is ensured. This means that the counseling approaches and forms of intervention explained in this book can be individually adapted and applied to the clients in this concept. Insights from psychoneuroendocrinology and related behavioral genetic insights are specifically implemented in the various pillars or phases of the coaching. This coaching approach is intended to follow the premise that individual people and individual problems and experiences also require individual tools. This, in turn, means for the counselors/therapists to definitely acquire a "toolbox." The individually adapted tools are further linked with the psychoneuroendocrinological insights. Even though the tools can be freely chosen by the psychosocial counselors and psychotherapists, the maxims of person-centered, life-world and biography-oriented, cooperative, and resource-oriented approaches must be anchored in this eclectic-integrative counseling approach, otherwise, the concept is not feasible.

Person-Centered or Client-Centered Approach This approach is based on Carl Rogers. The design of the relationship is considered a decisive factor for changes.

The approach is based at the interface of person and environment (life or work world) and assumes that individual behavior is triggered by the organism to satisfy its needs. This approach is therefore person-centered, holistic, and context-bound. Individual resources and social competencies are activated.

The **cooperative counseling approach** is a non-instructive approach in which clients and counselors/therapists are considered equal. A cooperative and understanding interaction is formed. The development of the clients' activity is promoted and supported. Impulses and assistance are given, but no advice is provided; instead, solutions to problems are sought together and worked on for implementation. Cooperative counseling is characterized by client-centered, resource-oriented, and systematic communication as well as a trusting, accepting, empathetic, and congruent relationship between counselors/therapists and clients.

PNES Coaching requires openness to interdisciplinarity, biopsychosocial concepts, and multimodal therapy forms. However, the most important foundation of PNES Coaching is a good relationship or successful alliance between counselors/therapists and clients/patients.

I have named the concept "PNES Coaching" because it carries the most significant abbreviations of this concept in its name: **P-Psycho; N-Neuro; E-Endocrinology; S-Social.** The term coaching is appropriate because the clients are "coached" by the counselors/therapists to make use of the knowledge about hormones in psychosocial everyday life, in difficult and challenging life situations, or to explain the connection between hormones and mental disorders. This biopsychosocial coaching approach can be used both for mentally healthy individuals and for people with mental disorders, in various crisis situations, in psychosocial everyday life, to maintain mental health, but also to improve mood. It is important to mention that there is no "promise of healing," but the goal of this coaching is to facilitate psychosocial everyday life or to promote coping with life, to promote emotional control, to strengthen resilience, to positively influence mood, and general well-being, as well as to support individual goal achievement. It is a biopsychosocial coaching that specifically uses psychoneuroendocrinological insights.

The concept consists of 13 pillars, which do not run linearly, with the pillars or phases being implemented partially simultaneously and can also be individually adapted to the clients' problem situations. The following will now explain these pillars or phases of PNES coaching.

4.2.1 "PNES Coaching": The 13 Pillars

As already mentioned, the biopsychosocial coaching approach is based on 13 pillars that represent the phases or steps of the coaching. The course of the coaching or the implementation of these pillars does not always proceed in the same way, as the counselors/psychotherapists must individually adapt the course of the coaching to the clients. The psychological stability, illnesses, psychological disorders, or even an initial reticence of the clients must be taken into account in the approach or implementation of the pillars. The following will explain the 13 pillars and reinforce them with some facts from the previous chapters; practical tips will be highlighted.

► **Biopsychosocial Diagnostics**

At the beginning of the coaching, there is a biopsychosocial diagnostic. This is of enormous importance for the further work or the entire coaching approach.

> **Biopsychosocial Diagnostics** Biological, psychological, and social factors are analyzed, and their interactions are observed. The concept of **biopsychosocial diagnostics** makes it possible to closely observe, analyze, and explain the problem constellations of the clients. Physiological and psychological disorders are recorded, as well as crises, conflicts, and stresses, and also the resources and motivation of the clients. The interactions between body, psyche, and social situation are analyzed on different system levels of the clients.

Thyroid findings, a general hormone profile, and other blood findings, for example, to determine possible deficiencies and diseases as well as inflammation values, are relevant here. Since nutrients or vitamins are needed as co-factors in hormone synthesis, corresponding blood tests are important. Findings and information on diseases, psychiatric reports, and information on medication intake are also of importance.

► It is advisable to cooperate with an endocrinologist to refer clients/patients if necessary. The endocrinologist should be informed about this coaching. Based on this background knowledge, he/she can then create the findings and order specific examinations.

It should also be decided based on the results of the biopsychosocial diagnostics whether the client might need additional (medical/psychiatric/therapeutic) assistance or should be recommended to them. Cooperation with psychiatrists and experts in various psychological disorders is also advantageous. In this pillar, it is already evident that a willingness for interdisciplinary cooperation must be present to successfully apply this coaching approach.

Psychoeducation

Psychoeducation is also at the beginning of the coaching. This concept is based on the clients implementing or integrating what they have learned in coaching into their everyday lives. For this, it is important that the clients are simply and understandably explained what hormones are, how they work, and what role they play in connection with their psyche, behavior, experiences, and environmental influences.

> It is important to mention here that the clients should not be cognitively overwhelmed and that the entire psychoneuroendocrinology should be taught to them. It is advisable to adopt a simple explanatory form for the clients: What are hormones? How are they related to psyche/behavior? Simple, practical examples can be helpful here.

Without an understanding of the importance of hormones, the implementation of the coaching will be difficult, and the motivation might not be sufficient to implement the learned things into life management. It is comparable to a diet and a change in diet. If I only implement this concept for a short time or only deal with it once a week in counseling/therapy, the successes will neither be long-term nor profound. Therefore, the implementation of this coaching approach is more comparable to a change in diet than to a diet.

> The clients are informed and educated about hormones and their connections to their problems. Depending on the reason for the counseling/therapy, the education takes place to varying degrees. In the case of a psychological disorder, it is important for the success of the therapy that the clients not only understand their illness but also the psychoneuroendocrinological connections of their disease well.

Especially for patients/clients with psychological disorders, I recommend detailed and interactive psychoeducation that includes guidance on self-observation. They should pay attention to their psychosocial everyday life and experiences, their activities, their moods/mood swings, and triggers, as well as their sleep-wake rhythm.

To sustainably benefit from this coaching approach, both in crisis and stress situations and to maintain psychological and psychosocial health or as resilience training, it is important to implement the insights of this approach into the psychosocial everyday life. Psychoeducation is to be regarded as the foundation for this. An understanding on the part of the clients promotes both the quality of implementation in the psychosocial everyday life and the motivation to implement and apply the interactive part of this coaching approach.

▶ "Alliance": the Relationship Level between Counselor/Therapist and Client

The relationship between psychosocial counselors/psychotherapists and clients is, as mentioned several times in this book, of enormous importance. The effectiveness of the alliance is empirically proven (neurobiologically as well as psychoneuroendocrinologically).

Alliance The effectiveness of psychological/psychosocial counseling and psychotherapeutic orientations has been extensively studied. Research has shown that only a good counselor/therapist-client relationship (alliance) has consistently shown an effect. Any success of psychological or psychosocial counseling/psychotherapy is based on this. The most skillful use of methods is not effective if there is no relationship characterized by trust and positive collaboration between clients and counselors/therapists. Alliance enables approaching problem-solving without fear and with confidence.

A trusting relationship not only means that the client fully opens up, but it can also lead to the release of oxytocin.

If the relationship is trusting enough, the client finds the sessions pleasant, feels secure, safe, and comfortable within the setting, they benefit from a tremendously important hormone release. OXY, as already mentioned, is significant for clients in extreme stress situations, anxiety, psychological trauma, or depressive moods. To promote the relationship level, the realization of the basic variables according to Rogers and the associated conversation techniques can be seen as guidelines.

The **realization of the basic variables** according to Rogers: These basic variables according to Rogers are considered classic characteristics of a supportive counselor/therapist-client relationship.

1) **Empathy:** Counselors/therapists have a fundamentally sensitive attitude and possess the ability to empathize with clients (thoughts, feelings, worldview). It requires the effort to understand clients in their world and to comprehend their actions.
2) **Warmth or acceptance:** Clients are respected and valued. It means showing them positive regard and conveying to them that they are taken seriously. Unconditional positive regard provides security, enables openness, and can prevent the development of fears. This attitude can enable the restructuring of cognitions, emotions, and actions.

3) **Genuineness or authenticity:** This means unadulterated authentic communication. An attitude that is self-honest and where actions match emotions. Counselors/therapists show an open and direct approach, which in turn allows clients to reveal real emotions and cognitions without fear.

As research has repeatedly empirically proven, even in biopsychosocial coaching like PNES coaching, a good alliance is the foundation.

The "Gene Compass"

As already extensively explained in this book, genetic individuality can be stimulated and altered by environmental influences and learning. Furthermore, physiological reactions and behaviors as well as physical and psychological illnesses can be based on a combination of gene configurations and environmental influences. Behavior is therefore always attributable to the interplay of genes and environmental influences or environmental factors. Environmental factors to be mentioned and causes of significant or targeted questions within this pillar include, for example, intrauterine factors (such as prenatal stress), nutrition, parenting style, peer attachment, accidents and illnesses, traumatic experiences (such as abuse, war experiences, assaults, etc.), chronic stress, and climate.

Gene-environment interaction Environmental factors or influences from the surroundings can influence our genetic potential. This can lead to an enhancement of realization.

The so-called Gene Compass is to be seen as a method that can function as a diagnostic tool to identify suitable individual interventions and acute tools. With targeted questions (see PNES coaching, Gene Compass - documentation sheet in the appendix), more individualized and targeted coping strategies and help plans can be created. This does not mean that this method corresponds to a diagnosis in which the exact polymorphisms of the clients are revealed, but rather, as the name Gene Compass already suggests, this method shows a direction to individually suitable interventions, coping strategies, and acute tools through the combination of behavioral genetic-epigenetic findings with the knowledge of counselors/psychotherapists about gene-environment interaction.

To make this method more understandable, an example is provided below, which is also explained in Chap. 2 ("Psychoneuroendocrinology").

Example: Oxytocin as an Intervention

Oxytocin (OXY) or the effect of oxytocin and how it can vary depending on genotype or depending on gene-environment interactions and experiences is well suited as an example here.

As already mentioned in Chap. 2 ("Psychoneuroendocrinology"), the effect of OXY does not positively influence all people equally, which is why oxytocin release cannot be considered a suitable acute tool for all clients, as early negative experiences can also weaken the effect of OXY. In particular, early childhood contact/relationship/bonding with the mother and father as well as possible abuse have an enormous influence on oxytocin function, oxytocin secretion, and the significant oxytocin concentration in cerebrospinal fluid.

- **Example 1: OXY and the A/A Genotype**
  - The A/A genotype is associated with lower levels of prosociality, empathy, trust, positive affect, optimism, mastery, and self-esteem.
  - This genotype is more sensitive to stress and has difficulty understanding other people against a background of noise.
  - A/A genotypes are less likely to seek social support in stressful situations (which would lead to OXY release), and their stress response is not inhibited by social interaction (OXY release).
  - Mothers with this gene tend to respond less empathetically to their infant.
  - It seems that these mothers are less sensitive to messages from the baby. This shows a lower physiological reactivity in response to the baby's crying.
  - However, it should be mentioned that the A allele can produce resilience to the effects of early negative experiences.
- **Example 2: OXY and the G/G Genotype**
  - People with the G allele benefit from social support from their partner in stressful situations.
  - Furthermore, they exhibit only low subjective stress sensitivity and lower cortisol release in response to stress.
  - The G allele could be a genetic variant that is more affected by the effects of environmental influences.
  - They also have a greater risk of developing emotional dysregulation and a disorganized attachment representation as a result of child abuse.

(Several examples of this can be found in Chap. 2 "Psychoneuroendocrinology".)

To obtain information about the clients that is valuable for the gene compass, a good alliance and professional conversation techniques are indispensable.

▶ As already mentioned in the "Alliance" pillar, I also recommend here the conversation approach of Carl Rogers. Based on the person-centered and motivational interviewing according to Rogers, the counselors/therapists not only obtain information relevant for a biopsychosocial diagnosis, but this conversation approach also functions as an intervention and strengthens the alliance between counselors/therapists and clients.

Once again, the enormous importance of the perinatal phase of the mother, early childhood experiences, and the (early childhood) bond with the mother/caregiver should be mentioned with this method. The gene-environment interaction must be present, meaning the clients must have had triggering experiences. Based on this method or with this knowledge about the clients, one can determine which targeted hormonal influences would particularly benefit the affected clients (for example, increased OXY release). It is also important to mention here that heritability is only one factor and that humans can indeed influence their genetics.

The "gene compass" method is based on a biography-oriented counseling approach, as, as frequently mentioned in previous chapters, the gene-environment interaction or biographical influences (experiences) are important. Furthermore, it is important to note here that if the clients have early childhood experiences associated with (complex) trauma, it is of enormous importance that the clients are psychologically stable enough and that the psychosocial counselors/psychotherapists are familiar with trauma counseling/trauma therapy and related methods. If this is not the case, I recommend that counselors/therapists cooperate with a trauma counselor/trauma therapist.

▶ If psychosocial counselors/psychotherapists detect resistance from clients to those diagnostic questions, especially questions about early childhood experiences and questions concerning parents, I recommend skipping this method/pillar (for now) and focusing on the psychological stability and resilience of the affected individuals in the coaching.

You can see what a documentation sheet for the gene compass might look like in the appendix.

▶ Psychoneuronal Basic Systems

It is also advisable to implement the findings about the psychoneuronal basic systems into psychosocial and psychotherapeutic practice. Questions about the psychoneuronal systems can, for example, function as diagnostic tools. Are the client's anxiety states based on a disturbed development of the stress processing system? Or does the client not complete any training because he/she has a disorder in the evaluation and reward system? Is the calming system impaired? These are just some of the issues that can be clarified here.

Psychoneuronal Basic Systems

The psychoneuronal basic systems are the stress processing system, the internal calming system, the internal evaluation and reward system, the impulse inhibition system, the attachment system, the system of reality sense and risk assessment.

All 6 psychoneuronal systems consist, to varying degrees, of innate reactions and temperament traits, emotional conditioning, socialization, as well as the level of cognitive-rational behavior. The levels are shaped by early childhood experiences with the mother and primary caregivers, as well as social experiences with family members and peers in school and kindergarten. The development of these systems influences our personality, our behavior and our psyche, our actions and our resilience.

These levels can be implemented into coaching as follows:

1) The stress processing system
How stress-resistant is the client? How quickly can excitement be dampened? How well can the stress management system handle physical and psychological stress?

2) The internal calming system
How quickly is a stress reaction dampened? How quickly does the client return to a state of calm?

3) The internal evaluation and reward system
By what motives and reasons is the client's behavior determined? What reward and punishment expectations does he/she have? How does he/she deal with reward delay? Does he/she prefer immediate reward instead of delay with the prospect of something greater (e.g., sweets now instead of optimal body weight later)?

4) The impulse inhibition system
How quickly does the client become aggressive/impulsive? To what extent is he/she able to actively control his/her impulses? To what extent does the client perceive his/her environment as threatening?

5) The attachment system
To what extent does the client long for closeness? Is something preventing him/her from emotionally engaging with other people? Can the client approach others?

6) The system of reality sense and risk assessment
To what extent is the client able to assess a risk or the negative consequences of a behavior? Does the individual have a pronounced sense of reality and good risk assessment?

Does the client ignore the consequences of a risk or are they underestimated? Is the client willing to fail?

Based on the insights that the counselor/therapist gains through this pillar, he/she can not only select individual forms of intervention but can also determine which hormone releases would be particularly valuable for the client.

> ▶ It should be mentioned here that a current hormone level is important to be able to detect a deficiency, for example, and to react appropriately!

Example: Stress Processing System—Anxiety—GABA If an impairment of the stress processing system leads to anxiety states, for example, GABA can be a suitable support.

Example: Internal Calming System—Return to Calm Mode—Serotonin and OXY In situations of social interaction, the release of serotonin and OXY dampens the mood again.

Example: Internal Evaluation and Reward System—Reward—Dopamine and Endogenous Opioids In the case of rewards, the system is also connected with the release of endogenous opioids.

Example: Impulse Inhibition System—Impulsive Actions—Dopamine and Serotonin Impulsive actions are connected with the dopamine and serotonin system. High impulsivity leads to a high dopamine level, extraversion, and high risk-taking. Reactive impulsivity leads to constant distress or fear. Here, the challenge is to distinguish between threatening and non-threatening.

Example: Attachment System—Inhibition of the Stress System—Oxytocin and Serotonin The attachment system develops in the first weeks after birth. For the attachment system, oxytocin (OXY) is particularly relevant. An increased release inhibits the stress system, and serotonin release is enhanced.

Example: Sense of Reality and Risk Assessment—Realistically Assessing Risks—Noradrenaline and Acetylcholine The competence to realistically assess risks is associated with noradrenaline (NA) and acetylcholine. Noradrenaline increases attention and focus, while acetylcholine enhances concentration and the targeted retrieval of memory contents.

Additionally, in this pillar, gene-environment interaction and related questions are also significant. Through various previously mentioned conversation techniques, much can be learned about the individual psychoneuronal basic systems of the clients. This method, when applying an appropriate conversation technique, should not merely be seen as a diagnostic tool but can also already be a significant intervention. As with every pillar or phase in this concept, the emotional level must never be neglected; not overwhelming the clients with cognitive knowledge, and the foundation, a good alliance, are indispensable.

For long-term success, it is important that clients implement exercises, homework, and transfer tasks into their daily lives. Appropriate behaviors must first be deepened/practiced in everyday life. If neuronal networks are involved in a problem, it cannot be "overwritten" in a short time, and the clients would soon fall back into an old pattern. Additionally, it must always be distinguished whether it is about minor stressors/small impairments or (severe) psychological disorders.

The insights into the individual characteristics or impairments of the psychoneuronal basic systems lead to a multidimensional or multimodal psychosocial/psychotherapeutic work, where it is especially important to have a diverse repertoire of tools/intervention forms.

▶ **Vulnerability Factors**

Vulnerability factors also play a significant role in this biopsychosocial coaching approach. The individual vulnerability of the clients is of enormous importance. The factors must be identified, especially if the clients themselves (still) do not know exactly what they are. Here, too, a biographical approach is recommended, and life-world-oriented principles are, in my view, indispensable.

A **biographical approach** creates opportunities for reflection as well as the exchange of individual experiences and events. With the perspective of turning problems into opportunities, various individual future concepts can be developed for the clients.

Working in a life-world-oriented manner means addressing people's problems and working together towards a successful life. The problems and difficulties of everyday life are illuminated. Self-help possibilities are focused on, and living environments are strengthened to optimize everyday coping.

Depending on the psychological stability or instability of the clients, meaning if there is no or only low resilience, it is important at the beginning of the coaching to rather avoid those vulnerability factors and jointly analyze protective factors. Here, psychological as well as social protective factors are particularly important. Initially, clients should learn to deal with the positive influences of hormones and learn to use them purposefully or even recognize that one can influence hormones. This primarily means many positive hormone releases that strengthen the clients and build psychological stability, and then gradually train resilience (see pillar: resilience training).

The results of the gene compass and the knowledge about the individually pronounced psychoneuronal basic system levels provide the foundation to "use" the appropriate or needed hormones as protective factors. The aim is to show the clients their individual protective factors and teach them how to apply or use their protective factors. The goal of this coaching is, based on the idea of the empowerment approach, that the clients can consciously react to all individual vulnerability factors. They should be able to use the influence of hormones, what lifts their mood, promotes their general well-being, or calms them, specifically in crisis situations. This means, for example, being able to calm themselves during a panic attack or lack of self-control, or to create a stress balance through the release of the individually needed hormones and to be aware of their individual protective factors.

In general, it should be mentioned here that homeostasis, i.e., a balance of hormone balance, serves as a protective factor. The body can thus react adequately in crisis situations. Regarding vulnerability factors and their frequent occurrence, it is particularly valuable for clients if they can specifically influence the release of the so-called "happiness hormones."

"Happiness Hormones": The so-called happiness hormones are scientifically undisputedly involved in the regulation of our mental-emotional balance. Various emotions, our basic psychological mood, and our psychological well-being are inevitably linked to our hormone levels. Examples are: serotonin, dopamine, GABA, and oxytocin.

When identifying vulnerability factors, the social aspects or the social network of the clients must not be overlooked. Stress or stress complaints, for example, are also based on interaction with the social environment, societal pressure, or professional difficulties. These stress or stress complaints can lead to disturbances in both psychological and physical functions.

▶ Vulnerability factors can be associated with psychological, health, and social factors. Genetics, personality, cultural, and societal aspects are also linked to them. Vulnerability factors trigger and maintain complaints, which is why it is important to identify these factors.

However, avoiding vulnerability factors alone does not lead to reduced vulnerability. Building resilience is essential to achieve sustainable positive effects on mental and physical functions.

▶ **Resilience Training**

The entire coaching should be seen as resilience training because resilience means being resistant to stress and crises, and each of these steps or pillars of this coaching contributes to that. Here, the resilience or the resilience and stability of the clients are examined and trained.

▶ It is important to know the individually different factors that lead to stress in the client in order to specifically increase stress resilience.

Of particular importance for promoting resilience are: strengthening self-esteem, training mindfulness, consciously allowing recovery times, internalizing positive beliefs, strengthening perception or self-perception, promoting self-acceptance, engaging in sports and exercise (movement therapy) in an individually appropriate scope and with regular breaks.

It is important to explain to clients the goal of adequately dealing with distress (negative, threatening, or overwhelming stress, prolonged or chronic stress). It is important to offer exercises that are easy to implement in practice and resource-oriented. It is important that clients understand that the stress processing system is a firmly anchored system and is not merely judged according to the norms of the psychosocial counselor or psychotherapist.

Additionally, as mentioned, it is important to pay attention to a good hormone balance and the release of hormones that have a positive effect on the psyche, especially in difficult life phases.

Serotonin An adequate amount of serotonin contributes to our mental well-being, our mental health, and a positive and balanced basic mood. Additionally, serotonin influences our social behavior, nerve signal transmission, and our feeling of satiety. A lack of serotonin can be associated with depression, anxiety, tension, and inner restlessness, aggressive moods, sleep disorders, cognitive performance problems, chronic headaches and migraines, chronic muscle pain, and disturbances in the feeling of satiety. A serotonin deficiency also physically affects the regulation of the cardiovascular system, the blood flow to the skeletal muscles and organs, and the nervous system of the intestines. Serotonin must be produced by the body itself, with the starting material for the body's own serotonin synthesis being the amino acid L-tryptophan, which is supplied through food (more details in the pillar "Nutrition": Significant starting materials and co-factors).

Dopamine The neurotransmitter dopamine is particularly associated with the "reward effect" and conveys positive feelings. Dopamine also promotes motivation and energy. It has a significant function in cognitive performance, and it is the precursor of the neurotransmitters norepinephrine and adrenaline, which are considered to increase drive. Since the consumption of dopamine and norepinephrine increases in stressful situations in healthy people, it is important to ensure adequate dopamine production. The body synthesizes dopamine from the amino acid L-tyrosine, which is ingested through food (more details in the pillar "Nutrition": Significant starting materials and co-factors). The amino acid L-tyrosine is therefore particularly used to restore stress resilience (for example, after burnout) or in particularly stressful situations.

GABA A lack of GABA causes inner restlessness, anxiety, and it promotes depression. A balanced GABA level balances out insecurities and feelings of anxiety and ensures natural relaxation. GABA is considered the body's natural tranquilizer. It reduces anxiety, aggression, and irritability, wandering thoughts, and inner tensions, calming and relaxing the body and mind. Thus, GABA strengthens the psyche and naturally reduces anxiety and inner restlessness. The starting material for the body's own GABA synthesis is the amino acid L-glutamine, which is ingested through food (more details in the pillar "Nutrition": Significant starting materials and co-factors).

Oxytocin Oxytocin is the so-called bonding hormone. It plays a role in the mother-child relationship, in couple relationships, sexual behavior, and trusting close social contacts. An increased release of the hormone inhibits the stress system and enhances serotonin release. Oxytocin strengthens the ability to recognize social and emotional signals, supports social motivation, and reduces feelings of anxiety. It has positive effects on all kinds of social emotions and behaviors. It promotes trust, empathy, and social contacts. Oxytocin is particularly important in children/infants (breastfeeding/trusted interaction). It is released in relationships with strong bonds, i.e., in partnerships and social interactions with friends. The effect of oxytocin often coincides with the release of endogenous opioids. For example, a trusting couple relationship, physical contact (hugs, cuddling, etc.), and close social contacts can specifically trigger the release of oxytocin.

Endogenous Opioids They have different functions and effects depending on their site of action. For example, if they act in the hypothalamus and limbic system, they reduce stress through induced isolation. If they act in the ventral tegmentum and striatum, they cause euphoria and regulate locomotor behavior.

When clients have achieved a certain level of psychological stability during the course of coaching and have internalized the use of acute tools or the targeted use of hormones that are positive for the psyche, they should be gradually motivated to cope with more/larger stress situations.

▶ **No stress is also not healthy!**

Here, I refer to Birbaumer's and Schmidt's approach as the basis for the "advanced training," namely that no stress at all is also not healthy. This means that when clients are psychologically stable and can use endogenous hormones in a targeted or conscious manner, the stress level and the associated cortisol secretion can be increased step by step. In this pillar or phase, stress resilience should be trained. This means gradually subjecting clients to more stress and teaching them to deal with increasing (natural/everyday) stress situations, thereby adequately increasing stress resilience. It is important that clients feel comfortable with each step.

▶ Here, it can be beneficial to keep a—I call it a **"sunshine diary"**. This diary does not document factors that went poorly, were difficult, or stressful, but rather records: What did I do well? What did I accomplish today? What am I grateful for? If clients are not feeling well or have not immediately achieved an individual goal, they can read this "sunshine diary" to remind themselves of what they have already managed and achieved. Photos of beautiful memories also have a positive hormone release effect when viewed.

▶ **Social Resource Activation and Bonding**

The "social" aspect is so important in this biopsychosocial coaching approach that the letter "S" appears in the name of the coaching. Why? Not only because relevant hormones are released through social interactions, which can be significant in any crisis situation, but also because regular social contacts should be integrated for the successful, sustainable implementation of this approach. These should not merely be life partners/spouses whom one sees daily at home, but also, for example, parents/relatives and good friends. Social contacts are considered resources because they may be needed for the implementation of various ideas or individual protective factors. Additionally, hormone secretions occur during social interactions.

Social Interactions that Trigger Hormone Secretions Close skin contact, hugging, spending time together ("feeling secure"), laughing, cuddling, kissing, sexual activities, communication (mutual exchange), etc.

It is important to mention that, although positive hormones are generally released through friends and social interactions, there are always individual exceptions, and some people avoid social contacts in every respect, feel uncomfortable, or even experience aggressive emotions during social interactions. For these clients, it is important not to push them, as the desired positive hormone secretion will not occur and may even have the opposite effect. Therefore, intervention forms or methods must be individually tailored for the clients, and a plan must be created to achieve the necessary hormone releases. However, it is important to make clients aware of the benefits of social resources and to work with them on their social interactions and social competence. For this, it is crucial to have sufficient biopsychosocial information (insufficient social competence can also be due to pathophysiological causes) about the clients. Additionally, detailed psychosocial diagnostics, such as resource diagnostics and network maps, are beneficial.

Resource Diagnostics To achieve resource activation, a resource diagnosis is first needed. Only this diagnosis enables a methodologically sound case conception, which is indispensable for this approach. The individual resources of the clients are the foundation of successful everyday and life management. Additionally, the usable resources promote the psychological and physical health as well as the general well-being of the clients. Important are: personal/intrapersonal resources (e.g., physical and psychological resources, inter- and intrapersonal resources, economic [personal] resources), environmental/external resources (e.g., psychosocial, social, and cultural resources, as well as social state and legal, physical-technical, and natural aids in the individuals' environment). To identify these resources, there are various resource procedures, as explained in detail in Chap. 3.

Network Map It is a diagnostic tool that records the social relationships of the clients. Relationship contexts and structures are integrated into the analysis. The focus is on recognizing relationship patterns. Friends and acquaintances, family, school, and/or professional/occupational relationships are important.

The goal is for clients to have a functioning bonding system and a social network from which their resilience and psychological stability also benefit. These do not have to be parents or life partners; they can also be individual reference persons. But social, stable resources are of enormous relevance for long-term success.

▶ The **activation of social resources** is a proven and sustainable concept in psychosocial fields of action. Especially in crisis situations/difficult life phases, it is important to consciously activate social resources or to be able to use them in a targeted manner. Often, it is a learning process for clients to be able to use/accept an already stable social network or bonding system for themselves. For PNES coaching, it is also important to be able to accept support and help from the social network and, beyond that, to specifically utilize the positive hormone secretions that social resources can trigger. Social resources include both socio-emotional relationship resources as well as contacts, relationships, and social integration in extended networks. Especially for adolescents and clients who are very active on social media, it is also important not to overlook online networks.

The various methods of resource diagnostics can be used not only as diagnostic tools but also as forms of intervention.

▶ **The "Indie Flower"**

In this pillar or method, the solution-oriented approach, the resource-oriented approach, and the systemic approach are particularly reflected.

The solution-oriented approach The problem-relevant context is not focused on; instead, a change of perspective is sought to move from the problem to the non-problem. Solution-oriented cognitions and perceptions as well as solution-oriented actions are strengthened, thereby promoting the solution.

The resource-oriented approach The strengths and potentials of the clients are focused on. The interactions of individual strengths and forces as well as resources based on social networks are of importance. The empowerment approach is guiding.

The solution is constructed based on individual and intrapersonal resources. The implementation of the Indie Flower means change. It can be seen as a plan with which the lives and everyday routines of the clients are intervened in or a self-dynamic change process is initiated. Additionally, the systemic approach is clearly evident in the "Indie Flower".

The systemic approach In the systemic approach, the focus is on the disturbance and deconstruction within the system, as well as the intertwined behavior and relationship patterns and beliefs, together with the system. More positive solutions, patterns, and constructs within the system are to be explored.

With this system, a change of perspective and (in many cases) a change of priorities is sought to strengthen biopsychosocial health and to facilitate individual well-being and everyday life or life management. It is an activity build-up that promotes the collection of positive and mood-enhancing experiences (based on hormone secretions). Solution-oriented actions are thus consciously intertwined with the power of endogenous hormones.

▶ Here, I recommend designing their "Indie Flower" (individual flower) together with the clients and creating a plan with them ("What do you need for this?") on how they can manage to transfer the "Indie Flower" into their everyday life. Using conversation techniques and adequate psychoeducation, the motivation of the clients can be promoted.

The flower can be seen as a visualized symbol to make clear what a flower (the client) needs to bloom. Additionally, each petal is a system in itself, but only all systems together form a complete, blooming flower. Together with the clients, those things (resources, protective factors, activities) that have a positive impact on the biopsychosocial health, resilience, and everyday management of the clients in stressful or burdensome life situations are worked out. These can be individually different things, such as artistic hobbies, music, sports and exercise, nature, social contacts, and much more; everything that brings joy to the clients and strengthens them or promotes their coping represents a petal (Fig. 4.1).

Operationalized goals are created and worked out, determining when and how they are feasible. This created flower should be hung up at the clients' homes (in a place where it is seen as often as possible). Hanging up the flower serves as a reminder; the poster should remain hung until the goals are achieved or the implementation of the recorded activities, resources, and protective factors are firmly integrated into everyday life and life management/life design. The goal is to create an individual and sustainable toolbox for the clients to use at home.

▶ Especially for adolescents, it can be helpful if the flower is not only hung up at home but also digitized and, for example, saved on the phone. Adolescents also like to save goals and reminders on their phones.

What helps me when I feel bad? What do I need regularly to maintain/improve my biopsychosocial health?

Examples of the Indie Flower Bonding/partnership/caregiver, security/safety/home/safe place, social interactions/friends, mindfulness-based methods, sports/exercise, music, art, sexual activities, healthy nutrition, sleep, pets, hobbies, nature...

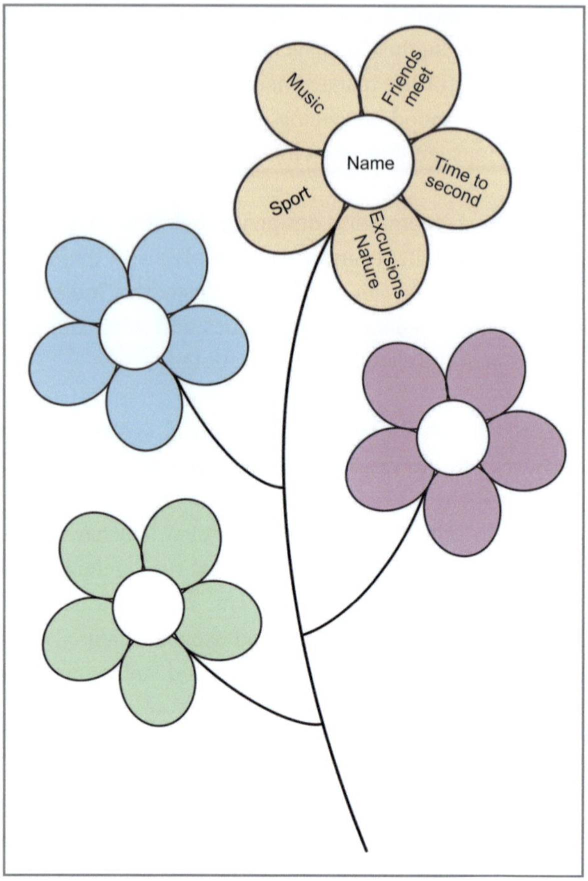

Fig. 4.1 Example Indie Flower: In each petal, individual activities, resources, protective factors, and plans for implementation are entered

▶ Sleep-Wake Rhythm

The findings presented in this book show that healthy sleep is indispensable for a functional immune system, good immune competence, and mental health.

> **Sleep-Wake Rhythm** Healthy, regular sleep is indispensable for both physical and mental health. Therefore, a healthy person sleeps at least once in 24 hours. The average sleep duration is 5–10 hours, with 8 hours being the recommended duration.

Sleep disorders inevitably lead to a change in the immune system, reduced immune competence, as well as a negative impact on mental disorders, increased pain sensitivity, and many other organic and functional diseases. It is not only important to take a nap of 1–2 hours in the afternoon after sleepless nights to lower the IL-6 level, but also to adhere to sleep hygiene and pharmacological recommendations. Additionally, mindfulness-based methods and Tai Chi have a positive effect on sleep. Interventions for healthy sleep are indispensable to promote and maintain both physiological and psychological health.

Hormones in Sleep The endocrine systems are indispensable for regular sleep, which in turn is indispensable for the immune system. Many endocrine systems show higher activity during sleep, such as growth hormone (GH, "growth hormone"), as well as melatonin, prolactin, catecholamines, and cortisol. The task of sleep is to stimulate endocrine processes that cannot be triggered during the day. By changing the sleep rhythm or getting too little sleep, both physiological and psychological regulatory processes and the immune system are affected. Since sleep regulates endocrine and immunological processes, it is understandable why sleep deprivation can have life-threatening to fatal consequences.

Melatonin Melatonin is considered the actual timekeeper for sleep. It is released in the dark (light suppresses melatonin secretion). About 2 hours after the onset of melatonin production, a person feels an increase in sleepiness. The peak of melatonin production is reached in the middle of the night, and the level drops again towards morning. A deficiency in melatonin can lead to sleep disorders and mental health issues. An overproduction can, for example, lead to jet lag. Externally supplied melatonin shortens the time to fall asleep and induces sleepiness and can reduce stress effects.

Sleep is therefore a very important pillar of this program. Sleep is not only indispensable for maintaining physiological health but also essential for our mental health. Sleep is particularly relevant for our stress processing system. The hormones released during sleep are of enormous importance for both our physiological and mental health.

Sleep is connected to our mental well-being, resilience, and overall behavior. Therefore, from the beginning of the coaching, there is a focus on sufficient (also pre-midnight) sleep, which should average 8 hours. If clients have sleep problems, the cause must be clarified and initially addressed with various proven training, methods, nutrition, sports, and similar approaches to achieve natural sleep without medication.

L-Tryptophan Tryptophan can promote natural and healthy hormone secretion during sleep. L-Tryptophan can be supplied to the body through diet or as a dietary supplement, which is biosynthesized into serotonin and then into melatonin, which is particularly important for the core sleep phase.

Furthermore, sleep protocols are recommended. Sleep-wake activity should be documented for at least one week with additional notes on behavior, daily routine, or anything unusual. This is helpful to identify causes of sleep disorders and find individual interventions for healthy sleep.

▶ Nutrition: Important Precursors and Co-Factors

In the section "Happiness Hormones and the Importance of Precursors and Co-Factors," it was already explained how enormously important nutrition, sufficient intake of precursors and co-factors, and a healthy gut are for hormone synthesis and both mental and physiological health and well-being. With appropriate nutrition that particularly considers precursors and co-factors, one can support hormone synthesis.

> So-called **co-factors** (micronutrients) are essential for our hormone synthesis. For the body to carry out the synthesis steps, it needs vitamins, minerals, and trace elements. Significant co-factors include B vitamins, magnesium, zinc, and vitamin D. If the body has an insufficient amount of co-factors or a nutrient deficiency, this also affects the formation of serotonin, dopamine, and GABA, which are of enormous importance for human psyche. Studies have shown a correlation between vitamin B_6 and the severity of depression.

This pillar focuses on the systemic connection between our diet and our mental and physical well-being. As starting materials for hormone synthesis, amino acids are of enormous importance, as most hormones are composed of amino acid chains.

> **Starting materials** Starting materials are supplied with food. In connection with the co-factors, hormones can then be formed in the respective synthesis steps. For example, the amino acid L-tryptophan is the starting material for the body's own serotonin synthesis.

From the amino acid tryptophan, the hormones serotonin and melatonin are formed in the absence of light stimuli (tryptophan → serotonin → melatonin), which regulate the circadian rhythm. In addition, melatonin is important for maintaining homeostasis (i.e., balance or hormone balance) to prevent or counteract deficiencies in the body.

Tryptophan → 5-HTP → Serotonin → Melatonin

Starting material: L-tryptophan in 5-HTP

Co-factors: Vitamin B_3, B_6, magnesium, and zinc

People with depression often have a reduced tryptophan plasma level. Supplementation with tryptophan leads to an increase in positive emotions. It also positively influences memory and leads to an improvement in resilience to negative moods and depressive episodes. It also improves sleep quality, extends sleep duration, and leads to increased cognitive performance in the morning. The significant effect of 5-HTP has also been demonstrated in various studies, for example, in depression, insomnia, eating disorders, and chronic headaches.

The amino acid L-tyrosine is converted into catecholamines (tyrosine → dopamine → norepinephrine → adrenaline), which then serve as both hormones and transmitters.

L-TYROSINE → L-DOPA → DOPAMINE

Starting material: L-tyrosine

Co-factors: Vitamin B_6, zinc, vitamin D

Studies show that increased stress conditions lead to changes in dopamine metabolism. Particularly due to post-traumatic stress disorders and addiction diseases, but also in healthy people, the consumption of catecholamines increases in stressful situations. This reduces cognitive performance and mood. Supplementation with L-tyrosine can stimulate dopamine production again.

In addition, L-glutamine (L-glutamine → glutamate → GABA) is an important starting material. The neurotransmitter GABA, which is formed from the starting material L-glutamine, is an important calming neurotransmitter that has a balancing effect and promotes stress reduction. The body forms glutamate from the starting material L-glutamine with the required co-factor vitamin B_6, from which GABA is then formed.

L-GLUTAMINE → GLUTAMATE → GABA

Starting material: L-glutamine

Co-factor: Vitamin B_6

Glutamate is a stimulating-exciting neurotransmitter (beware of glutamate-containing foods!). With a vitamin B_6 deficiency, more glutamate and less GABA are produced. This disrupts the natural hormone balance and leads to less relaxation and more excitement.

Promoting a nutrient- and vitamin-rich diet for clients is therefore of considerable importance in this biopsychosocial coaching approach. Nutrition provides us with nutrients that are synthesized into hormones. With balanced hormone synthesis, one can influence their mental and physical health as well as their behavior. The goal of this pillar is for clients to understand that nutrition is not only valuable for physical fitness, appearance, or the immune system but also for sleep, mental state, behavior, and our hormone balance, which in turn is linked to mental and physical well-being. It is therefore essential in a biopsychosocial approach like this to recommend a healthy, nutrient-rich diet.

▶ A blood test can precisely determine whether or what deficiencies the client has. By compensating for these deficiencies, mild to moderate depressive symptoms can be treated, for example. Interdisciplinary cooperation is recommended here.

This pillar is also intended to be an alternative to medications with side effects, to promote a natural hormonal balance or a healthy supply of the necessary starting materials and co-factors.

▶ If clients who are taking medication or have a mental disorder are considering supplementation with dietary supplements, this should always be discussed with a doctor.

In addition to the recommended interdisciplinary cooperation with doctors regarding the blood test, it may also be useful for some clients to consult nutritionists to promote and/or maintain mental and physical health.

▶ Psychoneuroimmunology

Psychoneuroimmunology is a neighboring discipline of psychoneuroendocrinology. In my view, these two scientific disciplines, especially in a biopsychosocial approach like this one, cannot be separated from each other, which is why the findings of psychoneuroimmunology also represent a pillar of this biopsychosocial coaching. Psychoneuroimmunology has gained increased attention during the last years of the COVID-19 pandemic, which is important because it is of enormous significance for both physical and mental health. Endocrine secretions influence our immune system. Physical health influences our mental health and vice versa.

Psychoneuroimmunology is the science that deals with the interactions between the immune system, the nervous system, and behavior.

To promote or maintain people's health, it is therefore important to make clients understand how important a healthy body and a strengthened immune system are for our behavior and psyche (and vice versa). In particular, sufficient sleep and a healthy diet, i.e., the intake of sufficient raw materials and co-factors, are important for a good stable immune system. This pillar is therefore intertwined with the pillar of sleep, nutrition, and psychoeducation. Clients should gain an understanding of the biopsychosocial approach, of which psychoneuroimmunology is definitely a part. Methods to strengthen the immune system include, for example, a regular sleep-wake rhythm, a healthy nutrient- and vitamin-rich diet, exercise, nature, walks in the fresh air, mindfulness-based methods/exercises, and much more.

A regular sleep-wake rhythm (melatonin production) is considered a prerequisite for adequate immune competence. Disturbances of a normal sleep-wake rhythm inevitably lead to changes in the immune system.

Changes in the neuroendocrine-immune system can negatively affect, for example, cardiovascular diseases and depressive disorders. Additionally, increased pain in organic and functional diseases can be the result.

Unfortunately, the possibilities for interventions are limited. Clients should be motivated to take care of themselves, their bodies, and thus their psyche. Keeping a journal can be supportive here, to make clients aware of whether and how much they pay attention to sleep, nutrition, exercise, etc. Above all, night sleep seems to be a simple method to promote physiological and psychological health. Interventions in this area are therefore of enormous importance.

▶ Coaching Evaluation—Successfully Concluding PNES Coaching

At the end of this biopsychosocial coaching approach, an evaluation is important to ensure quality assurance.

Evaluation means that the coaching is systematically, data-based, and criteria-related evaluated. The evaluation serves to optimize the coaching offer.

However, the evaluation of PNES coaching does not only focus on whether the clients were satisfied or not, or whether the set goals were achieved, but the evaluation or the final phase of the coaching also serves relapse prevention and the promotion of the development process of the counselors/therapists.

It is important that this evaluation does not simply happen in the last session, but that there is a final phase of this coaching. In this final phase, the methods and techniques used are evaluated and it is determined to what extent they are integrated into everyday coping. The agreed operationalized goals are broken down, and it should be openly discussed what worked well and what clients still find difficult. Additionally, it is important to deepen the application of acute tools. Clients should be taught how to manage to get out of a possible low on their own or to master difficult crisis situations on their own. Here it is important that clients know that it is not a shame if they have a relapse and that follow-up appointments can be arranged. This knowledge can provide clients with additional security. It is also advisable to create a structured individual action and thought list as a self-help aid.

▶ Creating a detailed biopsychosocial documentation sheet can be of particular importance for creating a self-help list. Additionally, a biopsychosocial documentation contributes to the reflection of the entire coaching process. It is important for quality assurance as well as for relapse prevention. An example of a documentation sheet for PNES coaching can be found in the appendix.

It can also be helpful to reenact various problem situations, for example in the form of role-playing. Clients should be able to practice and deepen their learned knowledge. Additionally, it is important (especially after longer coaching processes) to discuss the clients' feelings due to the end of the alliance.

▶ It is helpful if the coaching sessions do not end suddenly, but the sessions gradually taper off, for example from once a week to every 2 weeks, to once a month, etc.

Such reflection or evaluation of the coaching process contributes to quality assurance and quality management. It is part of relapse prevention and also the development processes of the counselors/therapists. A good evaluation of this eclectic-integrative approach shows to what extent the methods and techniques or multimodal therapy forms chosen by the counselors/therapists were successful and whether it would be helpful for the counselors/therapists to further expand their "toolbox".

4.2.2 "PNES Coaching": Conclusion

Thus, the most significant pillars for the maintenance and preservation of biopsychosocial health have been established in the form of a biopsychosocial eclectic-integrative coaching approach, which implements findings from psychoneuroimmunology as well as findings from (behavioral) genetics and serves both to promote health and to maintain health. It is an approach that transfers modern, undisputed scientific findings into psychosocial and psychotherapeutic practice. This approach demonstrates a way in which the insights presented in this book for our soul, psyche, and physical health can be implemented in practice. It is a coaching approach that can help both mentally healthy people in crisis situations or difficult life circumstances and people with mental disorders to successfully manage everyday life and life challenges.

Much of this knowledge has been "heard somewhere before," yet the significance of this knowledge is not known to many people. In addition to proven psychological and psychotherapeutic interventions, it is primarily about making individuals (again) aware of what the human body is actually capable of handling and how we can support it in doing so. The coaching approach is intended to support individuals in mobilizing their body's own forces or messengers and to convey an understanding of the enormous significance of the effects of hormones, both mentally and physically, coaching them to influence their own hormones and thus be more mentally stable and able to manage their lives in a healthier, more conscious, and happier way. Whether healthy people or people with mental disorders, whether for maintaining health or promoting health, the goal of this approach is to make it (easier) to manage psychosocial everyday life and to make life naturally (even) more worthwhile. As mentioned earlier, there is no promise of healing here; rather, clients should (re)learn to benefit from their body's own hormones and emotions and to optimize themselves, their own resilience, their leisure time, their physiological health, and their psychosocial everyday life through the endocrine system. With the knowledge of our endocrine system, our psyche, our brain, with the use of social resources and positive environmental influences, as well as an eclectic-integrative biopsychosocial coaching approach or multimodal therapy forms, I am convinced that I have presented a modern, scientifically based coaching approach for both psychosocial counseling and psychotherapy, which can contribute to an increase in quality in practice. Moreover, it is important that these modern scientific findings are not ignored. To ensure, guarantee, and ideally improve the quality of psychosocial counseling and psychotherapy, it is, in my view, important to individually adapt and implement the presented findings into psychological/psychosocial/psychotherapeutic practice tailored to the clients.

Appendix

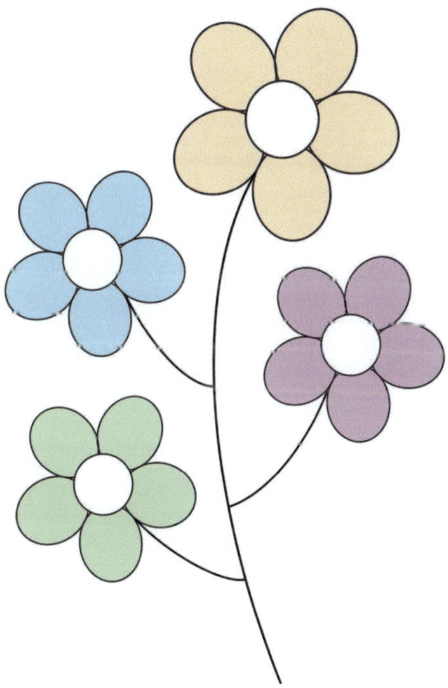

Indie flower.

PNES Coaching—Documentation Form

Client: Expected coaching duration:
Date of birth:
Tel.:
Email:
Address:

J. Wiederhofer, *Psychoneuroendocrinology in Psychosocial and Psychotherapeutic Practice,* https://doi.org/10.1007/978-3-658-46275-8

Other involved helpers/doctors:
School/Education/Profession:
Marital status:

	Case documentation	Notes
Coaching occasion, description of the problem or problematic behavior Problem development Problem description		
Biographical life situation Living conditions Development history, economic situation		
Motivation analysis Motivation for change Self-responsibility Problem awareness Ability to open up		
Biology		
Physical health Pre-diagnosis(es), test results Medical findings Medication intake Blood count/hormone levels Deficiencies (vitamins, minerals…) Smoker/non-smoker Alcohol/drug consumption		
Psychoneuroimmunology Common diseases Duration of diseases Medication intake, antibiotics, cortisol … Health-promoting motivation		
Sleep-wake rhythm Sleep disorders Sleep log Sleep-promoting interventions		
Nutrition and Gut Health Special Considerations (e.g., vegan, vegetarian, food intolerances ….) Weight (Special Considerations) Healthy Nutrition, (Starting Materials and Cofactors) Nutritional Counseling		
Psycho		

	Case documentation	Notes
Problem behavior Psychological basic needs Psychopathological abnormalities Psychopathological abnormalities in the family Social deviations Noticeable habits		
Psychoneuronal basic systems 1) Stress processing system 2) Internal calming system 3) Internal evaluation and reward system 4) Impulse inhibition system 5) Attachment system 6) System of reality sense and risk assessment		
Social		
Resource diagnostics (Personal resources & environmental resources)		
Social network, online network Family/bond(s): mother/father/caregiver Siblings Partnership Friendships		
Relationship analysis, relationship competencies, openness, building trust, proximity-distance regulation		
Operationalized Objectives		
Intervention Planning		
Resource activation		
Indie Flower		
Transfer tasks		
Consultation of the environment		
Methods/Therapies		
Referral to other helpers/doctors		
Coaching evaluation		
Coaching process		
Goal achievements		
Reflection of the coaching/feedback conversation		

PNES Coaching Documentation Form
GEN-COMPASS

Client:

Expected coaching duration:

Date of birth:
Tel.:
Email:
Address:
Other involved helpers/doctors:
School/Education/Profession:
School/Marital status:

Gene Compass	Case Documentation	Notes
Perinatal phase of the mother (Mother: Anxiety disorders? Trauma? Situation of the mother? Family situation? Professional?)		
Early childhood (0–3) mother-child relationship (caring mother)		
Sensitivity of the mother		
Bonds/Caregivers		
Traumatic childhood experiences		
Negative experiences/traumas in the past (after adolescence)		
Personality traits		
Prosocial/antisocial		
Openness		
Empathy		
Self-esteem		
Optimism		
Imaginative/artistic/intellectual		
Risky behavior		
Desire for sensations		
Fun in gambling		
Anxiety-related personality traits/increased anxiety?		
Stress resilience/Stress sensitivity		
Social interaction in stressful situations helpful (e.g., partner) yes/no		
Understanding against background noise		
Emotion regulation		
Impulse control		
Increased irritability?		
Aggressions/Criminality		
Reaction to threatening stimuli		
Depressions/depressive episodes		
Anxiety states/Panic attacks		
(only for mothers): Emotion when the baby cries?		
Psychopathological abnormalities within the family		

Glossary

Term	Definition/Explanation
A	
Adenohypophysis (anterior pituitary gland)	The adenohypophysis or anterior pituitary gland is the hormone-producing part of the pituitary gland (hypophysis). It is part of the hypothalamic-pituitary system and produces hormones with a wide range of effects. The adenohypophyseal hormones have a significant regulatory function for other hormone glands (endocrine glands), which is why they are referred to as glandotropic hormones. In addition to the regulatory hormones, effector hormones are also produced, which have an immediate effect. The production and release of adenohypophyseal hormones are controlled by the releasing and inhibiting hormones of the hypothalamus. The following adenohypophyseal hormones are distinguished: ACTH (corticotropin, adrenocorticotropic hormone), CS (chorionic somatomammotropin, placental lactogenic hormone), FSH (follicle-stimulating hormone), LPH (lipotropin, lipotropic hormone), LH (lutropin, luteinizing hormone), MSH (melanocortin, melanocyte-stimulating hormone), LTH (prolactin, lactotropic hormone, luteotropic hormone), STH (somatropin, somatotropic hormone, growth hormone), TSH (thyrotropin, thyroid-stimulating hormone) (cf. Spektrum Lexikon der Neurowissenschaft 2000a, n.p.).
Adrenalectomy	The surgical removal of the adrenal gland is referred to as adrenalectomy. The procedure is used, among other things, for the treatment of adrenal tumors (cf. Spektrum Lexikon der Neurowissenschaft 2000b, n.p.).
Amnesia	Amnesia is a quantitative memory disorder in which there is a temporal or content-related impairment of memory. The causes can be organic or psychogenic (cf. Dittmann 2022, n.p.).
Amygdala	The amygdala is a nucleus of the telencephalon (forebrain); it is located on the inner side of the temporal lobe. It is part of the limbic system and significant for memory processes, learning, and emotions, especially fear (cf. Maier 2016a, n.p.).
Anxiolytic	Anxiolytic means anxiety-relieving. Pharmaceutics with anxiolytic effects are referred to as anxiolytics. They are used in conditions of anxiety and tension (cf. Spektrum Lexikon der Neurowissenschaft 2000c, n.p.).

J. Wiederhofer, *Psychoneuroendocrinology in Psychosocial and Psychotherapeutic Practice,* https://doi.org/10.1007/978-3-658-46275-8

Term	Definition/Explanation
Apathy	Apathy is described as a state characterized by indifference and lack of passion, as well as an absence of emotions and drive. Apathy is often associated with loss of appetite, sleep disturbances, and a depressive mood. Additionally, there is usually an insensitivity to external stimuli (cf. Hollstein 2022a, n.p.).
Atrophy	In pathology, atrophy is defined as the reduction in size of tissue or organs, based on decreased cell function (cf. Bobbert and Mai 2022a, n.p.).
Axon	An axon is referred to as the extension of a nerve cell (neuron). It transmits nerve impulses to other cells. Axons transport excitations and pass them on to, for example, muscle cells via synapses (cf. Pschyrembel Redaktion 2019a, n.p.).
B	
Basal ganglia	The basal ganglia are understood to be a functional unit of nuclei in the cerebral white matter, which particularly regulate movement patterns and coordination. Additionally, they also fulfill cognitive and limbic functions (cf. Spektrum Lexikon der Neurowissenschaft 2000d, n.p.).
Basolateral	Cells that possess polarity have a lower (basal) and lateral (lateral) region. The end of cells facing the lumen, on the other hand, is referred to as the apical cell side. Thus, basolateral encompasses all sides except the apical (luminal) cell side (cf. Pschyrembel Editorial 2019b, n.p.).
Benzodiazepine	Benzodiazepine is a psychotropic drug that has an anxiolytic, anticonvulsant (effective against epilepsy), muscle-relaxing, and generally calming effect. Due to the high potential for dependence, a maximum intake of 4 weeks is recommended. It is used as a medication for a variety of indications, such as anxiety disorders, sleep disorders, and states of tension, as well as an antiepileptic and for muscle spasms. Benzodiazepines are medications from the group of tranquilizers (cf. Pschyrembel Editorial 2019c, n.p.).
Biochemistry; biochemical	Biochemistry is a natural science that deals with chemical processes and biological phenomena or life processes as well as functions. Biochemistry emerged as physiological chemistry from physiology (cf. Walther 2022a, n.p.).
Biogenic Amine	Biogenic amines are formed through a chemical reaction (decarboxylation) of amino acids. They have diverse physiological functions. They act as neurotransmitters, hormones, or co-factors. Important biogenic amines include, for example, dopamine, norepinephrine, adrenaline, GABA, and carnitine as well as melatonin, histamine, serotonin, spermine, and spermidine (cf. Walther 2022b, n.p.).
Biomarker	Biomarkers are understood to be objectively recognizable and determinable characteristics. The presence or increased occurrence of these characteristics can serve as a reference for processes or disease states in the body (cf. Heinzow/Jaehde 2023, n.p.).
Blood-brain barrier	The blood-brain barrier is a selectively permeable barrier between blood and brain substance. It controls the exchange of substances in the CNS and acts as a protection for nervous tissue against harmful substances and pathogens. The harmful substances are prevented from passing through the capillary wall (cf. Krause 2020a, n.p.).

Term	Definition/Explanation
C	
Optic chiasm	The optic chiasm is an important part of the visual pathway. It is located in the region of the sella turcica. Here, the nerve fibers of the two optic nerves meet, which then continue as the optic tract (cf. Diener 2019a, n.p.).
Surgery	Surgery is a medical specialty that, in addition to conservative methods for the diagnosis and treatment of diseases, particularly focuses on operative therapy. Through operations, a shortening of the healing process or an improvement in the functional outcome is to be achieved (cf. Pfitzmann 2020, n.p.).
Chromosome	Chromosomes are small bodies that consist of DNA and proteins and carry genetic information. In eukaryotes, they are present in the cell nucleus and appear looped or thread-like. In humans, there are a total of 46 chromosomes. Chromosomes are microscopically visible only during cell division (cf. Schöller 2021a, n.p.).
Corpus luteum	The corpus luteum (yellow body) is a collection of cells that produces hormones. It forms after ovulation from the ruptured follicle. In the corpus luteum, estrogens are produced as well as the corpus luteum hormone progesterone (cf. Schöller 2018d, n.p.).
Cortex	Cortex or Kortex means bark, shell. In medicine, it refers to the tissue portion that lies on the outside of certain organs. Most commonly, cortex refers to the cortex cerebri (cerebral cortex). Additionally, there is, among others, the cortex cerebelli (cerebellar cortex) or the cortex renalis (outer layer of the adrenal gland) (cf. Pschyrembel Editorial 2016a, n.p.).
Cortisol	The so-called stress hormone (because it leads to a significant increase in cortisol production during severe stress situations) is produced in the adrenal cortex. The release of the natural glucocorticoid cortisol is stimulated by ACTH. It is subject to negative feedback regulation (cf. Pschyrembel Editorial 2020a, n.p.).
D	
Dendrite	Dendrites are referred to as short, branched cytoplasmic extensions of a nerve cell. The nerve cell can have multiple dendrites. They serve to receive electrical signals and transmit them to the soma or perikaryon (cell body) (cf. Fanghänel 2016, n.p.).
Diencephalon	The diencephalon (synonym: interbrain) is a vital part of the brain. It is necessary for numerous life processes and consists of the thalamus, subthalamus, epithalamus, metathalamus, and hypothalamus. The interbrain-pituitary system influences all important metabolic functions as well as the testes or ovaries (gonads, sex glands) through the hormones released (cf. Falkai 2022a, n.p.).
Dilatation	Dilatation means the expansion of a hollow organ such as the heart (cardiac dilatation) or the pupil (mydriasis). Dilatation is also used as a therapeutic procedure, for example, a balloon dilatation (dilation in the gastrointestinal tract) (cf. Pschyrembel Editorial 2016b, n.p.).
Dopamine agonist	A dopamine agonist is a substance that stimulates dopamine receptors. The active ingredient is used, for example, to inhibit prolactin release as well as in Parkinson's syndrome (movement disorder) (cf. Schöller 2018a, n.p.).

Term	Definition/Explanation
Gland	Glands are referred to as organs or epithelial cells that release active substances (secretions) with physiological significance. In this context, a distinction is made between endocrine glands and exocrine glands, depending on the site of secretion. Exocrine glands release their secretion onto internal or external surfaces, whereas endocrine glands secrete into the blood (cf. Pschyrembel Editorial 2018a, n.p.).
E	
Eminentia mediana	The Eminentia mediana is a transition zone or interface between the pituitary gland and the hypothalamus, where contacts between the endocrine and nervous systems occur. It plays a significant role in the release of regulatory hormones. The hypothalamo-hypophyseal tracts terminate in the area of the Eminentia mediana. In these tracts, the releasing and inhibiting factors from the hypothalamus are conveyed. When these factors reach the portal system of the pituitary gland (hypophyseal portal system), they influence the secretion of hormones from the adenohypophysis. Axons run through the internal zone of the Eminentia mediana, in which neurotransmitters, vasopressin, and oxytocin are transported to the pituitary gland (hypothalamus-pituitary system) (cf. Spektrum Lexikon der Neurowissenschaft 2000e, n.p.).
Endocrine	Endocrine refers to a mechanism of secretion from hormone glands. This secretion mechanism causes the products to be directly secreted into the bloodstream (cf. Ganse 2022a, n.p.).
Endocrinology	Endocrinology is the study of the morphology and function of endocrine glands as well as of hormones and their mechanisms of action and regulation (cf. Schöller 2016a, n.p.).
Enteric Nervous System	The enteric nervous system is a complex network of nerves in the gastrointestinal tract. It is part of the autonomic nervous system and influences digestion. It consists of 2 large nerve plexuses (the myenteric plexus and the submucosal plexus) as well as several smaller plexuses. While it controls the functions of the gastrointestinal tract, it is influenced by the sympathetic and parasympathetic nervous systems (cf. Pschyrembel Editorial 2016c, n.p.).
Epigenetics; epigenetic	Epigenetics is a science that deals with hereditary genetic modification affecting the phenotype without changing the DNA sequence. Epigenetic changes can be detected in various diseases. Epigenetics is the molecular basis for the effect of environmental factors on the genome as well as for the gene-environment interaction in disease development (cf. Pschyrembel Editorial 2021a, n.p.).
Epiphysis (pineal gland, pineal organ, or glandula pinealis)	The epiphysis is an endocrine gland that produces melatonin in a light-dependent manner. It is a protrusion of the roof of the diencephalon, consisting of astrocytes, pinealocytes, and noradrenergic nerve fibers. In particular, pinealocytes produce melatonin in addition to polypeptides. Melatonin is produced in darkness, and it is believed to influence the rhythm of biological processes such as the sleep-wake cycle or the light-dark cycle (cf. Giebel 2020. n.p.).

Term	Definition/Explanation
Epithalamus	The epithalamus is a part of the diencephalon that adjoins the thalamus. It consists of the pineal gland (epiphysis) as well as the habenula, and also the two habenular nuclei (habenular nuclei; nucleus group in the habenula). The epithalamus is considered a relay station for olfactory impulses and regulates circadian changes in biological functions (the circadian rhythm) (cf. Chao 2016a, b, n.p.).
F	
Adipose tissue	Adipose tissue is a form of connective tissue that consists of fat cells. Adipose tissue has hormonal or endocrine activity, whereby it is important to distinguish between white adipose tissue and brown adipose tissue. White adipose tissue primarily serves as a carbon source, energy reservoir, and structural fat. It forms and secretes adipokines (influencing glucose and fat metabolism as well as the feeling of hunger). Brown adipose tissue primarily serves thermogenesis (heat production to maintain body temperature) and is particularly found in newborns and infants. The stimulation of thermogenesis (through cold stimuli) causes the release of catecholamines (cf. Fanghänel et al. 2020, n.p.).
G	
Gastrointestinal	Gastrointestinal means that something affects the stomach and intestines (cf. Pschyrembel Redaktion 2016d, n.p.).
Gene	A gene is the functional unit within the genome (the entirety of the genetic material of an organism or a cell). It contains the genetic (hereditary) information for a gene product. Genes exist in the organism as single or double strands and consist of DNA (eukaryotes, prokaryotes) or RNA (viruses). They contain information for the development of individuals and the expression of traits. Exogenous as well as endogenous factors can alter genes, with these changes potentially having positive, negative, or no effects on the individual. Additionally, genes are often the cause of hereditary (genetically determined) diseases (cf. Schöller 2018b, n.p.).
Genetics	Genetics is the science of the laws and fundamentals of heredity. It deals with the transmission and expression of genetically determined traits. In a broader sense, this also includes ontogenesis (development of the organism from the egg cell to its final form) and phylogenesis (evolutionary development of organisms through evolution). Gregor Mendel is considered the founder of (classical) genetics (cf. Schöller 2021b, n.p.).
Gluconeogenesis	Gluconeogenesis is the synthesis of glucose in the liver and kidney, glucoplastic amino acids, lactate, and glycerol. Stimulation of gluconeogenesis occurs through glucagon, while inhibition occurs through insulin (cf. Walther 2022c, n.p.).
Cerebrum (Synonyms: Telencephalon, Endbrain, Cerebrum)	The cerebrum forms the largest and most differentiated part of the brain as well as the central nervous system and is thus responsible for many of the human thinking and action processes. It consists of the two hemispheres (cerebrum), with the surface covered by the cerebral cortex (allocortex and isocortex) and enlarged and characterized by convolutions and furrows (cf. Maier 2019a, n.p.).

Term	Definition/Explanation
Gynecology	Gynecology is the study of diseases, prophylaxis, and therapy of the female reproductive organs or the female sexual and reproductive tract. It also implies obstetrics (cf. Schöller 2018c, n.p.).
Gyrus dentatus	The Gyrus dentatus are the tooth-like appearing brain convolutions made of gray matter (tissue mostly composed of nerve cell bodies). It is located between the hippocampus and the parahippocampal gyrus and is a part of the limbic system (cf. Krieglstein 2016, n.p.).
H	
Hippocampus	The hippocampus is part of the limbic system and is particularly involved in memory formation. It also plays a central role in certain forms of epilepsy (Ammon's horn sclerosis) as well as schizophrenia. In various diseases, a reduction in the volume of the hippocampus can be detected using MRI. This applies to diseases such as dementia (especially Alzheimer's disease), depression, trauma, and stress (see Chao 2016a, n.p.).
Brain ventricles	Brain ventricles are cavities filled with cerebrospinal fluid inside the brain. The cerebrospinal fluid protects the central nervous system from external influences, such as impacts. The ventricular system consists of four ventricles (see Diener 2019b, n.p.).
Homeostasis	The term homeostasis describes in physiology the maintenance of a state of equilibrium of a dynamic system, such as blood pressure, body temperature, metabolism, or the balance of bases, acids, water, and electrolytes. This maintenance functions through internal self-regulation with the help of control loops between the hypothalamus, hormone, and nervous systems. Disturbances of homeostasis, which are mostly caused by central disturbances, manifest in organ dysfunctions (cf. Hackermeier 2020, n.p.).
Hormone	Hormones are signaling substances or messenger molecules that are produced in endocrine organs (except tissue hormones). They reach their target organs in free or bound form via the blood and thus serve to regulate various body functions (cf. Schöller 2016b, n.p.).
Hormone receptor	A hormone receptor is a receptor to which usually a specific hormone binds. Through the reversible binding of the hormones, their effect is mediated into the cell via various biochemical secondary reactions (cf. Schöller 2016c, n.p.).
Human physiology	„Science of the normal life processes in humans" (Duden 2023, n.p.).
Hypercortisolism (Cushing's syndrome)	Hypercortisolism, or the so-called Cushing's syndrome, is a metabolic disorder that is characterized by an increased concentration of cortisol or synthetic glucocorticoid in the plasma (cf. Hollstein 2022b, n.p.).
Hyperprolactinemia	Hyperprolactinemia refers to an elevated serum concentration of prolactin in the blood. A distinction is made between a physiological increase during pregnancy and lactation and a pathological (e.g., prolactinoma) increase. Treatment is usually pharmacological, for example with dopamine receptor agonists (cf. Bobbert/Mai 2022b, n.p.).

Term	Definition/Explanation
Hypertension	In medicine, hypertension refers to the increase in tension or pressure beyond the physiological norm, for example, intracranial pressure, muscle tension, or pressure in blood vessels. The opposite of hypertension is hypotension (cf. Meyer 2016, n.p.).
Hypocortisolism	Hypocortisolism refers to a deficiency of cortisol due to primary or secondary adrenal insufficiency (cf. Hollstein 2022c, n.p.).
Hypophysis (pituitary gland)	The hypophysis is a cherry pit- to hazelnut-sized endocrine organ in the sella turcica of the bony skull base. It consists of the anterior pituitary (adenohypophysis) and the posterior pituitary (neurohypophysis). Through the pituitary stalk, it is connected to the hypothalamus, and together they control the (autonomic) nervous system. The anterior pituitary (adenohypophysis) produces hormones such as FSH, LH, and prolactin, and the posterior pituitary (neurohypophysis) secretes hypothalamic hormones (cf. Schöller 2019a, n.p.).
Pituitary stalk	The connection between the hypothalamus and the glandular body pituitary is referred to as the pituitary stalk (cf. Pschyrembel Editorial 2019d, n.p.).
Hypothalamus	The hypothalamus is a vital part of the diencephalon (interbrain). It is the highest regulatory center for all autonomic as well as endocrine processes and is considered the interface between the neural and endocrine systems. Among other things, it controls breathing, fluid and food intake, body temperature, circulation, and sexual behavior (cf. Schöller 2016d, n.p.).
I	
Immunosuppression	Immunosuppression refers to the weakening or suppression of the immune response. Immunosuppression can be the result of diseases, infections, medications, medical treatments, and also excessive physical or mental stress. Due to immunosuppression, there is an increased risk of particularly specific infections (cf. Krause 2020b, n.p.).
Infertility	Infertility is the term for the inability of a woman to carry a pregnancy to a viable child, although natural fertilization is possible (Impotentia gestandi). Additionally, the term is usually used in men as a synonym for sterility (inability to procreate) (cf. Schöller 2019b, n.p.).
Inhibiting hormone	Inhibiting hormones (inhibitory hormones) or releasing-inhibiting hormones are neurohormones that are produced in the hypothalamus. Through the hypophyseal portal system, they reach the adenohypophysis (anterior pituitary), where they inhibit the release of other hormones (cf. Spektrum Lexikon der Biologie 1999a, n.p.).
Internal Medicine	Internal medicine is a branch of human medicine that deals with the diagnosis, conservative therapy, rehabilitation, and prevention of diseases of internal organs. Subfields of internal medicine include, for example, endocrinology, cardiology, internal intensive care medicine, and gastroenterology (cf. Pschyrembel Editorial 2016e, n.p.).
Intensive care medicine	Intensive care medicine is a medical specialty that deals with the diagnosis and therapy of life-threatening diseases and conditions, as well as the treatment and monitoring after surgeries (cf. Lüdi et al. 2022, n.p.).

Term	Definition/Explanation
Intrauterine	Intrauterine means within the uterus (Uterus) (cf. Pschyrembel Editorial 2019e, n.p.).
K	
Cardiovascular	Cardiovascular means relating to the heart and the vascular system (cf. Pschyrembel Editorial 2016f, n.p.).
Catecholamine	Catecholamines are hormones as well as neurotransmitters that, among other things, have a blood pressure-increasing and catabolic effect. The primary catecholamines are referred to as norepinephrine and dopamine; secondary catecholamines are adrenaline as well as their derivatives. They are subject to a circadian rhythm and are elevated in anxiety and also after alcohol consumption (cf. Walther 2022d, n.p.).
Cerebellum (Cerebellum)	The cerebellum is the part of the brain that lies behind the cranial fossa below the occipital lobe of the cerebrum and controls the fluidity of movement. It consists of two hemispheres, and together with the cerebrum, it regulates balance and muscular tone (cf. Krieglstein 2018a, n.p.).
Cybernetics; cybernetic	Cybernetics is a branch of modern natural sciences. It deals with the control and regulatory relationships in biology, medicine, and technology as well as with the control and communication between machines and living beings. Additionally, the theory of functional possibilities in informational systems is discussed under abstraction from psychological, physiological, or physical peculiarities. It is the theoretical foundation for systemic psychotherapy and led to the elucidation of many biological processes (cf. Jähn 2016, n.p.).
L	
Liver	The liver is located in the right upper abdomen and is the largest and most important metabolic organ of the human body. In addition to its significant role in metabolism, it has a central role in detoxification (biotransformation). The liver receives blood from the digestive organs and synthesizes bile acids as well as steroids and many essential plasma proteins and coagulation factors. One of its tasks is therefore the synthesis of precursors for hormone production. It also stores vitamins (cf. Schulze-Schleithoff 2019a, n.p.).
Leydig cells	The Leydig cells are epithelioid cell groups in the interstitial connective tissue of the testis that produce androgens. The Leydig cells are stimulated by the luteinizing hormone (LH), which leads to the synthesis of testosterone (6–8 mg per day in adult men) (cf. Pschyrembel Editorial 2016g, n.p.).
Limbic System	The limbic system is a phylogenetically very old part of the brain, which is composed of several structures. It plays a significant role in the endocrine and autonomic nervous regulatory system. Together with other brain areas, it triggers and influences innate drive and instinctive actions. It is of great importance for overall behavior, emotional reactions such as fear, anger, or affection, as well as for memory and learning functions. Additionally, it is attributed with functions or the autonomic regulation of food intake, digestion, and reproduction (cf. Krieglstein 2018b, n.p.).

Term	Definition/Explanation
Locus caeruleus	The *Locus caeruleus* is a neurophysiological structure that is considered a major production site of norepinephrine in the brain. The Locus caeruleus regulates the interaction between the noradrenergic and serotonergic systems and plays a significant role in various physiological, emotional, and behavioral processes. For example, it influences the orientation response and attention control, the regulation of sleep stages, sexual behavior, and emotional mood. Overactivity is associated with anxiety disorders, and impairments of the Locus caeruleus are observed in conditions such as Alzheimer's disease, Down syndrome, and Parkinson's syndrome (cf. Pschyrembel Editorial 2018b, n.p.).
M	
Medial forebrain bundle (Fasciculus telencephalicus medialis)	The Fasciculus telencephalicus medialis (medial forebrain bundle) is a bundle of nerve fibers that connect the olfactory cortex with the reticular formation. The nerve pathways run through the hypothalamus and the limbic system. They contain noradrenergic and dopaminergic nerve fibers (cf. Maier 2018a, n.p.).
Melatonin	Melatonin is a neurosecretory hormone that is secreted almost exclusively in the pineal gland (epiphysis) as well as in cells of the retina. The secretion depends on the light-dark cycle (10 to 100 times more is secreted at night). Melatonin is involved in the regulation of the circadian rhythm (cf. Pschyrembel Editorial 2020b, n.p.).
Mesencephalon (midbrain)	The mesencephalon (midbrain) is a part of the brain that belongs to the brainstem and lies between the metencephalon (hindbrain) and the diencephalon (interbrain) (cf. Maier 2019b, n.p.).
Mesolimbic System	The mesolimbic system is a system in the CNS that serves the evaluation of emotional states. It consists of parts of the limbic system as well as the nucleus accumbens and is responsible for positive rewards. Additionally, it is involved in the generation of joy. The dopaminergic neurons of the mesolimbic system are connected with structures of the forebrain, which modulate them. Hyperactive dopaminergic neurons of the limbic system are also a cause of the symptoms in schizophrenia (cf. Pschyrembel Editorial 2018c, n.p.).
Molecular biology; molecular biological	Molecular biology is a sub-discipline of biology that was only established in the mid-20th century. It examines life phenomena at the molecular level and attempts to explain life processes (life, metabolism) at the level of structure, function (structure-function relationship), as well as the transformation of these molecules. According to J. Monod, the goal of molecular biology is "the interpretation of the essential properties of organisms based on their molecular structures." Molecular biology is an interdisciplinary science both in terms of content and methodology (cf. Spektrum Lexikon der Biologie 1999b, n.p.).
Monoamine	Monoamines are chemical substances that are formed by the decarboxylation of mostly aromatic amino acids. They act as neurotransmitters (such as dopamine) or as tissue hormones (such as histamine) (cf. Walther 2022e, n.p.).

Term	Definition/Explanation
Monoamine oxidase (MAO)	Monoamine oxidase, abbreviated as MAO, is an enzyme that catalyzes the breakdown of monoamines. MAO deaminates and thereby inactivates amines such as adrenaline, noradrenaline, dopamine, serotonin, tyramine, and histamine. Inhibition of MAO leads to an increase in the synaptic concentration of serotonin, adrenaline, and noradrenaline, which is used for the treatment of depression (cf. Walther 2022f, n.p.
Morphology	„Study of the form and structure, e.g., of body, organ, cell, or cell organelle" (Pschyrembel Editorial 2016h, n.p.).
Motoneuron	Motoneurons are nerve cells of the CNS that exert direct or indirect control over a muscle within motor cranial nerve nuclei or in the anterior horns of the spinal cord (motor anterior horn cells). They trigger a contraction of the muscle fibers via the transmitter acetylcholine (cf. Maier 2018b, n.p.).
Myopathy	The term myopathy refers to all primary diseases of the muscles that are not based on neuronal causes. They primarily originate from the muscle itself and are always characterized by a weakness of the affected muscle. A distinction is made between acquired (secondary) myopathies and hereditary myopathies (cf. Lücke 2020, n.p.).
N	
Adrenal gland (Glandula suprarenalis, Epinephron)	The adrenal gland is an endocrine organ that lies cap-like and paired above the kidneys. A distinction is made between the adrenal medulla and the adrenal cortex, as they synthesize different hormones. The adrenal cortex synthesizes steroid hormones (particularly mineralocorticoids, glucocorticoids, and sex hormones), and the adrenal medulla releases the neurohormones norepinephrine and epinephrine. Due to the high number of hormones produced, various clinical pictures arise in the event of adrenal disorders (cf. Schöller 2018e, n.p.).
Adrenal medulla (Medulla glandulae suprarenalis)	The adrenal medulla (AM) is a reddish-brown tissue inside the adrenal gland. It is the site of production of the catecholamines norepinephrine and epinephrine. These are released directly into the blood as needed. The adrenal medulla is therefore functionally regarded as a peripheral sympathetic ganglion (cf. Pschyrembel Editorial 2016i, n.p.)
Parathyroid gland (Epithelial bodies, Glandulae parathyroideae)	The parathyroid glands of humans are 4 lentil-sized and vital endocrine organs. They play a crucial role particularly in the regulation of calcium balance, as the parathyroid gland produces parathyroid hormone, which is important for calcium metabolism. Known disorders include, for example, an overactive parathyroid gland (hyperparathyroidism) and an underactive parathyroid gland (hypoparathyroidism) (cf. Schöller 2016e, n.p.).
Neocortex (Isocortex)	The neocortex is the phylogenetically youngest and largest part of the cerebral cortex. It has a 6-layered structure (see Isocortex) and consists of gray matter that surrounds the underlying white matter of the brain. The visual cortex, the primary auditory cortex, and the primary somatosensory cortex are located in the neocortex (see Pschyrembel Editorial 2016j, n.p.).

Term	Definition/Explanation
Neuroendocrinology	Neuroendocrinology is a subfield of endocrinology. It deals with the interactions, relationships, regulatory, and action mechanisms between the nervous and hormonal systems (cf. Margraf 2016a, n.p.).
Neurohypophysis (posterior pituitary, Lobus posterior hypophysealis)	The neurohypophysis or posterior pituitary is a part of the pituitary gland. It is an outpouching of the diencephalon and is considered part of the central nervous system. It is a part of the brain and is connected to the hypothalamus. The hormones produced in the hypothalamus (oxytocin and antidiuretic hormone) are stored by the neurohypophysis and released into the bloodstream as needed (cf. Schöller 2019c, n.p.).
Neurology	Neurology (nervous system medicine) refers to the science or medical field that deals with the diagnosis, therapy, and research of the nervous system as well as the muscles (cf. Diener 2016, n.p.).
Neuron (nerve cell)	Nerve cells are specialized cells that have the ability to process and transmit nerve impulses, receive stimuli, respond to them, and generate excitation. They consist of an axon and one or more dendrites. The dendrites receive the nerve impulses, and the axons transmit them via synapses to a target organ or downstream neurons (cf. Pschyrembel 2019f, n.p.).
Neuropeptide	Neuropeptides are neurotransmitters, hormones with peptide structure, or neuromodulators. They are formed in the CNS as well as in cells of other organ systems. Neuropeptides include, for example, endorphins, TSH, somatostatin, VIP, hypothalamic hormones, cholecystokinin, and bradykinin (cf. Walther 2022g, n.p.).
Neurotransmitter	Neurotransmitters are substances or chemical compounds that mediate the transmission of stimuli at the synapses from nerve to nerve. Through the exchange among themselves, signals are transmitted, thereby controlling feelings, thinking, and actions. Likewise, neurotransmitters are not only found in the brain; they are also involved in the regulation of blood vessels. Chemically, neurotransmitters are biogenic amines such as dopamine, serotonin, adrenaline, noradrenaline, etc., as well as amino acids like glutamate, GABA, peptides (e.g., opioids), etc. (cf. Walther 2022h, n.p.).
Neuroscience	Neuroscience is a scientific discipline that deals with all neural mechanisms and cognitive functions. In this context, the function and structure of the nervous system are summarized and interpreted integratively. Cognitive neuroscience relies on experimentally proven concepts of cognitive psychology. Furthermore, it is a central research strategy for all mental disorders (cf. Maier 2016b, n.p.).
Kidney (Ren, Nephros)	The kidney is a paired bean-shaped organ. Its main task is the formation of urine through ultrafiltration, reabsorption, and concentration. Additionally, it regulates the acid-base balance as well as the water and electrolyte balance. Furthermore, it secretes the hormones renin for systemic blood pressure regulation and erythropoietin for blood formation (cf. Pschyrembel Editorial 2016k, n.p.).

Term	Definition/Explanation
Nucleus accumbens	The Nucleus accumbens is a nucleus region in the basal forebrain and serves as a link between the basal ganglia, the limbic system, and the psychomotor system. The Nucleus accumbens is part of the reward system and is partly responsible for the development of addiction. Additionally, it is involved in the conversion of motivation and emotion into movement and action (cf. Pschyrembel Editorial 2018d, n.p.).
Nucleus arcuatus (Nucleus infundibularis)	The arcuate nucleus is a nucleus (nucleus) at the lower end of the infundibulum of the hypothalamus. It is located at the base of the third ventricle and surrounds the pituitary stalk in a horseshoe shape. The neurons present here produce regulatory hormones for the adenohypophysis. They are involved in the regulation of food intake (hunger, anorexia, etc.) as well as energy balance (cf. Chao 2019a, n.p.).
Nucleus paraventricularis	The Nucleus paraventricularis is a vegetative nucleus in the hypothalamus and is located on the lateral wall of the third ventricle. The axons of the neurons from the Nucleus paraventricularis extend to the posterior pituitary (neurohypophysis), where they secrete the hormone oxytocin into the bloodstream. This process is also referred to as neurosecretion (here secretion of hypothalamic hormones) (cf. Chao 2018, n.p.).
Nucleus suprachiasmaticus	The suprachiasmatic nucleus is a core area in the ventral hypothalamus. It is located below the third brain ventricle and above the optic chiasm. The suprachiasmatic nucleus plays a crucial role in the regulation of the circadian rhythm. It is involved in the control of several processes, such as the sleep-wake cycle, body temperature, and melatonin secretion (cf. Pschyrembel Editorial 2018e, n.p.)
Nucleus supraopticus	The Nucleus supraopticus is a significant vegetative nucleus in the hypothalamus. Here, the hormones oxytocin and ADH are produced. It is located cranial to the optic chiasm. The axons of the neurons from the Nucleus supraopticus extend to the posterior pituitary (neurohypophysis), where they are released as part of neurosecretion (cf. Chao 2019b, n.p.).
Nuclear Medicine	Nuclear medicine is a branch of medicine that deals with the diagnostic and therapeutic application of radioactive substances. The radioactive substances are either specifically introduced into the body to produce imaging of organs or to destroy organs or defined target tissue (cf. Lindner 2022, n.p.).
O	
Orbitofrontal cortex	The orbitofrontal cortex is a part of the frontal lobe (Lobus frontalis) in the prefrontal cortex of the brain. It integrates viscerosensory and somatosensory perceptions with innate and learned information as well as behaviors. In case of disorders or injuries to the orbitofrontal cortex, an adequate response (concerning both emotions and behavior) to internal or external stimuli may be impaired. Additionally, disorders of learning and motivation can occur, a change in personality traits and also social behavior can be affected (cf. Pschyrembel Editorial 2018f, n.p.).

Term	Definition/Explanation
Ovary (Ovaries = pl.)	The ovary is a female gonad and is considered one of the internal female reproductive organs. The ovary produces fertilizable eggs, which are expelled monthly during sexual maturity (ovulation). Additionally, the ovary secretes estrogens and progestogens, and in very small amounts, androgens (cf. Schöller 2018f, n.p.).
P	
Pancreas (Pancreatic gland)	The pancreas is a glandular organ that lies transversely in the upper abdomen and has both an endocrine function (produces hormones) and an exocrine function (produces digestive enzymes). The release of hormones (for example, insulin) is significant for the regulation of carbohydrate metabolism (cf. Schulze-Schleithoff 2019b, n.p.).
Paracrine	Paracrine means to release into the immediately adjacent environment. The meaning refers to the secretion mechanism, which means that, for example, certain cells produce a hormone and this hormone then directly affects the neighboring cells (without the interposition of the blood) (cf. Pschyrembel Redaktion 2016 l, o.S.).
Paraneoplastic syndrome (Paraneoplasia)	The paraneoplastic syndrome is a collective term for functional disorders and symptoms that occur in connection with tumor diseases. However, these do not occur due to the primary tumor or metastasis formation, nor due to mechanical and infiltrative processes or tissue interaction. The therapy here is the treatment of the underlying tumor disease (cf. Prochazka 2022, n.p.).
Pathophysiology	Pathophysiology is the study of pathological life processes and functional disorders and their origins (pathogenesis) in the human organism. Together with pathobiochemistry and pathomorphology, pathophysiology forms the general study of diseases (pathology). They deal, among other things, with molecular biological investigations within the cells to explain pathological deviations (cf. Blind 2016, n.p.).
Pediatrics (Pediatrics; Child and Adolescent Medicine)	Pediatrics or child medicine is a branch of medicine that deals with the diagnosis and treatment of diseases in infants, children, and adolescents (cf. Pschyrembel Editorial 2016m, n.p.).
Perimenopause	Perimenopause is a period that begins 2–4 years before menopause (the time of the last menstruation) with the onset of endocrinological, biological, and clinical signs of the approaching menopause. Perimenopause ends 1–2 years after menopause (cf. Schöller 2016f, n.p.).
Perinatal phase (Perinatal period)	Perinatal means around the time of birth. The perinatal phase or perinatal period refers in the narrow sense to the period between the onset of labor and (including) the 7th day after birth. In the broader sense, it refers to the period between the 24th week of gestation and the 7th day of life (the 24th week of gestation due to the empirically determined point of probable extrauterine viability) (cf. Pschyrembel Editorial 2022, n.p.).

Term	Definition/Explanation
Pharmacology; pharmacological	Pharmacology is the study of the interactions between active substances and the living organism. A distinction is made between general pharmacology and special pharmacology. Special pharmacology includes, among other things, pharmacodynamics, pharmacogenetics, and pharmacokinetics (cf. Ehnert 2016, n.p.).
Phenylalanine	Phenylalanine is an aromatic, proteinogenic, gluco- and ketoplastic amino acid. It is essential and is synthesized only by microorganisms and plants. Phenylalanine is a significant component of many proteins; additionally, it serves the synthesis of tyrosine or vice versa (cf. Walther 2022i, n.p.)
Physiology	„Science and teaching of the normal functional processes in cells, tissues, and organs of an organism" (Straube 2022, n.p.).
Pinealocyte (Pineal cell)	Pinealocytes are cells of the pineal gland that produce and release melatonin through neurosecretion. They contain proteins such as arrestin and opsin, and their activity, which is necessary for the sleep-wake cycle, is determined by light exposure (melatonin is primarily produced and secreted in darkness) (cf. Fanghänel 2019, n.p.).
Placenta (Afterbirth)	The placenta is an exchange organ between mother and child within the uterus during pregnancy. This means it supplies the embryo with nutrients and oxygen from the mother's metabolism. Additionally, the placenta produces various hormones. It develops from both maternal and embryonic parts and is expelled after birth (cf. Weingärtner 2022, n.p.).
Polymorphism	In genetics or biology, polymorphism refers to the occurrence of sequence variations in the genes of a population. Individuals differ due to differences in genotype. Genetic variability arises through changes in the sequence or the amount of DNA. The changes in sequence or the amount of DNA can be established in a population (polymorphism) (cf. Pschyrembel Editorial 2021b, n.p.).
Postpartum (post partum; postpartual)	„After birth" (Pschyrembel Editorial 2016n, n.p.).
Prefrontal cortex	The prefrontal cortex occupies the anterior cortical part of the frontal lobe. It plays a significant role in various cognitive functions or certain memory functions, in social behavior and psychological performances in terms of initiative and planning as well as emotionality (cf. Pschyrembel Editorial 2016o, n.p.).
Preganglionic	The term "preganglionic" is used to refer to when autonomic nerve fibers or neurons extend from the CNS to the ganglion. This means the term is used before the synaptic switch in a peripheral ganglion. The opposite of this is the term postganglionic (cf. Chao 2016b, n.p.).
Pregnenolone	Pregnenolone is an intermediate product (C21 steroid) of progesterone from cholesterol as well as androgens in the adrenal cortex (cf. Walther 2022j, n.p.).
Prohormone	Prohormones are inactive precursors of hormones. They are only converted into the active form when needed (cf. Spektrum Lexikon der Neurowissenschaft 2000f, n.p.).

Term	Definition/Explanation
Prostaglandin synthesis	Prostaglandin synthesis is the biosynthesis of prostaglandins, which are natural or partially synthetic hormones. They have diverse and sometimes opposing effects (cf. Pschyrembel Editorial 2020c, n.p.).
Psychiatry (Healing of the soul)	Psychiatry is a medical subfield that deals with the research, prevention, diagnosis, and therapy of mental disorders. Additionally, psychiatry includes rehabilitation as well as the interrelations of physical illnesses and psychotropic substances, as well as social conditions; likewise, the consequences of mental disorders and the investigation of disorder causes, therapy development, and disease distribution (cf. Maier 2016c, n.p.).
Psychoendocrinology	„The study of the relationships between psychological functions and endocrine glands, hormones, as well as their regulatory and action mechanisms" (Pschyrembel Editorial 2016p, n.p.).
Psychoneuroendocrinology	„Psychoneuroendocrinology (PNE) deals with the significance of hormones for psychological functions or characteristics. PNE has significance for almost all sub-disciplines of psychology (…)" (Henning and Netter 2000, n.p.).
Psychosomatics	Psychosomatics is a term for the interaction between body and mind. It is a doctrine of disease that relates to the connection between somatic (physical) disorders, symptoms, or disease patterns and the psyche. In somatic diseases, psychological influences are taken into account (cf. Bengel and de Zwaan 2020, n.p.).
R	
Raphe nuclei	The term Raphe nuclei refers to a serotonergic group of nuclei (serotonin as a neurotransmitter) on both sides of the midline of the brainstem (Raphe). They regulate pain perception as well as the state of consciousness and the cardiovascular system. Additionally, they are involved in mood regulation and sleep (cf. Pschyrembel Editorial 2018g, n.p.).
Hindbrain (Rhombencephalon)	Part of the brain consisting of the metencephalon and medulla oblongata (myelencephalon) (Falkai 2022b, n.p.).
Releasing hormone	Releasing hormones are neurohormones that are produced in the hypothalamus. They are peptide hormones that stimulate (releasing factors) or inhibit (release-inhibiting hormones) the production and release of anterior pituitary hormones. They reach the adenohypophysis via the hypothalamo-hypophyseal portal system, with their effect being mediated through hormone receptors (cf. Wurglics 2022, n.p.).
Retina (Netzhaut)	The retina is the inner layer of the eye. It is a tissue that lines the eye from the inside, between the choroid and the vitreous body. It receives light impulses, converts them into electrical currents, and transmits them to the visual centers of the brain (cf. Pschyrembel Redaktion 2016q, n.p.)
Receptor	Receptors (recipere, lat. = to accept, to receive) are understood to be cells or cell components that react to specific stimuli or signals and transmit them (signal transduction). This occurs after stimulation by a stimulus or after the receptor has bound with specific ligands such as neurotransmitters, hormones, mediators, or drugs. There are different forms of receptors that diverge in their mode of action (cf. Walther 2022k, n.p.).

Term	Definition/Explanation
Rostral	Rostral: "Located towards the front end of the body" (Pschyrembel Redaktion 2019g, n.p.).
S	
Thyroid gland (Glandula thyroidea; Glandula thyreoidea; Thyroidea; Thyreoidea)	The thyroid gland is a butterfly-shaped endocrine gland in the neck below the thyroid cartilage (part of the larynx). It is the largest pure hormone gland in the human body and, due to the synthesis and secretion of thyroid hormones—including triiodothyronine (T3), thyroxine (T4)—and calcitonin—a peptide hormone that influences calcium levels—it has an impact on energy metabolism as well as on phosphate and calcium balance (cf. Füeßl 2020, n.p.).
Secretion	Secretion is the release of important body substances, such as hormones or digestive enzymes, into an organ, into the blood, or onto the skin surface. Various forms of secretion are distinguished, such as: endocrine (internal) secretion = release inward, e.g., into the blood; exocrine (external) secretion = release outward, e.g., onto the skin; paracrine secretion = release to neighboring cells; or autocrine secretion = acts back on the secreting cell (cf. Ganse 2022b, n.p.).
Sex hormone	Sex hormones „serve the development of sexual characteristics and reproduction. In addition, they exert further, non-sex-specific effects. There are female and male sex hormones (…)" (Ostendorf 2021b, n.p.). Sex hormones are steroid hormones that serve reproduction and the development of sexual characteristics. In addition, they exert further non-sex-specific effects. There are female (estrogens and progesterone) and male (androgens, primarily testosterone) sex hormones. The biosynthesis and secretion are controlled in the hypothalamus-pituitary system (cf. Schöller 2016g, n.p.).
Secrete	„Separate" (Pschyrembel Editorial 2016r, n.p.).
Soma	Soma is a term in medicine for the human body (cf. Pschyrembel Editorial 2016s, n.p.).
Spermatogenesis	Spermatogenesis serves the formation of mature sperm, from the male primordial germ cell through spermatogonia, spermatocytes, and spermatids to sperm. It takes place from puberty onwards in the seminiferous tubules (Tubuli seminiferi) of the testis (cf. Schöller 2016h, n.p.).
Steroid receptor	Steroid receptors belong to the intracellular receptors, whose activation is mediated by steroid hormones. Steroid receptors are nuclear receptors that are located in the cytoplasm, migrate to the cell nucleus after activation, and function there as transcription factors (cf. Pschyrembel Editorial 2018h, n.p.).
Striatum (Corpus Striatum)	The striatum belongs to the basal ganglia and is part of the extrapyramidal system. It is a nucleus region in the white matter of the telencephalon and consists of the ventral striatum, putamen, and caudate nucleus. The striatum primarily influences postural motor control and voluntary motor control (cf. Pschyrembel Editorial 2020d, n.p.).

Term	Definition/Explanation
Substantia nigra (black substance; Nucleus niger)	The substantia nigra is a nucleus located in the mesencephalon. It is part of the basal ganglia system and has a blackish color (hence the name) due to the presence of melanin (a pigment that is, among other things, responsible for the dark coloration of the skin after sun exposure). The melanin is produced as a byproduct during the synthesis of dopamine. In addition to dopamine, other neurotransmitters can also be found in the neurons of the substantia nigra. While the dopamine-producing nerve cells are located in the pars compacta, the nerve cells of the pars reticulata (this part is not black-colored) produce GABA as a neurotransmitter. Clinically, the substantia nigra is especially significant in Parkinson's syndrome. The dopaminergic neurons of the substantia nigra thus have a particular effect on the initiation and planning of movements (cf. Spektrum Lexikon der Neurowissenschaft 2000g, n.p.).
Superior	Superior means the one that is situated higher up (cf. Pschyrembel Redaktion 2016t, n.p.).
Synapse	Synapses are switching points or a contact structure for the transmission of an electrical or chemical signal from one neuron to another or to another target cell (muscle cell, gland cell, sensory cell). The transmission of excitation occurs primarily via neurotransmitters. Synapses play a significant role in the action of many drugs. In particular, synapses are the main site of action for psychotropic drugs. Electrical synapses play an important role in epileptic seizures. It should also be mentioned that the receptor sensitivity for excitation transmission between synapses increases or decreases due to harmful substance use (cf. Chao 2019c, n.p.)

T

Tachycardia	Tachycardia is an increased, not age-appropriate heart rate (over 100 beats per minute in adults). The diagnosis is made using an ECG, and the symptoms depend on frequency, duration, origin, and existing preconditions (cf. Kirchner 2021, n.p.).
Tegmentum	The tegmentum is a layer in the area of the brainstem that borders the inner cerebrospinal fluid space ventrally. The tegmentum can be divided into: tegmentum myelencephali, medulla oblongata, see medulla oblongata; tegmentum pontis, pons, see pons; tegmentum mesencephali, midbrain, see mesencephalon (Antwerpes 2013c, n.p.). Tegmentum (from Latin: tegmentum—hood) is considered a general term for hood-like anatomical structures in the brain. The tegmentum is a layer in the area of the brainstem that can be divided into the following areas: tegmentum rhombencephali (lateral wall of the anterior rhombencephalon), tegmentum mesencephali (midbrain, refers to the floor and lateral walls of the mesencephalon), tegmentum metencephali (hindbrain, refers to the floor and lateral walls of the mesencephalon) and tegmentum pontis (pons) (cf. Spektrum Lexikon der Neurowissenschaft 2000h, n.p.).

Term	Definition/Explanation
Temporal lobe (Lobus temporalis; temporal lobe)	The temporal lobe is a lobe of the cerebrum (telencephalon). It includes, among other things, the temporal cortex and the medial temporal lobe with the hippocampus, the entorhinal cortex, perirhinal and parahippocampal cortex as well as the amygdala. It plays a significant role particularly in the processing of experiences and emotions, in learning, as well as in the consolidation and retrieval of memories. The medial temporal lobe is involved in almost all mental disorders (cf. Maier 2018c, n.p.).
Testis (testicles)	The two testicles are germ glands as well as endocrine glands, which are located in the scrotum (multilayered skin sac). Spermatogenesis takes place in the testicles. Additionally, the testicles produce testosterone (sex hormone) in the Leydig interstitial cells (epithelioid cell groups between the seminiferous tubules) (cf. Pschyrembel Editorial 2016u, n.p.).
Thymus	The thymus is a lymphoepithelial organ that lies in the upper mediastinum behind the sternum. It is the primary organ of the lymphatic system and is of fundamental importance for the immunological imprinting of T-lymphocytes (which play an important role in the human immune system), among other things through the endocrinological formation of thymus factors (polypeptides formed by the thymus) (cf. Pschyrembel Editorial 2019h, n.p.).
Tryptophan (L-Tryptophan)	Tryptophan is an aromatic, proteinogenic, essential amino acid. It serves as a precursor for the biosynthesis of serotonin, melatonin, and nicotinic acid. Tryptophan is involved in the metabolism of vitamins B_1, B_2, and B_6 and is also used as a medication (especially for sleep disorders) (cf. Ammon 2018, n.p.).
T cell (T lymphocyte)	T cells belong to the group of lymphocytes, with the T standing for thymus, as T cells mature in the thymus. They play a significant role in the human immune system (cf. Spektrum Lexikon der Neurowissenschaft 2000i, n.p.).
U	
Urology	Urology is a field of medicine that deals with the research, prevention, diagnosis, and therapy of diseases of the male reproductive organs, the urinary tract, as well as diseases of the kidneys (cf. Dietrich 2016, n.p.).
V	
Vegetative Nervous System (Autonomic Nervous System)	The vegetative nervous system is an autonomous part of the nervous system, which is controlled without voluntary regulation by hormones and centers in the brain. The classification of the vegetative nervous system diverges between the sympathetic nervous system (responsible for the response to stress), the parasympathetic nervous system (responsible for energy buildup and relaxation as well as the enteric nervous system) and the enteric nervous system (responsible for the functions of the gastrointestinal tract). The vegetative nervous system is closely related to the central nervous system and serves the regulation of vital functions. Additionally, it controls the interaction of individual body parts. It forms a functional unit with the entirety of the endocrine glands as well as the body fluids (cf. Falkai 2022c, n.p.).

Term	Definition/Explanation
Behavioral Medicine	Behavioral medicine is a medical research field that is situated between medicine, psychology, physiology, and sociology. It uses experimental psychology as well as learning theory for the therapy and explanation of diseases and disease behavior. Behavioral medicine deals with the interactions between health, illness, health behavior, and disease behavior (cf. Schäffler 2017, n.p.).
Vulnerability (Susceptibility; Vulnerability)	Vulnerability means an individual disposition to be more susceptible to mental disorders due to genetic, psychological, social, or organic-biological factors (vulnerability factors). The occurrence of the mental disorder is explained by the interaction of stress and vulnerability as well as maintaining conditions of the disorder (cf. Margraf 2016b, n.p.).
Z	
Cell membrane (Plasma membrane; Cytoplasmic membrane)	The cell membrane is a biomembrane made of lipids and proteins (membrane proteins). It serves for substance exchange and signal transmission, surface tension as well as cell movement and contact with neighboring cells (cf. Pschyrembel Editorial 2018i, n.p.).
Central Nervous System (CNS)	The central nervous system (CNS) refers to the nerve structures located in the brain and spinal cord. In the central nervous system, the main mass of a person's nerve cells is concentrated. The CNS serves sensory-motor integration and coordination and is the seat of the initiation of voluntary motor activity, which enables targeted responses to environmental conditions. It is also the site of conscious and unconscious thinking. It receives nerve impulses from the body's periphery and sensory organs, processes these impulses, and then sends information to the effector organs (cf. Spektrum Lexikon der Neurowissenschaft 2000j, n.p.). In summary, the CNS is responsible for movement coordination, memory, logical thinking, consciousness, emotions, and feelings, as well as for the reception and transmission of information, for example, in the form of organ activity and behavior (cf. BMSGPK 2022, n.p.).
Cerebral Blood Flow (Cerebral Circulation, Brain Circulation)	The cerebral blood flow is the blood flow through the brain to supply it with oxygen and nutrients. It also serves to remove waste products such as carbon dioxide (cf. Pschyrembel Editorial 2018j, n.p.).
Circadian Rhythm	Circadian rhythm means daily rhythmic changes in biological functions such as sleep, endocrine functions, kidney function, or vigilance, as well as parameters such as blood pressure, pulse rate, or cortisol secretion. The sleep-wake rhythm can be considered the most important circadian rhythm. The circadian rhythm is regulated by light-dark cycles and social factors (cf. Walther 2022l, n.p.).
Circumventricular Organ (CVO; Neurohemal Organ)	Circumventricular organs (CVO) are areas in the wall of the II and IV brain ventricles where no blood-brain barrier is formed. The CVOs represent a connection between the central nervous system, blood, and endocrine system. Examples of CVOs include the posterior pituitary (neurohypophysis) and the area postrema (mediates nausea and vomiting) (cf. Pschyrembel Editorial 2018k, n.p.).

Term	Definition/Explanation
Cytokine (Cytokine)	Cytokines are a group of short-lived polypeptides that serve for signal transmission between cells. For example, they modulate the function of immune cells and thus regulate both the strength and the duration of the immune response. In a broader sense, neurotrophic factors as well as growth factors are also counted among the cytokines (cf. Spektrum Lexikon der Neurowissenschaft 2000k, n.p.).

References

Ammon, Hermann (2018): Tryptophan [Aminosäure] (Trp). In: Pschyrembel online. Berlin: Walter de Gruyter GmbH. https://www.pschyrembel.de/Tryptophan/K0N3H/doc/ [20.04.2023].

Bengel, Jürgen/de Zwaan, Martina (2020): Psychosomatik. In: Pschyrembel online. Berlin: Walter de Gruyter GmbH. https://www.pschyrembel.de/Psychosomatik/K0J26/doc/ [19.04.2023].

Blind, Christiane (2016): Pathophysiologie. In: Pschyrembel online. Berlin: Walter de Gruyter GmbH. https://www.pschyrembel.de/Pathophysiologie/K0GFR/doc/ [19.04.2023].

BMSGPK (2022): Zentrales Nervensystem. In: Bundesministerium für Soziales, Gesundheit, Pflege und Konsumentenschutz (BMSGPK), Sozialministerium (Hrsg.) (2022): Öffentliches Gesundheitsportal Österreichs. https://www.gesundheit.gv.at/lexikon/z/lexikon-zentrales-nervensystem [19.01.2022].

Bobbert, Thomas/Mai, Knut (2022a): Atrophie. In: Pschyrembel online. Berlin: Walter de Gruyter GmbH. https://www.pschyrembel.de/Atrophie/K0361/doc/ [13.04.2023].

Bobbert, Thomas/Mai, Knut (2022b). Hyperprolaktinämie. In: Pschyrembel online. Berlin: Walter de Gruyter GmbH. https://www.pschyrembel.de/Hyperprolaktin%C3%A4mie/K0ABB/doc/ [15.04.2023].

Chao, Ivo (2016a): Hippocampus. In: Pschyrembel online. Berlin: Walter de Gruyter GmbH. https://www.pschyrembel.de/Hippocampus/P017E/doc/ [15.04.2023].

Chao, Ivo (2016b): Präganglionär. In: Pschyrembel online. Berlin: Walter de Gruyter GmbH. https://www.pschyrembel.de/Pr%C3%A4ganglion%C3%A4r/K0HK1/doc/ [19.04.2023].

Chao, Ivo (2018): Nucleus paraventricularis. In: Pschyrembel online. Berlin: Walter de Gruyter GmbH. https://www.pschyrembel.de/Nucleus%20%20paraventricularis/K0FGQ/doc/ [18.04.2023].

Chao, Ivo (2019a): Nucleus arcuatus. In: Pschyrembel online. Berlin: Walter de Gruyter GmbH. https://www.pschyrembel.de/Nucleus%20arcuatus/K0FFW [18.04.2023].

Chao, Ivo (2019b): Nucleus supraopticus. In: Pschyrembel online. Berlin: Walter de Gruyter GmbH. https://www.pschyrembel.de/Nucleus%20%20supraopticus/K0FGV/doc/ [18.04.2023].

Chao, Ivo (2019c): Synapse. In: Pschyrembel online. Berlin: Walter de Gruyter GmbH. https://www.pschyrembel.de/Synapse/K0M1U/doc/ [20.04.2023].

Chao, Ivo (2020): Epithalamus. In: Pschyrembel online. Berlin: Walter de Gruyter GmbH. https://www.pschyrembel.de/Epithalamus/K073K/doc/ [15.04.2023].

Diener, Hans Christoph (2016): Neurologie. In: Pschyrembel online. Berlin: Walter de Gruyter GmbH. https://www.pschyrembel.de/Neurologie.%20/K0F5F/doc/ [18.04.2023].

J. Wiederhofer, *Psychoneuroendocrinology in Psychosocial and Psychotherapeutic Practice,* https://doi.org/10.1007/978-3-658-46275-8

Diener, Hans Christoph (2019a): Chiasma opticum. In: Pschyrembel online. Berlin: Walter de Gruyter GmbH. https://www.pschyrembel.de/Chiasma%20opticum/K0KP7/doc/ [14.04.2023].
Diener, Hans Christoph (2019b): Hirnventrikel. In: Pschyrembel online. Berlin: Walter de Gruyter GmbH. https://www.pschyrembel.de/Hirnventrikel/K09V5/doc/ [15.04.2023].
Dietrich, Joseph (2016): Urologie. In: Pschyrembel online. Berlin: Walter de Gruyter GmbH. https://www.pschyrembel.de/Urologie/K0NDV/doc/ [20.04.2023].
Dittmann, Alexander (2022): Amnesie. In: Pschyrembel online. Berlin: Walter de Gruyter GmbH. https://www.pschyrembel.de/Amnesie/K027F/doc/ [13.04.2023].
Duden (2023): Humanphysiologie. In: DUDEN. Berlin: Cornelsen Verlag GmbH.
https://www.duden.de/rechtschreibung/Humanphysiologie [15.04.2023].
Ehnert, Sabrina (2016): Pharmakologie. In: Pschyrembel online. Berlin: Walter de Gruyter GmbH. https://www.pschyrembel.de/Pharmakologie/K0GSX/doc/ [19.04.2023].
Falkai, Peter (2022a): Diencephalon. In: Pschyrembel online. Berlin: Walter de Gruyter GmbH. https://www.pschyrembel.de/Diencephalon/P004C/doc/ [14.04.2023].
Falkai, Peter (2022b): Rhombencephalon. In: Pschyrembel online. Berlin: Walter de Gruyter GmbH. https://www.pschyrembel.de/Rautenhirn/P06AJ/doc/ [19.04.2023].
Falkai, Peter (2022c): Vegetatives Nervensystem. In: Pschyrembel online. Berlin: Walter de Gruyter GmbH. https://www.pschyrembel.de/Vegetatives%20%20Nervensystem/K0F3H/doc/ [20.04.2023].
Fanghänel, Jochen (2016): Dendrit. In: Pschyrembel online. Berlin: Walter de Gruyter GmbH. https://www.pschyrembel.de/Dendrit/K05MR/doc/ [14.04.2023].
Fanghänel, Jochen (2019): Pinealozyt. In: Pschyrembel online. Berlin: Walter de Gruyter GmbH. https://www.pschyrembel.de/Pinealozyt/K0H1G/doc/ [19.04.2023].
Fanghänel, Jochen/Giebel, Jürgen/Weingärtner, Jens (2020): Fettgewebe. In: Pschyrembel online. Berlin: Walter de Gruyter GmbH. https://www.pschyrembel.de/Fettgewebe/K07PP/doc/ [15.04.2023].
Füeßl, Hermann (2020): Schilddrüse. In: Pschyrembel online. Berlin: Walter de Gruyter GmbH. https://www.pschyrembel.de/Schilddr%C3%BCse/K0KE5/doc/ [20.04.2023].
Ganse, Bergita (2022a): Endokrin. In: Pschyrembel online. Berlin: Walter de Gruyter GmbH. https://www.pschyrembel.de/Endokrin/K06TF/doc/ [15.04.2023].
Ganse, Bergita (2022b): Sekretion. In: Pschyrembel online. Berlin: Walter de Gruyter GmbH. https://www.pschyrembel.de/Sekretion%20/K0KPS/doc/ [20.04.2023].
Giebel, Jürgen (2020): Epiphyse. In: Pschyrembel online. Berlin: Walter de Gruyter GmbH. https://www.pschyrembel.de/Epiphyse/K072Q/doc/ [15.04.2023].
Hackermeier, Ursula (2020): Homöostase. In: Pschyrembel online. Berlin: Walter de Gruyter GmbH. https://www.pschyrembel.de/Hom%C3%B6ostase/N014W/doc/ [15.04.2023].
Heinzow, Birger/Jaehde, Ulrich (2023): Biomarker. In: Pschyrembel online. Berlin: Walter de Gruyter GmbH. https://www.pschyrembel.de/Biomarker/H0H6S/doc/ [13.04.2023].
Hennig, Jürgen/Netter, Petra (2000): Psychoneuroendokrinologie. In: Spektrum der Wissenschaft. Lexikon der Psychologie. Heidelberg: Spektrum der Wissenschaft Verlagsgesellschaft mbH., Springer Nature. https://www.spektrum.de/lexikon/psychologie/psychoneuroendokrinologie/12129 [19.04.2023].
Hollstein, Guido (2022a): Apathie. In: Pschyrembel online. Berlin: Walter de Gruyter GmbH. https://www.pschyrembel.de/Apathie/K02NT [13.04.2023].
Hollstein, Guido (2022b): Hyperkortisolismus. In: Pschyrembel online. Berlin: Walter de Gruyter GmbH. https://www.pschyrembel.de/Hypercortisolis-mus/K0A9N/doc/ [15.04.2023].
Hollstein, Guido (2022c): Hypokortisolismus. In: Pschyrembel online. Berlin: Walter de Gruyter GmbH. https://www.pschyrembel.de/Hypocortisolismus/K0AE7/doc/ [15.04.2023].

Jähn, Karl (2016): Kybernetik. In: Pschyrembel online. Berlin: Walter de Gruyter GmbH. https://www.pschyrembel.de/Kybernetik%3B/K0CDF/doc/ [16.04.2023].
Kirchner, Franz-Ferdinand (2021): Tachykardie. In: Pschyrembel online. Berlin: Walter de Gruyter GmbH. https://www.pschyrembel.de/Tachykardie/K0M60/doc/ [20.04.2023].
Krause, Ute (2020a): Blut-Hirn-Schranke. In: Pschyrembel online. Berlin: Walter de Gruyter GmbH. https://www.pschyrembel.de/Blut-Hirn-Schranke/K03XD/doc/ [13.04.2023].
Krause, Ute (2020b): Immunsuppression. In: Pschyrembel online. Berlin: Walter de Gruyter GmbH. https://www.pschyrembel.de/Immunsuppressi-on/K0AME/doc/ [16.04.2023].
Krieglstein, Kerstin (2016): Gyrus dentatus. In: Pschyrembel online. Berlin: Walter de Gruyter GmbH. https://www.pschyrembel.de/Gyrus%20dentatus/K097E/doc/ [15.04.2023].
Krieglstein, Kerstin (2018a): Kleinhirn. In: Pschyrembel online. Berlin: Walter de Gruyter GmbH. https://www.pschyrembel.de/Kleinhirn/K0BQB/doc/ [16.04.2023].
Krieglstein, Kerstin (2018b): Limbisches System. In: Pschyrembel online. Berlin: Walter de Gruyter GmbH. https://www.pschyrembel.de/Limbisches%20System/K0M56/doc/ [16.04.2023].
Lindner, Oliver (2022): Nuklearmedizin. In: Pschyrembel online. Berlin: Walter de Gruyter GmbH. https://www.pschyrembel.de/Nuklearmedizin/K0FH1/doc/ [18.04.2023].
Lücke, Catherina (2020): Myopathie. In: Pschyrembel online. Berlin: Walter de Gruyter GmbH. https://www.pschyrembel.de/Myopathie/K0ER4/doc/ [18.04.2023].
Lüdi, Markus/Stüber, Frank/Venetz, Philipp (2022): Intensivmedizin. In: Pschyrembel online. Berlin: Walter de Gruyter GmbH. https://www.pschyrembel.de/Intensivmedizin/K0AWH/doc/ [16.04.2023].
Maier, Wolfgang (2016a): Amygdala. In: Pschyrembel online. Berlin: Walter de Gruyter GmbH. https://www.pschyrembel.de/Amygdala/P05FG/doc/ [13.04.2023].
Maier, Wolfgang (2016b): Kognitive Neurowissenschaft. In: Pschyrembel online. Berlin: Walter de Gruyter GmbH. https://www.pschyrembel.de/Neurowissenschaft%2C%20kognitive/P05T9/doc/ [18.04.2023].
Maier, Wolfgang (2016c): Psychiatrie. In: Pschyrembel online. Berlin: Walter de Gruyter GmbH. https://www.pschyrembel.de/Psychiatrie/K0J1D/doc/ [19.04.2023].
Maier, Wolfgang (2018a): Fasciculus medialis telencephali. In: Pschyrembel online. Berlin: Walter de Gruyter GmbH. https://www.pschyrembel.de/Mediales%20Vor-derhirnb%C3%BCndel/P06MF/doc/ [17.04.2023].
Maier, Wolfgang (2018b): Motoneurone. In: Pschyrembel online. Berlin: Walter de Gruyter GmbH. https://www.pschyrembel.de/Motoneurone/P0243/doc/ [18.04.2023].
Maier, Wolfgang (2018c): Temporallappen. In: Pschyrembel online. Berlin: Walter de Gruyter GmbH. https://www.pschyrembel.de/Temporallappen/P05W2/doc/ [20.04.2023].
Maier, Wolfgang (2019a): Telencephalon. In: Pschyrembel online. Berlin: Walter de Gruyter GmbH. https://www.pschyrembel.de/Gro%C3%9Fhirn/P0096/doc/ [15.04.2023].
Maier, Wolfgang (2019b): Mesencephalon. In: Pschyrembel online. Berlin: Walter de Gruyter GmbH. https://www.pschyrembel.de/Mesencephalon/P051N/doc/ [17.04.2023].
Margraf, Jürgen (2016a): Neuroendokrinologie. In: Pschyrembel online. Berlin: Walter de Gruyter GmbH. https://www.pschyrembel.de/Neuroendokrinologie/P02W7/doc/ [18.04.2023].
Margraf, Jürgen (2016b): Vulnerabilität. In: Pschyrembel online. Berlin: Walter de Gruyter GmbH. https://www.pschyrembel.de/Vulnerabilit%C3%A4t/K0NWL/doc/ [20.04.2023].
Meyer, Gerd Peter (2016): Hypertension. In: Pschyrembel online. Berlin: Walter de Gruyter GmbH. https://www.pschyrembel.de/Hypertonie/K0AC2/doc/ [15.04.2023].
Pfitzmann, Robert (2020): Chirurgie. In: Pschyrembel online. Berlin: Walter de Gruyter GmbH. https://www.pschyrembel.de/Chirurgie/K04RJ/doc/ [14.04.2023].

Prochazka, Katharina (2022): Paraneoplastisches Syndrom. In: Pschyrembel online. Berlin: Walter de Gruyter GmbH. https://www.pschyrembel.de/Paraneoplastisches%20Syndrom/K0M3D/ [19.04.2023].

Pschyrembel Redaktion (2016a): Kortex. In: Pschyrembel online. Berlin: Walter de Gruyter GmbH. https://www.pschyrembel.de/Cortex/K059H/doc/ [14.04.2023].

Pschyrembel Redaktion (2016b): Dilatation. In: Pschyrembel online. Berlin: Walter de Gruyter GmbH. https://www.pschyrembel.de/Dilatation/K0601/doc/ [14.04.2023].

Pschyrembel Redaktion (2016c): Enterisches Nervensystem. In: Pschyrembel online. Berlin: Walter de Gruyter GmbH. https://www.pschyrembel.de/Enterisches%20%20Nervensystem/K0F3G/doc/ [15.04.2023].

Pschyrembel Redaktion (2016d): Gastrointestinal. In: Pschyrembel online. Berlin: Walter de Gruyter GmbH. https://www.pschyrembel.de/Gastrointestinal/K08GQ/doc/ [15.04.2023].

Pschyrembel Redaktion (2016e): Innere Medizin. In: Pschyrembel online. Berlin: Walter de Gruyter GmbH. https://www.pschyrembel.de/Innere%20Medizin/K0AU9/doc/ [16.04.2023].

Pschyrembel Redaktion (2016f): Kardiovaskulär. In: Pschyrembel online. Berlin: Walter de Gruyter GmbH. https://www.pschyrembel.de/Kardiovaskul%C3%A4r/K0BEC/doc/ [16.04.2023].

Pschyrembel Redaktion (2016g): Leydig-Zwischenzellen. In: Pschyrembel online. Berlin: Walter de Gruyter GmbH. https://www.pschyrembel.de/Leydig-Zellen/K0CU8/doc/ [16.04.2023].

Pschyrembel Redaktion (2016h): Morphologie. In: Pschyrembel online. Berlin: Walter de Gruyter GmbH. https://www.pschyrembel.de/Morphologie/K0EGU/doc/ [17.04.2023].

Pschyrembel Redaktion (2016i): Nebennierenmark (NNM). In: Pschyrembel online. Berlin: Walter de Gruyter GmbH. https://www.pschyrembel.de/Nebennierenmark/K0FAF/doc/ [18.04.2023].

Pschyrembel Redaktion (2016j): Neocortex. In: Pschyrembel online. Berlin: Walter de Gruyter GmbH. https://www.pschyrembel.de/Neocortex/K0F1N/doc/ [18.04.2023].

Pschyrembel Redaktion (2016k): Niere. In: Pschyrembel online. Berlin: Walter de Gruyter GmbH. https://www.pschyrembel.de/Niere/K0F7V/doc/ [18.04.2023].

Pschyrembel Redaktion (2016l): Parakrin. In: Pschyrembel online. Berlin: Walter de Gruyter GmbH. https://www.pschyrembel.de/Parakrin/K0GA5/doc/ [18.04.2023].

Pschyrembel Redaktion (2016m): Pädiatrie. In: Pschyrembel online. Berlin: Walter de Gruyter GmbH. https://www.pschyrembel.de/P%C3%A4diatrie/K0G4W/doc/ [19.04.2023].

Pschyrembel Redaktion (2016n): Postpartal (p. p.). In: Pschyrembel online. Berlin: Walter de Gruyter GmbH. https://www.pschyrembel.de/Postpartal/K0HHL/doc/ [19.04.2023].

Pschyrembel Redaktion (2016o): Präfrontalkortex. In: Pschyrembel online. Berlin: Walter de Gruyter GmbH. https://www.pschyrembel.de/Pr%C3%A4frontalkortex/P0237/doc/ [19.04.2023].

Pschyrembel Redaktion (2016p): Psychoendokrinologie. In: Pschyrembel online. Berlin: Walter de Gruyter GmbH. https://www.pschyrembel.de/Psychoendokrino-logie/P03T6/doc/ [19.04.2023].

Pschyrembel Redaktion (2016q): Retina. In: Pschyrembel online. Berlin: Walter de Gruyter GmbH. https://www.pschyrembel.de/Retina/K0JS0/doc/ [20.04.2023].

Pschyrembel Redaktion (2016r): Sezernieren. In: Pschyrembel online. Berlin: Walter de Gruyter GmbH. https://www.pschyrembel.de/sezernieren/K0KVE/doc/ [20.04.2023].

Pschyrembel Redaktion (2016s): Soma. In: Pschyrembel online. Berlin: Walter de Gruyter GmbH. https://www.pschyrembel.de/Soma/K0L5M/doc/ [20.04.2023].

Pschyrembel Redaktion (2016t): Superior. In: Pschyrembel online. Berlin: Walter de Gruyter GmbH. https://www.pschyrembel.de/Superior/K0LXF/doc/ [20.04.2023].

Pschyrembel Redaktion (2016u): Hoden. In: Pschyrembel online. Berlin: Walter de Gruyter GmbH. https://www.pschyrembel.de/Hoden/K09X8/doc/ [20.04.2023].

Pschyrembel Redaktion (2018a): Drüse. In: Pschyrembel online. Berlin: Walter de Gruyter GmbH. https://www.pschyrembel.de/Dr%C3%BCse/K0692/doc/ [14.04.2023].

Pschyrembel Redaktion (2018b): Locus caeruleus. In: Pschyrembel online. Berlin: Walter de Gruyter GmbH. https://www.pschyrembel.de/Locus%20coeruleus/K0D8S/doc/ [16.04.2023].

Pschyrembel Redaktion (2018c): Mesolimbisches/-kortikales Neuronensystem. In: Pschyrembel online. Berlin: Walter de Gruyter GmbH. https://www.pschyrembel.de/Mesolimbisches%20System/B0NN5/doc/ [17.04.2023].

Pschyrembel Redaktion (2018d): Nucleus accumbens. In: Pschyrembel online. Berlin: Walter de Gruyter GmbH. https://www.pschyrembel.de/Nucleus%20accumbens/P0424/doc/ [18.04.2023].

Pschyrembel Redaktion (2018e): Nucleus suprachiasmaticus (SCN). In: Pschyrembel online. Berlin: Walter de Gruyter GmbH. https://www.pschyrembel.de/Nucleus%20suprachiasmaticus/K00FW/doc/ [18.04.2023].

Pschyrembel Redaktion (2018f): Orbitofrontalkortex. In: Pschyrembel online. Berlin: Walter de Gruyter GmbH. https://www.pschyrembel.de/Orbitofrontalkortex/P056S/doc/ [18.04.2023].

Pschyrembel Redaktion (2018g): Raphekerne. In: Pschyrembel online. Berlin: Walter de Gruyter GmbH. https://www.pschyrembel.de/Raphe-Kerne/K0197/doc/ [19.04.2023].

Pschyrembel Redaktion (2018h): Steroid-Rezeptoren. In: Pschyrembel online. Berlin: Walter de Gruyter GmbH. https://www.pschyrembel.de/Steroidrezeptor/P02F4/doc/ [20.04.2023].

Pschyrembel Redaktion (2018i): Zellmembran. In: Pschyrembel online. Berlin: Walter de Gruyter GmbH. https://www.pschyrembel.de/Zellmembran/K0PAD/doc/ [20.04.2023].

Pschyrembel Redaktion (2018j): Hirndurchblutung. In: Pschyrembel online. Berlin: Walter de Gruyter GmbH. https://www.pschyrembel.de/Zerebraler%20%20Blutfluss/B0MX9/doc/ [20.04.2023].

Pschyrembel Redaktion (2018k): Zirkumventrikuläres Organ. In: Pschyrembel online. Berlin: Walter de Gruyter GmbH. https://www.pschyrembel.de/Zirkumventrikul%C3%A4-res%20Organ/B0GXK/doc/ [20.04.2023].

Pschyrembel Redaktion (2019a): Axon. In: Pschyrembel online. Berlin: Walter de Gruyter GmbH. https://www.pschyrembel.de/Axon/K03A2/doc/ [13.04.2023].

Pschyrembel Redaktion (2019b): Basolateral. In: Pschyrembel online. Berlin: Walter de Gruyter GmbH. https://www.pschyrembel.de/Basolateral/A0V9T/doc/ [13.04.2023].

Pschyrembel Redaktion (2019c): Benzodiazepine. In: Pschyrembel online. Berlin: Walter de Gruyter GmbH. https://www.pschyrembel.de/Benzodiazepin/K03LC/doc/ [13.04.2023].

Pschyrembel Redaktion (2019d): Hypophysenstiel. In: Pschyrembel online. Berlin: Walter de Gruyter GmbH. https://www.pschyrembel.de/Hypophysenstiel/K0GE4/doc/ [16.04.2023].

Pschyrembel Redaktion (2019e): Intrauterin. In: Pschyrembel online. Berlin: Walter de Gruyter GmbH. https://www.pschyrembel.de/Intrauterin/H07JS/doc/ [16.04.2023].

Pschyrembel Redaktion (2019f): Nervenzelle. In: Pschyrembel online. Berlin: Walter de Gruyter GmbH. https://www.pschyrembel.de/Nervenzelle/K0F3L/doc/ [18.04.2023].

Pschyrembel Redaktion (2019g): Rostral. In: Pschyrembel online. Berlin: Walter de Gruyter GmbH. https://www.pschyrembel.de/Rostral/K0K3V/doc/ [20.04.2023].

Pschyrembel Redaktion (2019h): Thymus. In: Pschyrembel online. Berlin: Walter de Gruyter GmbH. https://www.pschyrembel.de/Thymus/K0MJT/doc/ [20.04.2023].

Pschyrembel Redaktion (2020a): Kortisol. In: Pschyrembel online. Berlin: Walter de Gruyter GmbH. https://www.pschyrembel.de/Cortisol/K059R/doc/ [14.04.2023].

Pschyrembel Redaktion (2020b): Melatonin. In: Pschyrembel online. Berlin: Walter de Gruyter GmbH. https://www.pschyrembel.de/Melatonin/K0DXE/doc/ [17.04.2023].

Pschyrembel Redaktion (2020c): Prostaglandine (PG). In: Pschyrembel online. Berlin: Walter de Gruyter GmbH. https://www.pschyrembel.de/Prostaglandinsynthese/K0HTJ/doc/ [19.04.2023].

Pschyrembel Redaktion (2020d): Corpus striatum. In: Pschyrembel online. Berlin: Walter de Gruyter GmbH. https://www.pschyrembel.de/Striatum/K059B/doc/ [20.04.2023].
Pschyrembel Redaktion (2021a): Epigenetik. In: Pschyrembel online. Berlin: Walter de Gruyter GmbH. https://www.pschyrembel.de/Epigenetik/K00CC/doc/ [15.04.2023].
Pschyrembel Redaktion (2021b): Polymorphismus. In: Pschyrembel online. Berlin: Walter de Gruyter GmbH. https://www.pschyrembel.de/Polymorphismus/K0HEB/doc/ [19.04.2023].
Pschyrembel Redaktion (2022): Perinatalperiode. In: Pschyrembel online. Berlin: Walter de Gruyter GmbH. https://www.pschyrembel.de/Perinatalperiode/K0GM8/doc/ [19.04.2023].
Schäffler, Arne (2017): Verhaltensmedizin. In: Pschyrembel online. Berlin: Walter de Gruyter GmbH. https://www.pschyrembel.de/Verhaltensmedizin/K0NNX/doc/ [20.04.2023].
Schöller, Dorit (2016a): Endokrinologie. In: Pschyrembel online. Berlin: Walter de Gruyter GmbH. https://www.pschyrembel.de/Endokrinologie/K06TG/doc/ [15.04.2023].
Schöller, Dorit (2016b): Hormone. In: Pschyrembel online. Berlin: Walter de Gruyter GmbH. https://www.pschyrembel.de/Hormon/K0A1S/doc/ [15.04.2023].
Schöller, Dorit (2016c): Hormon-Rezeptoren. In: Pschyrembel online. Berlin: Walter de Gruyter GmbH. https://www.pschyrembel.de/Hormonrezeptor/K0A1V/doc/ [15.04.2023].
Schöller, Dorit (2016d): Hypothalamus. In: Pschyrembel online. Berlin: Walter de Gruyter GmbH. https://www.pschyrembel.de/Hypothalamus/K0AFR [16.04.2023].
Schöller, Dorit (2016e): Nebenschilddrüsen. In: Pschyrembel online. Berlin: Walter de Gruyter GmbH. https://www.pschyrembel.de/Nebenschilddr%C3%BCsen/K0F0K/doc/ [18.04.2023].
Schöller, Dorit (2016f): Perimenopause. In: Pschyrembel online. Berlin: Walter de Gruyter GmbH. https://www.pschyrembel.de/Perimenopause/K0QRF/doc/ [19.04.2023].
Schöller, Dorit (2016g): Sexualhormone. In: Pschyrembel online. Berlin: Walter de Gruyter GmbH. https://www.pschyrembel.de/Sexualhormon/K0KV6/doc/ [20.04.2023].
Schöller, Dorit (2016h): Spermatogenese. In: Pschyrembel online. Berlin: Walter de Gruyter GmbH. https://www.pschyrembel.de/Spermatogenese/K0L99/doc/ [20.04.2023].
Schöller, Dorit (2018a): Dopamin-Rezeptor-Agonisten. In: Pschyrembel online. Berlin: Walter de Gruyter GmbH. https://www.pschyrembel.de/Dopaminagonist/K0HRR/doc/ [14.04.2023].
Schöller, Dorit (2018b): Gen. In: Pschyrembel online. Berlin: Walter de Gruyter GmbH. https://www.pschyrembel.de/Gen/K08L4/doc/ [15.04.2023].
Schöller, Dorit (2018c): Gynäkologie. In: Pschyrembel online. Berlin: Walter de Gruyter GmbH. https://www.pschyrembel.de/Gyn%C3%A4kologie/K0971/doc/ [15.04.2023].
Schöller, Dorit (2018d): Corpus luteum. In: Pschyrembel online. Berlin: Walter de Gruyter GmbH. https://www.pschyrembel.de/Corpus%20luteum/K058X/doc/ [14.04.2023].
Schöller, Dorit (2018e): Nebenniere. In: Pschyrembel online. Berlin: Walter de Gruyter GmbH. https://www.pschyrembel.de/Nebenniere/K0F0A/doc/ [18.04.2023].
Schöller, Dorit (2018f): Ovar. In: Pschyrembel online. Berlin: Walter de Gruyter GmbH. https://www.pschyrembel.de/Ovar/K0G22/doc/ [18.04.2023].
Schöller, Dorit (2019a): Hypophyse. In: Pschyrembel online. Berlin: Walter de Gruyter GmbH. https://www.pschyrembel.de/Hypophyse/K0AF1/doc/ [16.04.2023].
Schöller, Dorit (2019b): Infertilität. In: Pschyrembel online. Berlin: Walter de Gruyter GmbH. https://www.pschyrembel.de/Infertilit%C3%A4t/K0ARX/doc/ [16.04.2023].
Schöller, Dorit (2019c): Neurohypophyse. In: Pschyrembel online. Berlin: Walter de Gruyter GmbH. https://www.pschyrembel.de/Neurohypophyse/K0F59/doc/ [18.04.2023].
Schöller, Dorit (2021a): Chromosomen. In: Pschyrembel online. Berlin: Walter de Gruyter GmbH. https://www.pschyrembel.de/Chromosomen/K04WR [14.04.2023].
Schöller, Dorit (Genetik. In: Pschyrembel online. Berlin: Walter de Gruyter GmbH. https://www.pschyrembel.de/Genetik/K08LK/doc/ [15.04.2023].

Schulze-Schleithoff, Anna-Elisa (2019a): Leber. In: Pschyrembel online. Berlin: Walter de Gruyter GmbH. https://www.pschyrembel.de/Leber/K0CMR/doc/ [16.04.2023].

Schulze-Schleithoff, Anna-Elisa (2019b): Pankreas. In: Pschyrembel online. Berlin: Walter de Gruyter GmbH. https://www.pschyrembel.de/Pankreas/K0G70/doc/ [18.04.2023].

Spektrum Lexikon der Biologie (1999a): Inhibiting-Hormone. In: Spektrum der Wissenschaft. Heidelberg: Spektrum der Wissenschaft Verlagsgesellschaft mbH., Springer Nature. https://www.spektrum.de/lexikon/biologie/inhibiting-hormone/34081 [16.04.2023].

Spektrum Lexikon der Biologie (1999b): Molekularbiologie. In: Spektrum der Wissenschaft. Heidelberg: Spektrum der Wissenschaft Verlagsgesellschaft mbH., Springer Nature. https://www.spektrum.de/lexikon/biologie/molekularbiologie/43525 [17.04.2023].

Spektrum Lexikon der Neurowissenschaft (2000a): Adenohypophyse. In: Spektrum der Wissenschaft. Heidelberg: Spektrum der Wissenschaft Verlagsgesellschaft mbH., Springer Nature. https://www.spektrum.de/lexikon/neurowissenschaft/adenohypophyse/139 [11.04.2023].

Spektrum Lexikon der Neurowissenschaft (2000b): Adrenalektomie. In: Spektrum der Wissenschaft. Heidelberg: Spektrum der Wissenschaft Verlagsgesellschaft mbH., Springer Nature. https://www.spektrum.de/lexikon/neurowissenschaft/adrenalektomie/165 [13.04.2023].

Spektrum Lexikon der Neurowissenschaft (2000c): Anxiolytika. In: Spektrum der Wissenschaft. Heidelberg: Spektrum der Wissenschaft Verlagsgesellschaft mbH., Springer Nature. https://www.spektrum.de/lexikon/neurowissenschaft/anxiolytika/762 [13.04.2023].

Spektrum Lexikon der Neurowissenschaft (2000d): Basalganglien. In: Spektrum der Wissenschaft. Heidelberg: Spektrum der Wissenschaft Verlagsgesellschaft mbH., Springer Nature. https://www.spektrum.de/lexikon/neurowissenschaft/basalganglien/1290 [13.04.2023].

Spektrum Lexikon der Neurowissenschaft (2000e): Eminentia mediana. In: Spektrum der Wissenschaft. Heidelberg: Spektrum der Wissenschaft Verlagsgesellschaft mbH., Springer Nature. https://www.spektrum.de/lexikon/neurowissenschaft/eminentia-mediana/3395 [15.04.2023]

Spektrum Lexikon der Neurowissenschaft (2000f): Prohormone. In: Spektrum der Wissenschaft. Heidelberg: Spektrum der Wissenschaft Verlagsgesellschaft mbH., Springer Nature. https://www.spektrum.de/lexikon/neurowissenschaft/prohormone/10308 [19.04.2023].

Spektrum Lexikon der Neurowissenschaft (2000g): Substantia nigra. In: Spektrum der Wissenschaft. Heidelberg: Spektrum der Wissenschaft Verlagsgesellschaft mbH., Springer Nature. https://www.spektrum.de/lexikon/neurowissenschaft/substantia-nigra/12484 [20.04.2023].

Spektrum Lexikon der Neurowissenschaft (2000h): Tegmentum. In: Spektrum der Wissenschaft. Heidelberg: Spektrum der Wissenschaft Verlagsgesellschaft mbH., Springer Nature. https://www.spektrum.de/lexikon/neurowissenschaft/tegmentum/12787 [20.04.2023].

Spektrum Lexikon der Neurowissenschaft (2000i): T-Lymphozyten. In: Spektrum der Wissenschaft. Heidelberg: Spektrum der Wissenschaft Verlagsgesellschaft mbH., Springer Nature. https://www.spektrum.de/lexikon/neurowissenschaft/t-lymphocyten/13000 [20.04.2023].

Spektrum Lexikon der Neurowissenschaft (2000j): Zentralnervensystem. In: Spektrum der Wissenschaft. Heidelberg: Spektrum der Wissenschaft Verlagsgesellschaft mbH., Springer Nature. https://www.spektrum.de/lexikon/neurowissenschaft/zentralnervensystem/14201 [20.04.2023].

Spektrum Lexikon der Neurowissenschaft (2000k): Cytokine. In: Spektrum der Wissenschaft. Heidelberg: Spektrum der Wissenschaft Verlagsgesellschaft mbH., Springer Nature. https://www.spektrum.de/lexikon/neurowissenschaft/cytokine/2585 [20.04.2023].

Straube, Sebastian (2022): Physiologie. In: Pschyrembel online. Berlin: Walter de Gruyter GmbH. https://www.pschyrembel.de/Physiologie/K0GXU/doc/ [19.04.2023].

Walther, Reinhard (2022a): Biochemie. In: Pschyrembel online. Berlin: Walter de Gruyter GmbH. https://www.pschyrembel.de/Biochemie/K03RG/doc/ [13.04.2023].

Walther, Reinhard (2022b): Biogene Amine. In: Pschyrembel online. Berlin: Walter de Gruyter GmbH. https://www.pschyrembel.de/Biogenes%20Amin/K026E/doc/ [13.04.2023].

Walther, Reinhard (2022c): Glukoneogenese. In: Pschyrembel online. Berlin: Walter de Gruyter GmbH. https://www.pschyrembel.de/Gluconeogenese/K08WX/doc/ [15.04.2023].
Walther, Reinhard (2022d): Kathecholamine. In: Pschyrembel online. Berlin: Walter de Gruyter GmbH. https://www.pschyrembel.de/Katecholamin/K0BGT/doc/ [16.04.2023].
Walther, Reinhard (2022e): Monoamine. In: Pschyrembel online. Berlin: Walter de Gruyter GmbH. https://www.pschyrembel.de/Monoamin/P05V1/doc/ [17.04.2023].
Walther, Reinhard (2022f): Monoaminooxidase (MAO). In: Pschyrembel online. Berlin: Walter de Gruyter GmbH. https://www.pschyrembel.de/Monoaminoxidase/K0EEP/doc/ [17.04.2023].
Walther, Reinhard (2022g): Neuropeptide. In: Pschyrembel online. Berlin: Walter de Gruyter GmbH. https://www.pschyrembel.de/Neuropeptide/K0F5T/doc/ [18.04.2023].
Walther, Reinhard (2022h): Neurotransmitter. In: Pschyrembel online. Berlin: Walter de Gruyter GmbH. https://www.pschyrembel.de/Neurotransmitter/K0F6D/doc/ [18.04.2023].
Walther, Reinhard (2022i): Phenylalanin. In: Pschyrembel online. Berlin: Walter de Gruyter GmbH. https://www.pschyrembel.de/Phenylalanin/K0GU4/doc/ [19.04.2023].
Walther, Reinhard (2022j): Pregnenolon. In: Pschyrembel online. Berlin: Walter de Gruyter GmbH. https://www.pschyrembel.de/Pregnenolon/K0HM8/doc/ [19.04.2023].
Walther, Reinhard (2022k): Rezeptoren. In: Pschyrembel online. Berlin: Walter de Gruyter GmbH. https://www.pschyrembel.de/Rezeptor%20/K0JU3/doc/ [20.04.2023].
Walther, Reinhard (2022l): Zirkadianer Rhythmus. In: Pschyrembel online. Berlin: Walter de Gruyter GmbH. https://www.pschyrembel.de/Zirkadianer%20%20Rhythmus/K0JW8/doc/ [20.04.2023].
Weingärtner, Jens (2022): Plazenta. In: Pschyrembel online. Berlin: Walter de Gruyter GmbH. https://www.pschyrembel.de/Plazenta/K0H5M/doc/ [19.04.2023].
Wurglics, Mario (2022): Releasing-Hormone. In: Pschyrembel online. Berlin: Walter de Gruyter GmbH. https://www.pschyrembel.de/Releasing-Hormon/K0JNE/doc/ [19.04.2023].